Chest MR

Guest Editor

MICHAEL B. GOTWAY, MD

MAGNETIC RESONANCE IMAGING CLINICS OF NORTH AMERICA

www.mri.theclinics.com

May 2008 • Volume 16 • Number 2

SAUNDERS an imprint of ELSEVIER, Inc.

W.B. SAUNDERS COMPANY
A Division of Elsevier Inc.

Elsevier Inc. ● 1600 John F. Kennedy Boulevard ● Suite 1800 ● Philadelphia, Pennsylvania 19103-2899

http://www.theclinics.com

MRI CLINICS OF NORTH AMERICA Volume 16, Number 2
May 2008 ISSN 1064-9689, ISBN 13: 978-1-4160-5849-6, ISBN 10: 1-4160-5849-4

Editor: Lisa Richman

The ideas and opinions expressed in *Magnetic Resonance Imaging Clinics of North America* do not necessarily reflect those of the Publisher. The Publisher does not assume any responsibility for any injury and/or damage to persons or property arising out of or related to any use of the material contained in this periodical. The reader is advised to check the appropriate medical literature and the product information currently provided by the manufacturer of each drug to be administered to verify the dosage, the method and duration of administration, or contraindications. It is the responsibility of the treating physician or other health care professional, relying on independent experience and knowledge of the patient, to determine drug dosages and the best treatment for the patient. Mention of any product in this issue should not be construed as endorsement by the contributors, editors, or the Publisher of the product or manufacturers' claims.

Magnetic Resonance Imaging Clinics of North America (ISSN 1064-9689) is published quarterly by Elsevier Inc., 360 Park Avenue South, New York, NY 10010-1710. Months of issue are February, May, August, and November. Business and Editorial Offices: 1600 John F. Kennedy Blvd., Suite 1800, Philadelphia, PA 19103-2899. Customer Service Office: 6277 Sea Harbor Drive, Orlando, FL 32887-4800. Periodicals postage paid at New York, NY and additional mailing offices. Subscription prices are $253.00 per year (US individuals), $376.00 per year (US institutions), $123.00 per year (US students), $283.00 per year (Canadian individuals), $463.00 per year (Canadian institutions), $167.00 per year (Canadian students), $345.00 per year (international individuals), $463.00 per year (international institutions), and $167.00 per year (international students). International air speed delivery is included in all *Clinics* subscription prices. All prices are subject to change without notice. **POSTMASTER:** Send address changes to *Magnetic Resonance Imaging Clinics*, Elsevier Periodicals Customer Service, 6277 Sea Harbor Drive, Orlando, FL 32887-4800. Customer Service: 1-800-654-2452 (US). From outside the United States, call 1-407-563-6020. Fax: 1-407-363-9661. E-mail: JournalsCustomerService-usa@elsevier.com.

Magnetic Resonance Imaging Clinics of North America is covered in the *RSNA Index of Imaging Literature, Index Medicus, MEDLINE*, and *EMBASE/Excerpta Medica*.

Printed in the United States of America.

Contributors

GUEST EDITOR

MICHAEL B. GOTWAY, MD
Scottsdale Medical Imaging, an affiliate
of Southwest Diagnostic Imaging, Ltd.,
Scottsdale, Arizona; Clinical Associate
Professor, Diagnostic Radiology and
Pulmonary/Critical Care Medicine,
Department of Radiology, University of
California, San Francisco, San Francisco,
California

AUTHORS

PHILIP A. ARAOZ, MD
Assistant Professor of Radiology, Department
of Radiology, Mayo Clinic, Rochester,
Minnesota

JEROME F. BREEN, MD
Assistant Professor of Radiology, Department
of Radiology, Mayo Clinic, Rochester,
Minnesota

JEREMY COLLINS, MD
Chief Resident, Department of Radiology,
Diagnostic Radiology Residency Program,
University of California, San Francisco, San
Francisco, California

DALI FENG, MD
Assistant Professor of Medicine, Department
of Cardiology, Mayo Clinic, Rochester,
Minnesota

J. PAUL FINN, MD
Professor of Radiology and Medicine; and
Chief of Diagnostic Cardiovascular Imaging;
and Director of Magnetic Resonance
Research, Department of Radiology, David
Geffen School of Medicine at the University of
California, Los Angeles, Los Angeles, California

VICTOR H. GERBAUDO, PhD
Lecturer and Director of Nuclear Medicine/PET
Program; and Senior Administrative Director,

Noninvasive Cardiovascular Imaging Program,
Department of Radiology, Brigham and
Women's Hospital, Harvard Medical School,
Boston, Massachusetts

RITU R. GILL, MBBS
Instructor, Department of Radiology, Brigham
and Women's Hospital, Harvard Medical
School, Boston, Massachusetts

CHRISTINE M. GLASTONBURY, MBBS
Associate Professor of Radiology, Division
of Neuroradiology, University of California,
San Francisco, San Francisco, California

JAMES GLOCKNER, MD, PhD
Assistant Professor in Radiology, Department
of Radiology, Mayo Clinic, Rochester,
Minnesota

ALLA GODELMAN, MD
Assistant Professor of Radiology, Albert
Einstein College of Medicine; Attending,
Division of Cardiothoracic Imaging,
Department of Radiology, Montefiore
Medical Center, Bronx, New York

LINDA B. HARAMATI, MD
Professor of Clinical Radiology, Albert Einstein
College of Medicine; Chief, Division of
Cardiothoracic Imaging, Department of
Radiology, Montefiore Medical Center, Bronx,
New York

SCOTT R. HARRIS, MD
Cardiac Imaging Fellow in Radiology,
Department of Radiology, Mayo Clinic,
Rochester, Minnesota

HIROTO HATABU, MD, PhD
Clinical Director, MRI Program; and Associate
Professor of Radiology, Department of
Radiology; and Medical Director, Center for
Pulmonary Functional Imaging, Brigham and
Women's Hospital, Harvard Medical School,
Boston, Massachusetts

CHARLES B. HIGGINS, MD
Professor of Radiology, Department of
Radiology, University of California, San
Francisco, San Francisco, California

ANDETTA R. HUNSAKER, MD
Assistant Professor, Department of Radiology,
Brigham and Women's Hospital, Harvard
Medical School, Boston, Massachusetts

FRANCINE L. JACOBSON, MD, MPH
Assistant Professor, Department of Radiology,
Brigham and Women's Hospital, Harvard
Medical School, Boston, Massachusetts

HANS-ULRICH KAUCZOR, MD
Department of Diagnostic Radiology,
University Hospital Heidelberg; and German
Cancer Research Center, Heidelberg, Germany

MAYIL KRISHNAM, MD
Assistant Professor, Department of Radiology,
David Geffen School of Medicine at the
University of California, Los Angeles, Los
Angeles, California

THEODORE J. LEE, MD
Associate Professor of Clinical Radiology,
Department of Radiology, University of
California, San Francisco; Chief, Thoracic
Radiology, San Francisco General Hospital,
San Francisco, California

SEBASTIAN LEY, MD
Department of Pediatric Radiology, University
Hospital Heidelberg, Heidelberg, Germany

JULIA LEY-ZAPOROZHAN, MD
Department of Pediatric Radiology, University
Hospital Heidelberg; Department of Radiology,
German Cancer Research Center, Heidelberg,
Germany

DEREK G. LOHAN, MD
Visiting Assistant Professor, Department of
Radiology, David Geffen School of Medicine at
the University of California, Los Angeles, Los
Angeles, California

MATTHEW W. MARTINEZ, MD
Instructor in Medicine, Department of
Cardiology, Mayo Clinic, Rochester, Minnesota

SHIN MATSUOKA, MD, PhD
Visiting Assistant Professor, Department of
Radiology, Brigham and Women's Hospital,
Boston, Massachusetts

DYLAN V. MILLER, MD
Assistant Professor of Laboratory Medicine
and Pathology, Department of Anatomic
Pathology, Mayo Clinic, Rochester,
Minnesota

ANDREW J. MISSELT, MD
Cardiac Imaging Fellow in Radiology,
Department of Radiology, Mayo Clinic,
Rochester, Minnesota

YOSHIHARU OHNO, MD, PhD
Associate Professor, Department of Radiology,
Kobe University Graduate School of Medicine,
Chuo-ku, Kobe, Japan

KAREN G. ORDOVAS, MD
Assistant Professor of Radiology, Department
of Radiology, University of California, San
Francisco, San Francisco, California

ELLEN E. PARKER, MD
Clinical Instructor of Radiology, Division of
Neuroradiology, University of California, San
Francisco, San Francisco, California

SAMUEL PATZ, PhD
Associate Professor, Department of Radiology;
and Director, Center for Pulmonary Functional
Imaging, Brigham and Women's Hospital,
Boston, Massachusetts

MICHAEL PUDERBACH, MD
Department of Radiology, German Cancer
Research Center, Heidelberg, Germany

SANDRA PUJADAS, MD
Staff Cardiologist, Unidad de Imagen
Cardiaca, Hospital de la Santa Creu i Sant Pau,
Barcelona, Spain

NAVID RAHMANI, MD
Cardiothoracic Radiology Fellow, Department
of Radiology, University of Maryland Medical
Center, Baltimore, Maryland

GAUTHAM P. REDDY, MD, MPH
Associate Professor of Radiology; and Chief of
Cardiac and Pulmonary Imaging; and Director of
the Diagnostic Residency Program, Department
of Radiology, University of California, San
Francisco, San Francisco, California

ROYA SALEH, MD
Research Fellow, Department of Radiology,
David Geffen School of Medicine at the
University of California, Los Angeles,
Los Angeles, California

DAVID J. SUGARBAKER, MD
Richard E. Wilson Professor of Surgical
Oncology; and Chief, Division of Thoracic
Surgery, Department of Surgery, Brigham and
Women's Hospital, Harvard Medical School,
Boston, Massachusetts

IMRAN S. SYED, MD
Instructor in Medicine, Department of
Cardiology, Mayo Clinic, Rochester,
Minnesota

ANDERANIK TOMASIAN, MD
Research Fellow, Department of Radiology,
David Geffen School of Medicine at the
University of California, Los Angeles, Los
Angeles, California

BEATRICE TROTMAN-DICKENSON, MBBS
Instructor, Department of Radiology,
Brigham and Women's Hospital,
Harvard Medical School, Boston,
Massachusetts

CHARLES S. WHITE, MD
Vice Chair and Professor of Diagnostic
Radiology; and Director of Thoracic Imaging,
Department of Radiology, University of
Maryland Medical Center, Baltimore,
Maryland

Contents

Cardiac MR imaging is the preferred method for assessment of cardiac masses. A comprehensive cardiac MR imaging examination for a cardiac mass consists of static morphologic images using fast spin-echo sequences, including single-shot techniques, with T1 and T2 weighting and fat suppression pulses as well as dynamic imaging with cine steady-state free precession techniques. Further tissue characterization is provided with perfusion and delayed enhancement imaging. Specific cardiac tumoral characterization is possible in many cases. When specific tumor characterization is not possible, MR imaging often can demonstrate aggressive versus nonaggressive features that help in differentiating malignant from benign tumors.

Cardiomyopathies, diseases of the myocardium associated with cardiac dysfunction, include hypertrophic, restrictive, and dilated forms and rare entities, such as arrhythmogenic right ventricular dysplasia, ventricular noncompaction, and apical ballooning syndrome. Many have similar presentations, but the underlying condition determines prognoses and treatment. Cardiac MR imaging plays a role in characterizing the range of entities and is crucial for evaluation and management. In addition, delayed enhanced imaging can allow differentiation among the forms of cardiomyopathy and offer prognostic information. As the speed and technical ease of cardiac imaging improve, MR imaging will assume an increasing role in the care of patients who have cardiomyopathy.

Imaging of the pericardium requires understanding of anatomy and the normal and abnormal physiology of the pericardium. MR imaging is well-suited for answering clinical questions regarding suspected pericardial disease. Pericardial diseases that may be effectively imaged with MR imaging include pericarditis, pericardial effusion, cardiac-pericardial tamponade, constrictive pericarditis, pericardial cysts, absence of the pericardium, and pericardial masses. Although benign and malignant primary tumors of the pericardium may be occasionally encountered, the most common etiology of a pericardial mass is metastatic disease.

When ischemic heart disease (IHD) is suspected or confirmed, the primary imaging modality is echocardiography. When appropriate, complementary examinations can be performed. These include stress perfusion scintigraphy, cardiac catheterization, coronary angiography, and CT. MR imaging techniques have developed rapidly over the past several years, and MR imaging has the ability to delineate myocardial perfusion, ventricular function, and myocardial viability in a single examination. Although coronary MR angiography is promising, in recent years it has been supplanted as a noninvasive imaging modality by coronary CT angiography. The other capabilities of MR imaging suggest that it will be performed more and more frequently for the assessment of IHD.

MR imaging has been incorporated into the diagnostic algorithm for suspected thoracic aortic pathology, challenging CT and invasive catheter angiography as investigations of choice. Techniques, including spin echo, 3-D steady-state free precession, cardiac cine imaging, phase-contrast flow quantification, and high-resolution contrast-enhanced magnetic resonance angiography, are poised to trump other single competitive modalities. The proliferation of 3-tesla systems has advanced the performance of magnetic resonance, aided by parallel imaging techniques, multiarray surface coils, and powerful gradient coils. This article considers the current status of MR imaging in evaluation of the thoracic aorta, with reference to common clinical indications in clinical practice.

Time-resolved magnetic resonance angiography (TR-MRA) has received considerable attention recently owing to its ability to provide a dynamic complement to otherwise "static" high-resolution 3-D contrast-enhanced MRA for a variety of clinical indications. Steady technologic advances, including ultrafast pulse sequences, phased multiarray surface coils, parallel data acquisition techniques, and the widespread availability of high-field magnetic resonance systems, have enhanced the clinical usefulness of TR-MRA. This article considers the current role of TR-MRA in thoracic imaging, illustrating many of its clinical applications, and potential future of this recent approach to noninvasive dynamic vascular evaluation.

The thoracic venous system can be visualized and characterized well with MR imaging. In this article, MR sequences that are suited for this purpose (including the more advanced techniques) are reviewed. The normal thoracic venous anatomy and a brief summary of its embryogenesis is provided. The appearances of congenital and acquired abnormalities of the systemic and pulmonary thoracic veins are described. This article also discusses recent applications of MR imaging in the evaluation of the pulmonary veins and the left atrium in patients who have atrial fibrillation.

MR Imaging/Magnetic Resonance Angiography of the Pulmonary Arteries and Pulmonary Thromboembolic Disease
263

Sebastian Ley and Hans-Ulrich Kauczor

Magnetic resonance angiography (MRA) of the pulmonary arteries still is a rapidly evolving technique with already proved high clinical usefulness. Contrast-enhanced and non–contrast-enhanced angiographic techniques are widely available for high spatial or real-time imaging of the pulmonary arteries. Multiple step protocols, such as perfusion MR imaging followed by high spatial resolution contrast-enhanced MRA, seem to be an optimal clinical approach for the assessment of different vascular diseases affecting the pulmonary arteries. This review article describes the MR imaging techniques available and their application in acute and chronic thromboembolic disease.

Functional MR Imaging of the Lung
275

Shin Matsuoka, Andetta R. Hunsaker, Ritu R. Gill, Francine L. Jacobson, Yoshiharu Ohno, Samuel Patz, and Hiroto Hatabu

Recent development of MR techniques has overcome many problems, such as susceptibility artifacts or motion artifact, allowing both static and dynamic MR lung imaging and providing quantitative information of pulmonary function, including perfusion, ventilation, and respiratory motion. Dynamic contrast-enhanced MR perfusion imaging is suitable for the evaluation of angiogenesis of pulmonary solitary nodules. ^{129}Xe MR imaging is potentially a robust technique for the evaluation of various pulmonary function and may replace ^{3}He. The information provided by these new MR imaging methods is proving useful in research and in clinical applications in various lung diseases.

MR for the Evaluation of Obstructive Pulmonary Disease
291

Julia Ley-Zaporozhan, Michael Puderbach, and Hans-Ulrich Kauczor

Obstructive lung diseases include emphysema, chronic bronchitis, chronic obstructive pulmonary disease, asthma, and cystic fibrosis. These diseases are a heterogeneous group of pulmonary disorders that share in common obstruction of air flow and deranged gas exchange. Traditionally these diseases are evaluated with clinical testing, such as pulmonary function tests, but such tests provide only global measures of respiratory function. MR techniques designed for obstructive lung disease have the capability of directly imaging the anatomic and pathophysiologic derangements and may prove useful for monitoring response to therapy.

MR Imaging in Diagnosis and Staging of Pulmonary Carcinoma
309

Alla Godelman and Linda B. Haramati

Lung cancer is the most common cause of cancer-related death for men and women in the United States. Accurate cancer staging is essential for determining appropriate management and predicting prognosis. CT, along with positron emission tomography with fluorodeoxyglucose, currently is the main imaging modality for staging lung cancer. The role of MR imaging is limited, although improvements in MR imaging technology and contrast media potentially will make MR imaging a viable ionizing-radiation-free alternative.

Magnetic Resonance Imaging Clinics of North America

THE CLINICS ARE NOW AVAILABLE ONLINE!

Access your subscription at:
www.theclinics.com

GOAL STATEMENT

The goal of *Magnetic Resonance Imaging Clinics of North America* is to keep practicing physicians up to date with current clinical practice by providing timely articles reviewing the state of the art in patient care.

ACCREDITATION

The *Magnetic Resonance Imaging Clinics of North America* is planned and implemented in accordance with the Essential Areas and Policies of the Accreditation Council for Continuing Medical Education (ACCME) through the joint sponsorship of the University of Virginia School of Medicine and Elsevier. The University of Virginia School of Medicine is accredited by the ACCME to provide continuing medical education for physicians.

The University of Virginia School of Medicine designates this educational activity for a maximum of 15 *AMA PRA Category 1 Credits*™. Physicians should only claim credit commensurate with the extent of their participation in the activity.

The American Medical Association has determined that physicians not licensed in the US who participate in this CME activity are eligible for 15 *AMA PRA Category 1 Credits*™.

Credit can be earned by reading the text material, taking the CME examination online at: http://www.theclinics.com/home/cme, and completing the evaluation. After taking the test, you will be required to review any and all incorrect answers. Following completion of the test and evaluation, your credit will be awarded and you may print your certificate.

FACULTY DISCLOSURE/CONFLICT OF INTEREST

The University of Virginia School of Medicine, as an ACCME accredited provider, endorses and strives to comply with the Accreditation Council for Continuing Medical Education (ACCME) Standards of Commercial Support, Commonwealth of Virginia statutes, University of Virginia policies and procedures, and associated federal and private regulations and guidelines on the need for disclosure and monitoring of proprietary and financial interests that may affect the scientific integrity and balance of content delivered in continuing medical education activities under our auspices.

The University of Virginia School of Medicine requires that all CME activities accredited through this institution be developed independently and be scientifically rigorous, balanced and objective in the presentation/discussion of its content, theories and practices.

All authors/editors participating in an accredited CME activity are expected to disclose to the readers relevant financial relationships with commercial entities occurring within the past 12 months (such as grants or research support, employee, consultant, stock holder, member of speakers bureau, etc.). The University of Virginia School of Medicine will employ appropriate mechanisms to resolve potential conflicts of interest to maintain the standards of fair and balanced education to the reader. Questions about specific strategies can be directed to the Office of Continuing Medical Education, University of Virginia School of Medicine, Charlottesville, Virginia.

The authors/editors listed below have identified no professional or financial affiliations for themselves or their spouse/partner:
Jerome F. Breen, MD; Jeremy Collins, MD; Eduard de Lange, MD (Test Author); DaLi Feng, MD; Paul Finn, MD; Victor H. Gerbuado, PhD; Ritu R. Gill, MBBS; James F. Glockner, MD, PhD; Alla Godelman, MD; Michael B. Gotway, MD (Guest Editor); Linda B. Haramati, MD; Scott R. Harris, MD; Hiroto Hatabu, MD, PhD; Charles B. Higgins, MD; Andetta R. Hunsaker, MD; Francine L. Jacobson, MD, MPH; Hans-Ulrich Kauczor, MD; Mayil Krishnam, MD; Theodore J. Lee, MD; Sebastian Ley, MD; Julia Ley-Zaporozhan, MD; Derek G. Lohan, MD; Matthew W. Martinez, MD; Shin Matsuoka, MD, PhD; Dylan V. Miller, MD; Andrew Misselt, MD; Yoshiharu Ohno, MD, PhD; Karen Gomes Ordovás, MD; Ellen E. Parker, MD; Samuel Patz, PhD; Michael Puderbach, MD; Sandra Pujadas, MD; Navid Rahmani, MD; Gautham P. Reddy, MD, MPH; Lisa Richman (Acquisitions Editor); Roya S. Saleh, MD; David J. Sugarbaker, MD; Imran S. Syed, MD; Anderanik Tomasian, MD; Beatrice Trotman-Dickenson, MBBS; and, Charles S. White, MD.

The authors/editors listed below identified the following professional or financial affiliations for themselves or their spouse/partner:
Philip A. Araoz, MD is an independent contractor for Medtronic.
Christine M. Glastonbury, MBBS is a consultant and owns stock in AMIRSYS.

Disclosure of Discussion of non-FDA approved uses for pharmaceutical products and/or medical devices:
The University of Virginia School of Medicine, as an ACCME provider, requires that all faculty presenters identify and disclose any "off label" uses for pharmaceutical and medical device products. The University of Virginia School of Medicine recommends that each physician fully review all the available data on new products or procedures prior to instituting them with patients.

TO ENROLL

To enroll in the Magnetic Resonance Imaging Clinics of North America Continuing Medical Education program, call customer service at 1-800-654-2452 or visit us online at: www.theclinics.com/home/cme. The CME program is available to subscribers for an additional fee of $99.95.

Preface

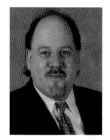

Michael B. Gotway, MD
Guest Editor

In recent years, there have been tremendous advancements in cardiopulmonary CT imaging—no doubt the readership of *Magnetic Resonance Imaging Clinics of North America* is aware of these advances. Simultaneously, cardiothoracic MR imaging has made substantial strides and continues to grow at a rapid rate. Recent developments in MR imaging technology provide shorter imaging times and improved resolution, providing improved tissue characterization and enhanced diagnostic accuracy. These improvements complement the strides made in CT imaging technology, and the two modalities provide very powerful and complementary methods for the investigation of cardiopulmonary disease.

During the last few years, as CT and MR imaging has become more common and image quality have improved dramatically, increasing recognition of the power of these methods for the investigation of cardiac disease, in particular, has stimulated great interest for the radiology community as a whole. Somewhat paradoxically, this interest actually has served to narrow the gap between those who consider themselves primary "pulmonary imagers" and those who would consider themselves exclusively "cardiac imagers." Radiologists are acknowledging that the anatomy and physiology of the cardiopulmonary system, while often addressed individually, should be considered as a whole, and the development of expertise in one anatomic area necessitates proficiency in the other. The common techniques that may be used with CT and MR imaging for the assessment of pulmonary and cardiovascular disease reinforces that a firm understanding of the technology used to investigate the cardiovascular and pulmonary systems should be accompanied by a strong grasp of the anatomy and physiology of both systems, and the interdependence of the cardiopulmonary system should be recognized.

This addition of *MRI Clinics of North America* is a thoracic issue, but a significant component is devoted to cardiovascular imaging. As one peruses these articles, some common themes (particularly MR imaging techniques) will become obvious. Although some techniques will be more specific to the cardiovascular system and others will be aimed toward the respiratory system, commonalities exist nonetheless.

A quick review of the contributing author list shows that this issue benefits from prominent experts in cardiopulmonary imaging. The first portion of this issue focuses more on the cardiac side of cardiopulmonary imaging and then transitions to more pulmonary-focused articles, with one article devoted to pulmonary arterial imaging (certainly a topic of interest to even the most subspecialized cardiac and pulmonary imagers). The issue concludes with articles devoted to the role of MR imaging in the evaluation of pulmonary disease, pleural abnormalities, and thoracic inlet and chest wall disorders.

While this issue is substantial, it is by no means exhaustive. Many areas of study, including thoracic trauma, details of MR imaging evaluation of lung nodules, MR imaging evaluation of the diaphragm and thoracoabdominal junction, and so forth were not included in this issue, but they certainly remain

Magn Reson Imaging Clin N Am 16 (2008) xiii–xiv
doi:10.1016/j.mric.2008.03.005

important considerations. There is no doubt such topics will be visited in future issues.

I express my gratitude to and sincerely thank the contributors of this thoracic focus issue of *MRI Clinics of North America*. I certainly found it to be a highly enlightening process to compile and edit this issue, and I am confident readers will find this issue to be a tremendous educational source for their practice.

Michael B. Gotway, MD
Scottsdale Medical Imaging—an affiliate
of Southwest Diagnostic Imaging, Ltd.
3501 North Scottsdale Road
Suite 130, Box 1573
Scottsdale, AZ 85251, USA

E-mail address:
mgotway@esmil.com (M.B. Gotway)

MR Imaging of Cardiac Masses

Imran S. Syed, MD[a], DaLi Feng, MD[a], Scott R. Harris, MD[b],
Matthew W. Martinez, MD[a], Andrew J. Misselt, MD[b],
Jerome F. Breen, MD[b], Dylan V. Miller, MD[c], Philip A. Araoz, MD[b],*

KEYWORDS
- Mass • Heart tumor • MR imaging

Primary cardiac tumors are rare with an autopsy incidence of only 0.02% and an echocardiographic incidence of 0.15%.[1,2] Among primary cardiac tumors, about 75% are benign, and 25% are malignant.[3] Cardiac metastases are by far more common than primary cardiac malignancies, with incidence rates 20 to 40 times that of primary cardiac tumors.[4,5] Autopsies in patients who have malignancy have demonstrated metastatic involvement of the heart in 10% to 12% of cases, although a much smaller proportion come to clinical attention.[6,7]

A comprehensive knowledge of the characteristics of cardiac tumors is essential for generating a meaningful differential diagnosis or even a specific diagnosis in some cases. Many tumors have specific predilections for certain cardiac chambers or valves. Other features, such as tumor mobility and attachment site, also may be helpful for offering a specific diagnosis. Furthermore, it is important to develop a sense of the aggressiveness of a cardiac tumor. Features such as invasion of extracardiac structures, involvement of more than one cardiac chamber, right-sided location, inhomogeneous tumor tissue, poor border definition, and the presence of a pericardial effusion are aggressive features and suggest a malignant tumor.[8–10] A detailed evaluation of these imaging characteristics is essential, regardless of the imaging modality used.

A variety of imaging modalities are available for the comprehensive evaluation of cardiac masses. Echocardiography often is the initial imaging modality because it is inexpensive, rapidly performed, ubiquitous, portable, and provides high-resolution real-time images. Echocardiography suffers from significant limitations, however, including limited acoustic windows, a restricted field of view that hinders visualization of adjacent mediastinal structures, difficulties in patients who have large body habitus resulting in degraded image quality, inadequate evaluation of the right heart, and limited ability to provide tissue characterization. CT, especially ECG-gated multislice CT, is developing an important role in the assessment of cardiac masses. Newer scanners allow multiplanar reconstructions using isotropic voxels, resulting in high-resolution imaging in virtually any plane, thus matching a previous advantage enjoyed by MR imaging. Dynamic cinematic displays of cardiac motion, usually reserved for echocardiography and MR imaging, are now possible, albeit with lower temporal resolution. CT can depict calcification (better than MR imaging) and fat and also allows excellent visualization of extracardiac anatomy. Significant limitations of CT include the use of ionizing radiation, which in the case of gated multislice CT can exceed the radiation dose of cardiac catheterization, and the need for iodinated contrast media, which carries a risk of nephrotoxicity and allergic reactions.

For various reasons, MR imaging presently is the modality of choice in evaluating cardiac masses. It offers direct multiplanar imaging, a large field of view, and high spatial and temporal resolution with newer cardiac sequences that allow good delineation of the anatomic extent of a mass and any associated functional consequences. Unlike

[a] Department of Cardiology, Mayo Clinic, 200 First Street SW, Rochester, MN 55905, USA
[b] Department of Radiology, Mayo Clinic, 200 First Street SW, Rochester, MN 55905, USA
[c] Department of Anatomic Pathology, Mayo Clinic, 200 First St SW, Rochester, MN 55905, USA
* Corresponding author.
E-mail address: paraoz@mayo.edu (P.A. Araoz).

Magn Reson Imaging Clin N Am 16 (2008) 137–164
doi:10.1016/j.mric.2008.02.009
1064-9689/08/$ – see front matter © 2008 Elsevier Inc. All rights reserved.

echocardiography, there are no limitations with regard to acoustic windows, field of view, or assessment of the right heart. Unlike CT, there is no requirement for radiation or iodinated contrast. The most important advantage of MR imaging is that it provides better tissue characterization than either echocardiography or CT.

MR IMAGING TECHNIQUES

A standard cardiac examination for cardiac masses should incorporate static morphologic images and dynamic imaging with high-resolution cine images of the heart. Administration of gadolinium is helpful, with perfusion and delayed enhancement (DE) imaging assisting in tissue characterization.

Static morphologic imaging usually is performed by means of ECG-gated fast spin-echo sequences that allow image acquisition in a single breath-hold. Newer (eg, single-shot fast spin-echo) sequences may allow significantly faster image acquisition, albeit with a slightly lower signal-to-noise ratio. In addition to morphologic information, fast spin-echo T1- and T2-weighted imaging is valuable in tissue characterization. For example, malignant cells generally are larger and have higher intracellular water content than normal cells, and malignant tissue also often has increased extracellular fluid. The higher free water content of malignant tissue results in longer T1 and T2 relaxation times, resulting in inherent contrast between tumors and normal tissue. Fat suppression prepulses can be added to these sequences to characterize further suspected fatty tumors such as lipomas or, when combined with T2 weighting, can be used to demonstrate the edema associated with aggressive malignant processes.

Dynamic assessment of cardiac masses and of their effect on cardiac and valvular structures can be performed with cine gradient-recalled echo techniques. Older gradient-recalled echo techniques, although still useful, largely have been supplanted by steady-state free precession (SSFP) techniques, which provide excellent contrast between the myocardium and blood pool that is relatively flow insensitive and which have the added advantage of very short repetition times, resulting in shorter breath-holds and faster acquisition times. Signal intensity in this technique depends on the T2/T1 ratio. Structures with a high T2/T1 ratio, such as fat, fluid, and blood, appear bright, whereas myocardium has low signal intensity. The excellent contrast between myocardium and blood pool is especially helpful in the assessment of small intracavitary lesions. Occasionally

sequences using myocardial tagging may be performed to evaluate noncontractile masses in the myocardium (eg, rhabdomyomas).[11]

Administration of gadolinium allows further tissue characterization. Perfusion sequences that are heavily T1 weighted can provide information regarding tumor vascularity. DE imaging, using segmented T1-weighted inversion-recovery, gradient echo, or SSFP sequences, can demonstrate areas of heterogenous enhancement resulting from regional variations in capillary permeability and distribution volumes (eg, increased inflammatory extracellular fluid or areas of necrosis within a tumor). Both these techniques also are helpful in detecting nonenhancing thrombus.

These techniques demonstrate the superior tissue characterization of MR imaging compared with CT and echocardiography. Nevertheless, specific tumoral characterization often is possible only in cases of myxoma, lipoma, fibroma, cysts, and hemangioma.[9]

Benign Cardiac Tumors

Although histologically benign, benign cardiac tumors often cause clinical symptoms related to hemodynamic obstruction, arrhythmias, embolization (of tumor or adherent thrombus), and altered myocardial contractility. MR imaging plays a vital role in early detection and characterization and in providing information that facilitates surgical removal. **Table 1** provides an overview of benign cardiac tumors.

Myxoma

Myxomas are the most abundant primary cardiac tumor, accounting for 50% of all cardiac tumors.[12,13] They primarily affect adults between 30 and 60 years old and have a higher prevalence in women (3:1).

Histologically these tumors consist of scattered cells within a mucopolysaccharide stroma. The tumor cell is thought to originate from multipotential mesenchymal cells that persist as embryonic residues during septation of the heart.[12,14] Macroscopically, they are gelatinous in consistency because of abundant myxoid matrix, with a smooth and lobular or villous and friable surface.[15] They vary considerably in size, ranging from 1 to 15 cm in diameter. They frequently have organized thrombi on the surface. Internally, myxomas are heterogenous and frequently contain cysts, necrosis, calcification, and hemorrhage.[13,16]

The classic triad for the clinical presentation of myxomas consists of constitutional symptoms (fever, malaise, arthralgias, and weight loss), embolic phenomenon (tumor fragments or thrombi), and cardiac obstructive symptoms (eg, prolapse of a pedunculated myxoma through the mitral valve in diastole, simulating mitral stenosis on physical examination), with one or more of these present in most patients.[12] Most myxomas are sporadic, although, rarely, they may be part of a heritable syndrome, the Carney complex. The Carney complex is distinct from Carney's triad (the association of gastrointestinal stromal tumor, extra-adrenal paraganglioma, and pulmonary chondroma). Carney's complex is an autosomal dominant condition that consists of cardiac myxomas and a variety of hyperpigmented skin lesions.[17] It is associated with the development of extracardiac tumors such as pituitary adenomas, breast fibroadenomas, and melanotic schwannomas. Patients who have Carney complex are likely to be younger than patients who have sporadic myxomas and to have multiple myxomas in atypical sites outside the left atrium, which may recur after resection.[18]

Myxomas typically are solitary tumors (90%) and usually are located in the left atrium (80%) or right atrium (15%–20%) and, rarely, in the ventricles.[13] They frequently are pedunculated masses that are attached to the interatrial septum, specifically the fossa ovalis, by either a broad base or a narrow stalk. They may arise from any endocardial surface, however. Occasionally they may extend across the fossa ovalis to involve both atria.[12] Lesions with a narrow stalk may demonstrate significant mobility and prolapse through the mitral or tricuspid valves during diastole, thus mimicking the clinical picture of mitral or tricuspid stenosis.

The imaging appearance of a myxoma varies, depending on its myxomatous components and on the presence of areas of calcification, hemorrhage, necrosis, or thrombus, which result in a heterogenous appearance. Dark-blood morphologic imaging typically demonstrates an intracavitary mass arising from the fossa ovalis and extending into the left atrium. In general, myxomas are hyperintense on T2-weighted images because of their myxoid stroma (high extracellular water content).[19] They usually appear isointense on T1-weighted images. The presence of calcification or hemorrhage may result in a heterogenous appearance on T1- and T2-weighted images, however.[20] SSFP cine images usually demonstrate higher signal intensity than myocardium (but lower signal intensity than blood) because of the higher T2/T1 ratio of myxoid stroma, although areas of internal calcification and overlying thrombus demonstrate lower signal intensity.[19] Cine imaging is especially helpful in visualizing the endocardial attachment of the myxoma and the hemodynamic effect of

a mobile lesion. DE images (using an inversion pre-pulse to null normal myocardium) usually demonstrate heterogenous enhancement, but intense enhancement may be seen. Overlying thrombus is intensely hypointense on DE images, even when long inversion times are used. **Figs. 1–3** demonstrate examples of myxomas.

Papillary Fibroelastoma

Papillary fibroelastoma is the second most common benign cardiac tumor after myxoma and represents 10% of all benign tumors in some series.[13,16,21] There is no gender predilection, and the mean age at presentation is 60 years.

Papillary fibroelastomas are composed of avascular fronds of dense connective tissue lined by endothelium. The pathologic origin remains unclear. Macroscopically they resemble a sea anemone and are composed of delicate, frondlike excrescences attached to the endocardium by a short pedicle. They typically are small tumors (usually < 1 cm in size), and 80% to 90% present on valve surfaces, making them the most common primary tumor to occur on valves.[21,22] Less commonly they may occur on the endocardial surface of the atria or ventricles. They are slightly more common on the aortic (44%) and mitral (35%) than on the tricuspid (15%) and pulmonary (8%) valves, although this reported predilection may be attributed to the increased prevalence of symptoms associated with left-sided lesions.[21] In contrast to Lambl's excrescences, which are smaller filiform structures, papillary fibroelastomas usually are found away from the free edges of the valve. They occur most commonly on the atrial side of atrioventricular valves and the aortic surface of the semilunar valves. These tumors usually are isolated, although multiple tumors have been reported.[23] They usually are detected incidentally on echocardiograms, but affected patients may present with neurologic symptoms related to embolic events resulting from tumor fragments or fibrin clots that develop on the surface of these tumors. The treatment is surgical excision with possible valve repair or replacement, if necessary. There are no reports of recurrences after surgical resection.

Papillary fibroelastomas usually are not visualized well on MR imaging because of their small size and their location on mobile valve leaflets. There are only a few descriptions in the MR imaging literature.[24–28] They are best appreciated on cine MR imaging sequences with high spatial and temporal resolution (eg, SSFP), where they appear as a mass on a valve leaflet or endocardial surface with peritumoral turbulence of blood flow.

Table 1
Benign cardiac tumors

Type of Tumor	Site	Location	Population	T1-weighted	T2-weighted	Cine-MR Imaging	Postcontrast Enhancement	Special Diagnostic Features/ Syndrome	Other Data
Myxoma	Intracavitary	Interatrial septum (left atrium, 80%; right atrium, 15%–20%)	Female: male ratio, 3:1 30–60 years	Isointense, heterogenous	Hyperintense, heterogenous	High signalintensity	Heterogenous enhancement	Carney complex, mobile left atrial tumor, commonly has a stalk, attachment to fossa ovalis	Areas of necrosis, calcification, and overlying thrombus may be present
Papillary fibroelastoma	Intracavitary	Cardiac valves (usually left-sided)	Middle-aged to elderly	Isointense	Isointense			Small (< 1 cm) frondlike sessile lesions attached to left-sided cardiac valves	Usually not well seen on MR imaging
Fibroma	Intramural	Ventricular septum, left ventricle free wall, right ventricle	Children, mean age 13 years	Isointense	Hypointense	Isointense	Enhancement	Gorlin syndrome, usually solitary intramural ventricular mass that distorts normal anatomy, commonly calcified	Lack of first-pass enhancement on perfusion imaging
Lipoma	Epicardial/ intramural/ endocardial	Variable	Adults	Hyperintense	Hyperintense	High signal intensity	None	Encapsulated homogenous masses that are commonly epicardial, suppression with fat saturation techniques	

Rhabdomyoma	Intramural	Left ventricle	Children	Isointense	Iso- or mildly hyperintense	Isointense	Homogenous enhancement	Tuberous sclerosis, multiple intramural masses	Tagging may demonstrate altered contractility; may undergo spontaneous regression
Paraganglioma	Intramural	Atrial walls (left atrium > right atrium), atrioventricular sulcus, aortic root	30–40 years	Isointense, heterogenous	Hyperintense ("light bulb" bright)	High signal intensity	Enhancement	Encapsulated hypervascular lesions that are hyperintense on T2-weighted and postcontrast images	Extensive enhancement on first-pass perfusion; usually sporadic
Hemangioma	Intramural/epicardial/pericardial	Variable	Variable	Hyperintense, heterogenous	Hyperintense, heterogenous	High signal intensity	Enhancement	Multicystic septated enhancing lesions with high signal intensity on T1- and, T2-weighted and postcontrast images	Extensive enhancement on first-pass perfusion, high signal intensity on T1-weighted images because of interspersed fat
Lymphangioma	Epicardial/pericardial	Pericardial space	Infants, children	Isointense, heterogenous	Hyperintense, heterogenous		None (single report)	Multicystic septated lesions with low signal intensity on T1-weighted images and high signal intensity on T2-weighed images	Low signal intensity on T1-weighted images because of extensive cystic fluid-filled spaces
Intravenous leiomyomatosis	Intracavitary	Right atrium	Middle-aged women	Isointense	Iso- or mildly hyperintense		Heterogenous enhancement	Originates from inferior vena cava	

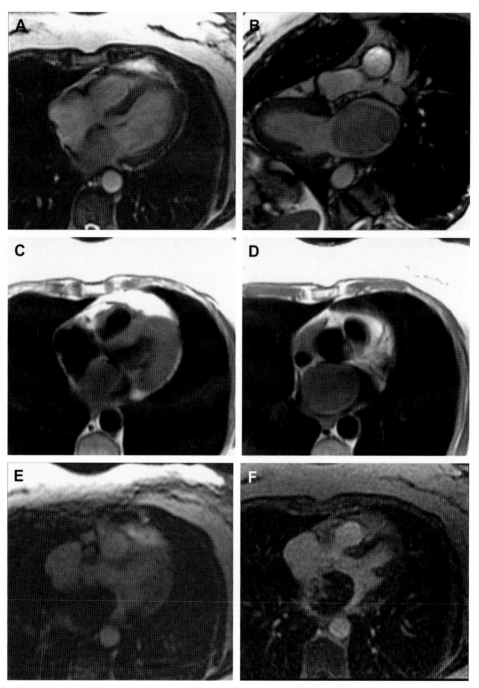

Fig. 1. Cardiac myxoma. (*A*) Four-chamber and (*B*) two-chamber SSFP images show a broad-based, smoothly contoured, sessile left atrial mass that is hyperintense relative to myocardium. (*C, D*) Axial T1-weighted black-blood images show the mass to be isointense relative to myocardium. The attachment site seems to be the interatrial septum. (*E*) First-pass perfusion imaging after contrast shows relative hypovascularity. (*F*) DE inversion-recovery image shows scattered foci of DE.

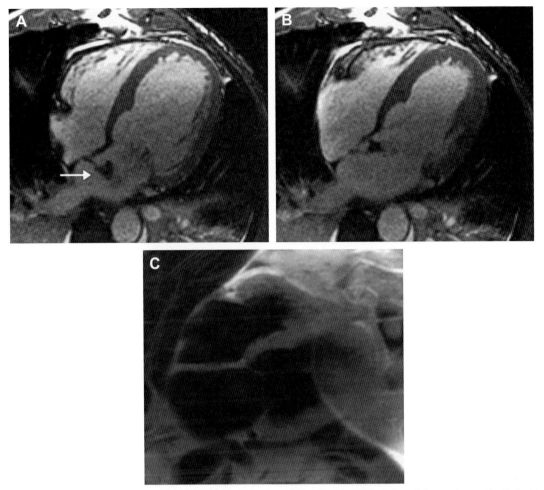

Fig. 2. Myxoma. (*A, B*) Four-chamber SSFP image shows a pedunculated, mobile left atrial mass (*arrow* in *A*) that is attached to the fossa ovalis via a narrow stalk and is relatively isointense to the myocardium. (*C*) T1-weighted black-blood image in a four-chamber view shows only a faint outline of the mass. Small, rapidly mobile lesions sometimes can be missed on black-blood imaging.

They are difficult to visualize on static fast spin-echo images, but when seen they have intermediate signal intensity on T1- and T2-weighted images.

Lipoma

Cardiac lipomas are benign tumors composed of mature adipocytes. Their exact incidence is unclear, because some series do not distinguish between lipomas and lipomatous hypertrophy of the interatrial septum, which is not a true neoplasm.[13] They probably are quite rare. They typically are found in adult patients but can affect patients of all ages. There is no gender predilection.

At gross examination, cardiac lipomas are encapsulated, homogenous collections of adipocytes. They usually originate from the epicardium and grow into the pericardial space, although myocardial or endocardial origins are also possible with growth into any of the cardiac chambers.[18] They usually are seen as solitary lesions, although multiple lipomas have been described in children who have tuberous sclerosis; however, they generally do not occur as part of a syndrome.[13] They often are quite large by the time they come to clinical attention and have weighed as much as 4800 g.[29]

Most patients who have cardiac lipomas are asymptomatic, and the tumors are detected incidentally.[30] Intracavitary lipomas have been reported to cause blood flow obstruction with related symptoms.[31] Lipomas in the pericardial space may cause dyspnea, either by ventricular compression or by displacing adjacent lung tissue.[32,33] Intramural tumors also have been

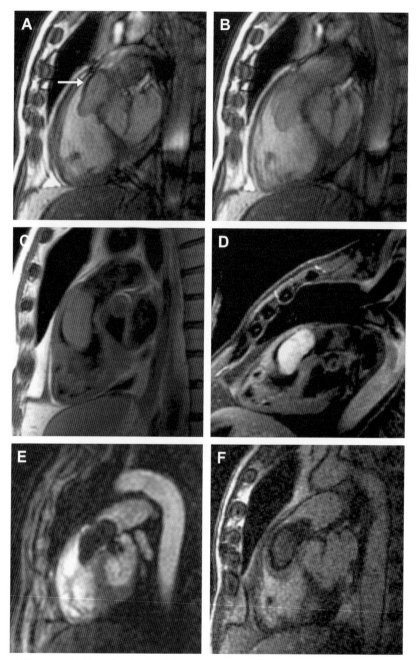

Fig. 3. Myxoma with an atypical location in the right ventricular outflow tract (RVOT). (*A, B*) Oblique sagittal SSFP images show a large, smoothly contoured, hyperintense mass in the RVOT (*arrow in panel 3A*), causing severe outflow obstruction. The smooth contour and lack of invasiveness favor a nonmalignant etiology. (*C*) The mass is mildly hyperintense on T1-weighted images and (*D*) is strongly hyperintense on T2-weighted images. (*E*) First-pass perfusion imaging after administration of contrast shows relative hypovascularity and a delay in enhancement. (*F*) DE inversion-recovery image shows some central DE.

associated with a variety of atrial and ventricular arrhythmias and conduction abnormalities.[34–37] Cardiac lipomas usually are treated by surgical resection, especially if symptoms are present. They may encapsulate or infiltrate the coronary vessels,

which is a significant factor in determining resectability.[30]

MR imaging is diagnostic and demonstrates encapsulated, smooth, homogenous lesions with high signal intensity on T1-weighted images, slightly less high signal intensity on T2-weighted images, and signal dropout on fat-saturated images (**Fig. 4**). They have high signal intensity on cine SSFP images (see **Fig. 4**A). The signal intensity is similar to that of adjacent epicardial and mediastinal fat. They do not demonstrate postcontrast enhancement.[18]

Fibroma

Cardiac fibromas are rare, congenital tumors that primarily afflict infants and children, being the second most common tumor in this age group. They are less frequently encountered in adolescents and adults. The mean age at presentation is 13 years.

These tumors represent collections of fibroblasts and collagen and frequently contain foci of calcification. Cystic change, hemorrhage, and necrosis usually are not seen.[38] They are thought to have a congenital origin, and many pathologists believe they represent a hamartoma rather than a neoplasm.[13] Macroscopically, they are firm, solid, usually well-circumscribed tumors that present as a solitary, discrete, focal mass within the myocardial wall. They often are quite large (mean diameter, 5 cm) and can obliterate the ventricular cavity. They typically are located in the ventricular

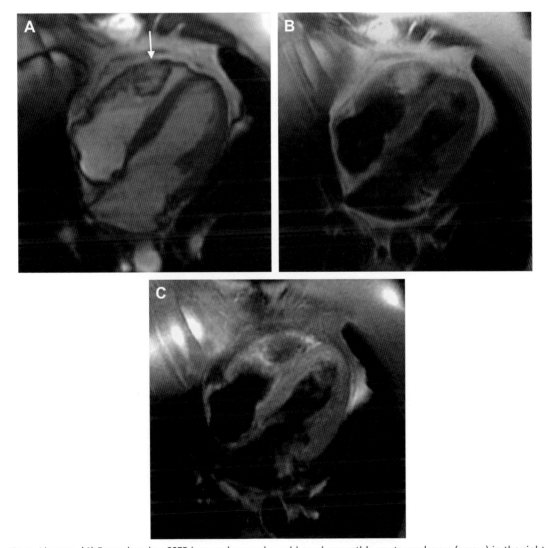

Fig. 4. Lipoma. (*A*) Four-chamber SSFP image shows a broad-based, smoothly contoured mass (*arrow*) in the right ventricle that is hyperintense with intensity similar to surrounding epicardial fat. Lipomas appear markedly hyperintense on SSFP images because fat has a high T2/T1 ratio. (*B*) Lipomas appear bright on T1-weighted images and (*C*) demonstrate signal drop-out with fat suppression prepulses.

septum or left ventricular free wall but less commonly occur in the right ventricle or the atria.[13]

Cardiac fibromas frequently are associated with arrhythmias and are the second most common primary cardiac tumor associated with sudden cardiac death after endodermal heterotopias of the atrioventricular node.[39] Patients also may present with symptoms related to heart failure, syncope, chest pain, and blood flow obstruction.[40] About a third of patients are asymptomatic.[13] Fibromas are associated with Gorlin syndrome, which is characterized by basal cell carcinomas of the skin, odontogenic keratocysts, skeletal anomalies,

and a tendency toward other neoplasms.[41,42] Treatment usually is surgical resection.

The primary differential diagnoses in an infant are rhabdomyoma and rhabdomyosarcoma. If there are multiple masses or signs of tuberous sclerosis, rhabdomyoma can be diagnosed confidently. If the tumor is solitary, ventricular, and calcified, the diagnosis of fibroma is likely. Rhabdomyosarcomas are rare, malignant tumors that differ from fibromas in that they do not calcify, frequently contain areas of cystic change, hemorrhage, and necrosis, and occur in all cardiac chambers with equal frequency.[10]

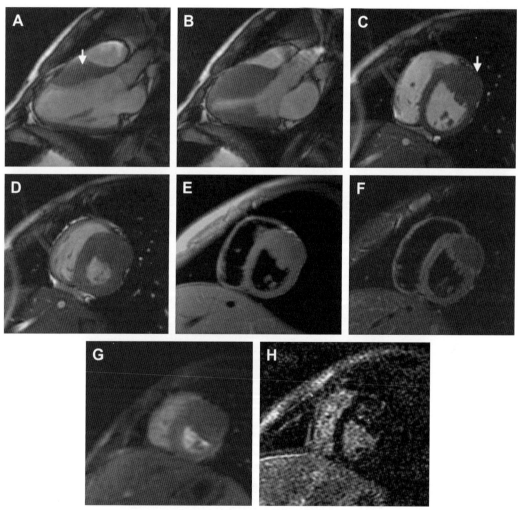

Fig. 5. Fibroma in the left ventricular myocardium. (*A, B*) Three-chamber SSFP images show focal thickening of the anterior ventricular septum (*arrow in panel A*). (*C, D*) Short-axis SSFP images also show focal thickening of the anterior ventricular septum and anterior ventricular wall (*arrow in panel C*). Because their intensity is similar to that of myocardium on SSFP images, fibromas easily can be mistaken for asymmetric ventricular hypertrophy. (*E*) Fibromas are isointense to myocardium on T1-weighted images but (*F*) are characteristically hypointense on T2-weighted images, in contradistinction to most cardiac tumors. (*G*) First-pass perfusion image after contrast shows hypovascularity compared with normal myocardium. (*H*) DE inversion-recovery image shows peripheral foci of hyperenhancement.

MR imaging allows fairly specific tumoral characterization of cardiac fibroma. It appears as a discrete intramural mass or area of focal myocardial thickening that often distorts ventricular anatomy (**Figs. 5 and 6**). Cardiac fibromas generally are isointense on T1-weighted images (see **Figs. 5E and 6B**) and, unlike most tumors, appear hypointense on T2-weighted images (because of their fibrous composition and low water content; see **Figs. 5F and 6C**).[18,19] The presence of calcification may make their appearance heterogenous. They are hypointense compared with the remaining myocardium on cine SSFP images (see **Figs. 5A–D and 6A**).[43] Because of their relative avascularity, they are hypovascular compared with normal myocardium on perfusion imaging (see **Fig. 5G**).

DE inversion-recovery imaging has been reported recently with intense hyperenhancement of these lesions, sometimes with a hypointense core that reflects their reduced vascularity (see **Figs. 5H and 6D**).[43,44]

Rhabdomyoma

Rhabdomyomas are the most common primary cardiac tumor in infants and children. Approximately 50% of rhabdomyomas occur in association with tuberous sclerosis. Although most infants who have tuberous sclerosis have cardiac rhabdomyomas, their prevalence decreases with age, in part because of spontaneous tumor regression, so fewer than 25% of adults who have tuberous sclerosis have cardiac tumors.[45]

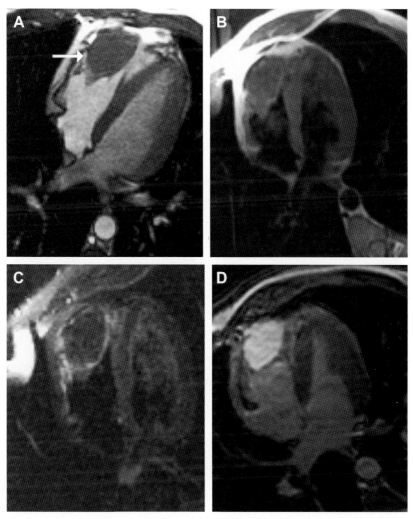

Fig. 6. Fibroma in the right ventricular myocardium. (*A*) Four-chamber SSFP image demonstrates a discrete intramural right ventricular mass (*arrow*) that distorts the shape of the right ventricular cavity and is isointense to normal myocardium. (*B*) Fibromas are isointense to myocardium on T1-weighted images and (*C*) are characteristically hypointense on T2-weighted images. (*D*) DE inversion-recovery image demonstrates marked hyperenhancement.

Histologically rhabdomyomas consist of enlarged, vacuolated cells with abundant glycogen and sparse cytoplasm that resemble altered myocytes. They are usually 1 to 3 cm in size. When associated with tuberous sclerosis, they occur as multiple intramural masses in the ventricular myocardium and usually are detected by prenatal ultrasonography. Prenatal MR imaging also can detect cardiac rhabdomyomas.[46] Because most of these tumors regress spontaneously, surgery is not required routinely. Sporadic rhabdomyomas, on the other hand, often are single lesions, usually do not regress, and may require surgery. Rhabdomyomas can produce life-threatening symptoms related to obstruction of the left ventricular outflow tract or arrhythmias, and these tumors require surgical excision.

On MR imaging rhabdomyomas usually present as multiple intramyocardial masses that are isointense to myocardium on T1-weighted images and are hyperintense on T2-weighted images. On cine MR imaging they appear as masslike regions of myocardium with focally altered contractility. These regions of altered contractility also can be differentiated from normal myocardium using myocardial tagging.[11] There is strong homogenous enhancement after contrast administration.[47]

Paraganglioma

Cardiac paragangliomas are extremely rare tumors that originate from neuroendocrine cells. Patients typically are young adults who present with symptoms of catecholamine excess such as hypertension, flushing, palpitations, and heart failure. Cardiac paragangliomas occur as sporadic lesions. Histologically, they consist of paraganglial cells surrounded by sustentacular cells and are identical to extracardiac paragangliomas. Macroscopically they tend to be large lesions (3 to 8 cm) that may be well encapsulated or infiltrative with areas of necrosis. They usually are located in the distribution of the normal cardiac ganglia, most frequently in the posterior wall of the left atrium, along the atrioventricular groove, and at the roots of the great vessels. Occasionally they may arise from the interatrial septum and must be distinguished from myxomas. Because of their vascularity and tendency to involve the coronary arteries, surgical resection often is quite difficult.

MR imaging of cardiac paragangliomas often shows a nonspecific intracardiac mass, appearing hypo- or isointense on T1-weighted images (**Fig. 7**A).[18,48] Paragangliomas, however, are characterized by marked hyperintensity on T2-weighted images (see **Fig. 7**B) and have been described as "light-bulb" bright.[18,48] Increased

signal intensity on T1-weighted images, probably caused by hemorrhage within the tumor, also has been described.[49] Because of their vascularity they demonstrate intense enhancement after contrast. The enhancement often is heterogenous, with central nonenhancing areas caused by tumor necrosis (see **Fig. 7**).[48,50,51]

Hemangiomas

Hemangiomas are benign vascular tumors that can affect patients of all ages (mean age at diagnosis, 43 years) and probably account for 5% to 10% of all benign tumors.[13] They are classified according to the size of their vascular channels as cavernous, capillary, or arteriovenous hemangiomas. Histologically they consist of endothelial-lined, thin-walled spaces, but they may contain other tissue elements such as fat, interspersed calcification, and fibrous tissue.[52] They can occur in any cardiac chamber and may be endocardial, intramural, or epicardial. Most hemangiomas are asymptomatic and are detected incidentally.

SSFP MR imaging in patients who have hemangioma often shows a mass with low signal intensity within the affected cardiac chamber (**Fig. 8**A and B). Hemangiomas are heterogeneously isointense compared with myocardium on T1-weighted MR images (see **Fig. 8**C) and are hyperintense on T2-weighted images (see **Fig. 8**D).[19] They demonstrate intense and prolonged enhancement after contrast administration, although this enhancement often is heterogenous because of interspersed calcium and fibrous septa (see **Fig. 8**E and F).[53–55]

Lymphangioma

Lymphangiomas are extremely rare benign tumors composed of endothelial-lined, thin-walled spaces that contain lymph. Most reported cases have occurred in children. These tumors most commonly involve the epicardial surface or the pericardial space, sometimes compressing adjacent structures. They have been known to cause arrhythmias, cardiac tamponade, and sudden cardiac death.

Most MR imaging reports of lymphangioma have described low-intermediate signal intensity on T1-weighted images and high signal intensity on T2-weighted images.[56,57] In a recent report, there was no enhancement with contrast.[58]

Intravenous Leiomyomas

Intravenous leiomyomas are rare, benign, smooth muscle tumors usually originating from a uterine myoma and extending via the inferior vena cava into the right atrium and sometimes through the

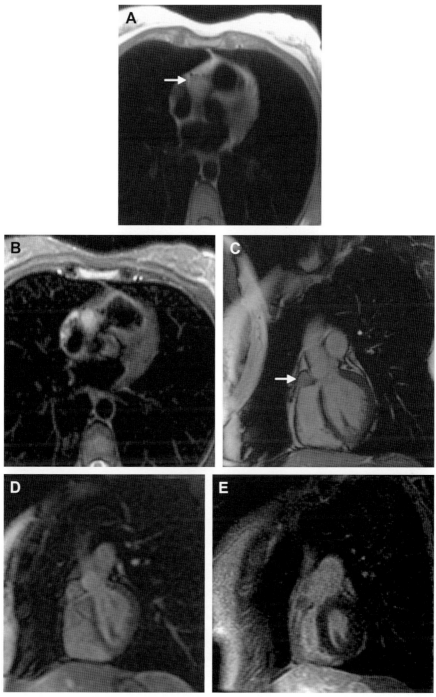

Fig. 7. Paraganglioma in the right atrioventricular (AV) groove. (*A*) Axial T1-weighted image demonstrates an isointense mass (*arrow*) in the right AV groove, immediately subjacent to the right coronary artery. Many of the imaging features of paragangliomas are a result of their high vascularity. (*B*) This vascularity gives them a characteristic "light-bulb" bright appearance on T2-weighted images. (*C*) Coronal SSFP image shows a hyperintense mass in the right AV groove (*arrow*), again a result of hypervascularity. (*D*) Paragangliomas appear as hypervascular structures on first-pass perfusion imaging. (*E*) DE inversion-recovery image demonstrates mild contrast retention but no real DE.

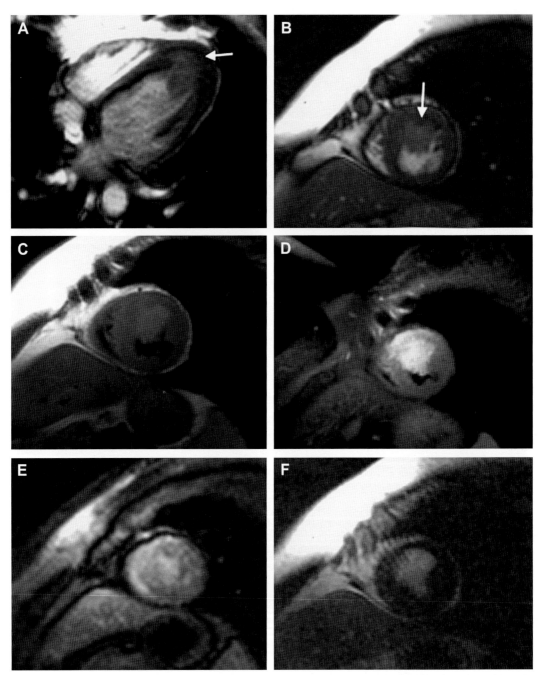

Fig. 8. Cavernous hemangioma. (*A*) Four-chamber SSFP image shows a well-defined hyperintense mass (*arrow*) in the left ventricular apex that seems to arise from the endocardial surface. (*B*) Short-axis SSFP image shows that the mass (*arrow*) involves the anterior and anteroseptal endocardial surface of the left ventricle. (*C*) The mass is mildly hyperintense on T1-weighted images and (*D*) is strongly hyperintense on T2-weighted images. (*E*) First-pass perfusion image shows the mass to be highly vascular. (*F*) DE inversion-recovery image shows marked contrast retention and hyperenhancement.

tricuspid orifice into the right ventricle. They usually occur in premenopausal women.

Intravenous leiomyomas usually appear on MR imaging as mobile right atrial masses that extend from the inferior vena cava. They are isointense on T1-weighted images and isointense to mildly hyperintense on T2-weighted images. They show enhancement after contrast administration.[59]

MALIGNANT CARDIAC TUMORS

Metastases are by far the most common cardiac malignancy. The most common primary cardiac tumors are sarcomas; the remainder are lymphomas.[13] Primary cardiac sarcomas, by definition, are confined to the heart or pericardium at the time of diagnosis with no evidence of an extracardiac primary tumor. The various cardiac sarcomas display a wide variety of morphologies because of their mesenchymal origin; the most common types are angiosarcoma (37%), undifferentiated (24%), malignant fibrous histiocytoma (11%–24%), leiomyosarcoma (8%–9%), and osteosarcoma (3%–9%).[13] MR imaging usually cannot provide a specific tissue diagnosis for the different malignancies but can demonstrate aggressive features that favor a malignant etiology: poor border definition, heterogenous appearance with foci of necrosis and hemorrhage, frequent involvement of the right-sided cardiac chambers or involvement of multiple chambers, extracardiac extension, and coexistent pericardial effusions.

Most cardiac sarcomas, with the exception of angiosarcoma (in the right atrium) and fibrosarcoma and rhabdomyosarcoma (generalized), usually are located within the left atrium. Thus, they may be mistaken for myxomas, which are more common and benign. This misidentification is especially likely for malignant fibrous histiocytomas, osteosarcomas, and leiomyosarcomas. A broad base of attachment, multiple attachment sites, nonseptal origin, and an aggressive growth pattern (such as extension into the pulmonary veins or infiltration of the epicardium) should raise concern for sarcoma. **Table 2** provides an overview of malignant cardiac tumors.

Angiosarcoma

Angiosarcoma is the most common primary cardiac tumor. It typically occurs in middle-aged men. It is a tumor of mesenchymal origin with ill-defined anastomotic vascular spaces lined by endothelial cells. In contradistinction to most sarcomas, which tend to arise in the left atrium, angiosarcomas have a predilection for the right atrium.[60] The gross morphologic appearance usually is of a bulky, heterogenous, infiltrative right atrial mass with large central areas of necrosis and hemorrhage that frequently invades other cardiac chambers, adjacent structures, and the pericardium. Sometimes, however, an angiosarcoma can present as an ill-defined infiltrative pericardial mass. Because of its location, patients usually present with right-sided heart failure or tamponade from a hemorrhagic pericardial effusion, often with superimposed signs such as fever and

weight loss. Pericardiocentesis may not always reveal tumor cells.[10] Presentation is late, with more than two thirds of patients exhibiting metastases, usually to the lungs.[60,61]

Angiosarcomas show a heterogenous appearance on T1-weighted MR imaging images with hyperintense foci corresponding to hemorrhage interspersed within isointense areas (**Fig. 9A**).[62–65] Necrotic areas may appear hypointense. Angiosarcomas have a heterogenous, predominantly hyperintense appearance on T2-weighted images. This heterogenous appearance on T1- and T2-weighted images has been likened to a "cauliflower" appearance.[63,64] This "cauliflower" appearance is also evident on cine-images with SSFP, which commonly demonstrate a polymorphic tumor that is partly hyperintense because of its highly vascular nature (see **Fig. 9B**).[64,66] After contrast administration, angiosarcomas demonstrate a heterogenous pattern of enhancement reflecting regions of hypervascularity and necrosis. Recently several authors have described such heterogenous enhancement on DE images.[64,66] In cases with diffuse pericardial infiltration, linear contrast enhancement at the surface with a hypointense necrotic core gives rise to a "sunray" appearance.[67]

Undifferentiated Sarcoma

Undifferentiated sarcomas have no specific histologic features. Their relative proportion has decreased over the years because of improved diagnostic techniques. They usually are located in the left atrium and often appear as intracavitary or infiltrating polypoid masses.[10]

There are no specific findings that allow the MR diagnosis of undifferentiated cardiac sarcoma. Undifferentiated sarcomas usually have been described as isointense lesions on T1- and T2-weighted images.

Malignant Fibrous Histiocytoma

Malignant fibrous histiocytoma is the second most common identifiable cardiac sarcoma. There is a slight female predilection, and the mean age at presentation is 47 years.[68] The cell of origin is a fibroblast or histioblast. On histology, a storiform pattern of spindle cells (fibroblasts) and round cells (histiocytic cells) cells is characteristic.[69] A histiocytoma is located in the left atrium in more than 80% of cases and must be distinguished from a myxoma.[68] Unlike a myxoma, it usually arises from the posterior wall of the left atrium and may cause pulmonary venous or mitral inflow obstruction. There is a high rate of metastasis and local recurrence after surgery.

Table 2
Malignant cardiac tumors

Type of Tumor	Location	Population	T1-weighted	T2-weighted	Cine-MR Imaging	Postcontrast Enhancement	Special Diagnostic Features	Other Data
Angiosarcoma	Right atrium	Males, mean age 42 years	Isointense with hyperintense areas (hemorrhage), "cauliflower" appearance	Isointense	Heterogenous, partly hyperintense	Strong enhancement, "sunray" appearance	Bulky, irregular right atrial mass that frequently infiltrates the pericardium	Most common primary malignancy; hemorrhagic areas; cardiac tamponade
Undifferentiated sarcoma	Left atrium	Variable	Isointense	Isointense		Nonspecific	Variable morphology: infiltrative or masslike	Possible pericardial origin
Osteosarcoma	Left atrium	Variable	Heterogeneously isointense (no detailed reports)	Heterogeneously hyperintense	Heterogenous, mostly isointense	Nonspecific	Calcification	Often involves the mitral valve; pulmonary venous obstruction
Rhabdomyosarcoma	Variable	Children	Isointense	Isointense, heterogenous	Isointense	Enhancement with central nonenhancing areas (necrosis)	Central necrosis	May arise from valves; may involve pericardium
Malignant fibrous histiocytoma	Left atrium	Slight female predilection, mean age 47 years	Isointense	Hyperintense		Limited reports, heterogenous enhancement	Posterior wall of the left atrium in > 80% of cases	Pulmonary venous obstruction; left atrial obstruction; distinguish from myxoma

Leiomyosarcoma	Left atrium	Variable	Isointense	Hyperintense	Nonspecific	Posterior wall of the left atrium in > 80% of cases	Pulmonary venous obstruction; left atrial obstruction; distinguish from myxoma
Fibrosarcoma	Left atrium	Variable	Isointense, heterogenous	Hyperintense	Central nonenhancement	Large areas of necrosis	Most common sarcoma to involve ventricles; pericardial involvement frequent (possible pericardial origin)
Liposarcoma	Left atrium	Variable	Not reported	Not reported	Nonspecific	Foci of macroscopic fat sometimes evident	
Lymphoma	Right atrium and ventricle	Immunocompromised patients	Iso- or hypointense	Hyperintense	Homogenous or heterogenous enhancement		Less likely than sarcomas to demonstrate necrosis and extend into cardiac chambers

Malignant fibrous histiocytoma usually is visualized on MR imaging as a bulky left atrial mass. The morphologic features described previously help distinguish it from myxoma.[70] Tumoral characterization is nonspecific. It appears isointense on T1-weighted images and hyperintense on T2-weighted images. Inhomogeneous enhancement has been reported after contrast administration.[71]

Rhabdomyosarcoma

Rhabdomyosarcomas, which are malignant tumors of striated muscle, account for only 4% to 7% of all sarcomas but are the most common primary cardiac malignancy in infants and children. There are two main histologic types: embryonal neoplasms, which occur in children and adults, and a rarer pleomorphic type, which occurs in adults. They arise from the myocardium, have no specific chamber predilection, are more likely than any other sarcoma to involve the cardiac valves, often are multiple, and may invade the pericardium.[10] At gross examination, they usually contain large areas of central necrosis.

Rhabdomyosarcomas appear isointense relative to myocardium on T1-weighted MR images.[72,73] They also appear isointense on cine-MR imaging.[19] When entirely intramyocardial, they may appear as focally hypertrophied myocardium.[74] After contrast administration they demonstrate enhancement, which may be heterogenous because of central necrosis within the tumor.[72,73]

Osteosarcoma

Cardiac osteosarcomas are rare malignant tumors composed of bone-producing cells of osteo-, chondro-, or fibroblastic differentiation. Unlike metastatic osteosarcomas, which often occur in the right atrium, primary cardiac osteosarcomas usually arise in the left atrium. They often have dense calcification, which is better appreciated by CT. Because of their left atrial location, they may be confused for myxomas, which are more common and are benign. Cardiac osteosarcomas are often aggressive tumors, with a very poor prognosis.

MR imaging features that suggest an osteosarcoma rather than a myxoma include a broad base of attachment, location away from the fossa ovalis, and evidence of invasive behavior (**Fig. 10**). There is no detailed description of MR imaging findings, but osteosarcomas generally appear heterogeneously isointense on T1-weighted images (see **Fig. 10C**) and hyperintense on T2-weighted images (see **Fig. 10D**).[75,76] An important feature is the presence of calcification, which can be confirmed by CT (see **Fig. 10E**).

Leiomyosarcoma

Leiomyosarcoma are rare tumors of smooth muscle origin. They usually present as sessile masses from the posterior wall of the left atrium.[13] They must be distinguished from left atrial myxomas. They tend to invade the pulmonary veins and mitral valves, and patients may

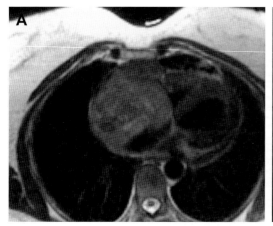
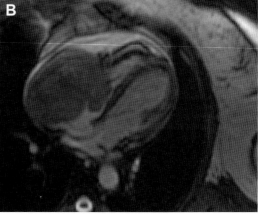

Fig. 9. Angiosarcoma. (*A*) Axial T1-weighted black-blood image shows a heterogenous "cauliflower" mass with bright areas corresponding to hemorrhage and dark areas corresponding to tumor necrosis. A small pericardial effusion is present. (*B*) Axial SSFP image shows a bulky, irregular, infiltrative right atrial mass that invades the pericardium and the tricuspid valve. It has a heterogenous appearance with hyperintense areas caused by tumor vascularity.

present with symptoms of congestive heart failure from mitral inflow obstruction. They may be multiple in 30% of cases.[13]

Limited MR imaging descriptions of leiomyosarcoma exist in the literature. Generally, these tumors appear as isointense on T1-weighted images and hyperintense on T2-weighted images[77,78] and demonstrate enhancement after contrast administration.[79]

Fibrosarcoma

Cardiac fibrosarcomas are rare malignant tumors that are primarily fibroblastic in origin. Although most common in the left atrium, they also may be seen on the right side of the heart and sometimes in the ventricles. They often contain necrotic areas. They are aggressive tumors and frequently invade the pericardium.[10]

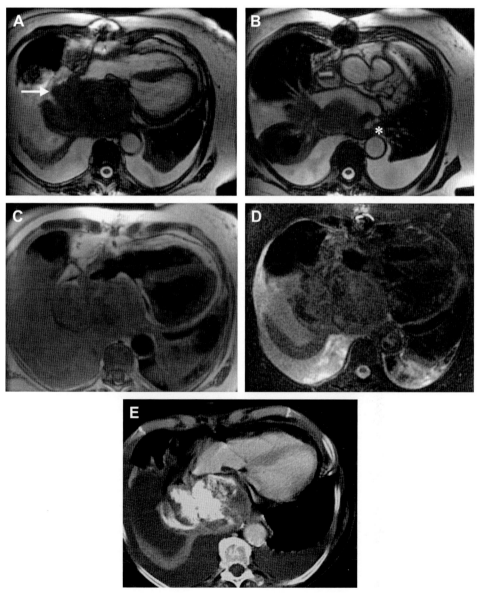

Fig. 10. Osteosarcoma. (*A*) Axial SSFP image shows a bulky, irregular, heterogenous, infiltrative left atrial mass (*arrow*) that invades the mitral annulus. (*B*) Axial SSFP image shows invasion and obstruction of the inferior pulmonary veins (*asterisk*). Bilateral pleural effusions are present. (*C*) Osteosarcomas often have a heterogeneously isointense appearance on T1-weighted and (*D*) a heterogeneously hyperintense appearance on T2-weighted images. (*E*) Axial contrast-enhanced CT scan demonstrates calcification within the left atrial mass.

Limited MR imaging descriptions of fibrosarcoma exist in the literature. They may be heterogenous or isointense on T1-weighted images and hyperintense on T2-weighted images.[80–82] Fibrosarcomas appear hyperintense relative to the myocardium on SSFP images.[81] Mild contrast enhancement has been described.[81]

CARDIAC LYMPHOMA

Primary cardiac lymphomas are aggressive B-cell lymphomas and are distinct from systemic lymphomas such as non-Hodgkin lymphomas, which also may involve the heart. The definition of primary cardiac lymphoma has been debated, with the strictest classical definition being an extranodal lymphoma that involves only the heart and pericardium. Today, massive cardiac involvement with only minimal infiltration of other sites also is accepted as having primary cardiac origin with early dissemination. The incidence of primary cardiac lymphoma is higher in immunocompromised patients, although immunocompetent persons can be affected also.[83] Clinical presentation is diverse, with dyspnea, arrhythmia, tamponade, chest pain, superior vena cava obstruction, and

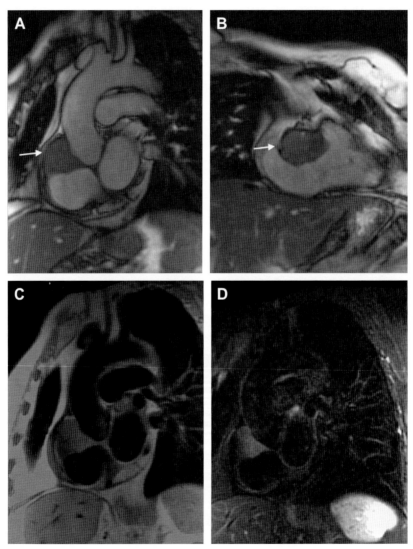

Fig. 11. Metastasis in a patient who has malignant melanoma. (*A*) Oblique sagittal SSFP image shows a mass (*arrow*) in the right atrioventricular (AV) groove. (*B*) Two-chamber right ventricular inflow view shows that the mass (*arrow*) encases the right coronary artery in the AV groove. (*C*) Oblique sagittal T1-weighted and (*D*) T2-weighted images demonstrate that the mass is isointense on T1 imaging (*panel C*) and hyperintense on T2 imaging (*panel D*).

vague systemic complaints reported.[10] At gross examination cardiac lymphomas appear as multiple masses of firm nodules, which frequently involve the epicardium. They most commonly arise in the right atrium and usually involve multiple cardiac chambers. Associated pericardial effusions, which usually are large and may produce symptoms, are seen frequently.[13] Primary lymphomas are less likely than sarcomas to involve the heart valves, to have necrosis, or to extend into the cardiac chambers.[10]

Primary lymphomas may appear on MR imaging as circumscribed polypoid or ill-defined infiltrative lesions typically affecting multiple cardiac chambers and usually with a large associated pericardial effusion. They typically are hypointense or isointense on T1-weighted images and are heterogeneously hyperintense on T2-weighted images. Contrast enhancement usually is present and varies from minimal to heterogenous to homogenous.[10]

METASTATIC HEART DISEASE

Secondary cardiac metastases have been reported to be 20 to 40 times more frequent than primary cardiac tumors.[4,5] The real incidence of metastases may be even higher, because autopsy studies demonstrate cardiac metastatic involvement in 10% to 12% of patients who have known malignant tumors.[6,7] It is estimated that up to 90% of cardiac metastases are clinically silent and are recognized only at autopsy.[84]

Cardiac metastases usually occur late in the course of a malignancy. Findings suggestive of cardiac metastases include the development of unexplained dyspnea, congestive heart failure, arrhythmias, or pericardial effusions in a patient with a known malignancy. Certain malignancies, such as malignant melanoma, have a particular propensity for metastasizing to the heart. More than half of all patients who have metastatic melanoma have cardiac deposits, which can affect any of the cardiac chambers.[7] Because of the relatively low prevalence of melanoma, however, more common malignancies such as lung and breast carcinoma are more likely to be the source of cardiac metastases. Leukemias and lymphomas also are common sources of cardiac metastases.

Malignant tumors can reach the heart by four pathways: lymphatic spread, hematogenous spread, direct extension, or transvenous extension. Lymphatic spread is the most common pathway and is encountered frequently with lung, breast, and esophageal malignancies. A retrograde route via mediastinal lymphatics results in epicardial tumor implants, which often are

associated with pericardial effusions. Hematogenous spread results in myocardial implants, usually via the coronary arteries. Melanoma and many sarcomas spread hematogenously to the heart. Direct extension to the heart and pericardium is seen commonly with lung, breast, and esophageal malignancies and with thymic neoplasms and mediastinal lymphomas. Because of pericardial invasion, a pericardial effusion usually is present also. Lung carcinoma also may invade the pulmonary veins and extend into the left atrium, leading to symptoms of congestive heart failure. Transvenous extension into the right atrium via the inferior vena cava is typical of renal cell carcinoma but also can occur with adrenal and hepatocellular carcinomas. MR imaging allows the delineation of tumor extension, which facilitates surgical planning.

MR imaging findings of metastases are highly variable, depending on the type of primary tumor and the pathway used to reach the heart. Pericardial effusions probably are the most common feature associated with cardiac metastases. These pericardial effusions often are complex or loculated and typically are hemorrhagic, thus demonstrating high signal intensity on T1-weighted images. Pericardiocentesis is required for definitive diagnosis. Tumors that directly invade the heart or pericardium from an adjacent noncardiac primary malignancy usually are self evident. Epicardial or intramyocardial nodular deposits or deposits within a cardiac chamber (**Fig. 11**) in a patient who has a known primary malignancy are suggestive of

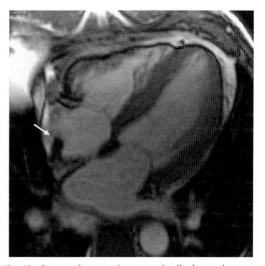

Fig. 12. A prominent crista terminalis (*arrow*) sometimes can be mistaken for a right atrial mass. The crista terminalis is a fibromuscular ridge that separates the embryologic sinus venosus from the primitive right atrium.

metastases, especially if there are other signs such as an infiltrative appearance or an associated pericardial effusion. Most malignant tumors have low to intermediate signal intensity on T1-weighted images and high signal intensity on T2-weighted images. One notable exception is metastatic melanoma, which appears bright on both T1- and T2-weighted images because of the presence of paramagnetic melanin (see **Fig. 11**C and D).[85,86] After the administration of contrast, most metastatic deposits demonstrate some degree of enhancement. DE imaging of cardiac metastases also may demonstrate hyperenhancement relative to surrounding myocardium.[87]

TUMOR MIMICS
Normal Cardiac Structures

Many normal cardiac structures can mimic cardiac tumors and sometimes can lead to referrals for cardiac MR imaging. The right atrium, especially, contains many such structures. A prominent crista

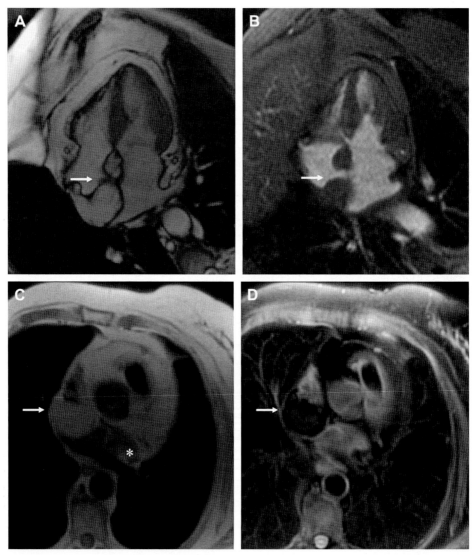

Fig. 13. Lipomatous hypertrophy of the interatrial septum. (*A*) Four-chamber SSFP image shows a characteristic dumbbell appearance (*arrow*) of the interatrial septum. The dumbbell shape results from the sparing of the fossa ovalis. (*B*) DE inversion-recovery image shows no enhancement of the interatrial septum (*arrow*). (*C*) Axial T1-weighted image shows a hyperintense appearance of the atrial septum (*arrow*) with (*D*) signal drop-out after application of a fat-suppression prepulse consistent with fatty tissue. Also shown in panel C is a "Q-tip" sign (*asterisk*) that is caused by an infolding of the left atrial wall at the junction of the left superior pulmonary vein and left atrial appendage, which sometimes can be mistaken for a left atrial mass.

terminalis can be confused for a mass in the posterior right atrial wall (**Fig. 12**).[88] Similarly, a prominent eustachian valve or Chiari network can be mistaken for a right atrial mass. In the right ventricle, prominent trabeculae or the moderator band may mimic masses. A "Q-tip" appearance at the junction of the entrance of the left upper pulmonary vein and left atrial appendage also may be mistaken for a mass on echocardiography. Lipomatous hypertrophy of the interatrial septum represents hyperplasia of normal fat cells within the interatrial septum and does not represent a cardiac tumor (**Fig. 13**). When it is prominent, it can be a source of referral for cardiac MR imaging based on the echocardiographic appearance of an atrial mass.[88] It is diagnosed when the interatrial septal thickness exceeds 2 cm. A characteristic distinguishing feature of lipomatous hypertrophy of the interatrial septum is that the fossa ovalis is spared from fatty infiltration, giving a dumbbell-shaped appearance. It parallels fat imaging characteristics on MR imaging sequences. This condition may be associated with atrial tachyarrhythmias.

Pericardial Cyst

Pericardial cysts (**Fig. 14**) are benign congenital structures that can occur anywhere along the margin of the pericardium, although they have a particular predilection for the right cardiophrenic angle. The echocardiographic appearance is of a cystic mass behind the right atrium. Pericardial cysts

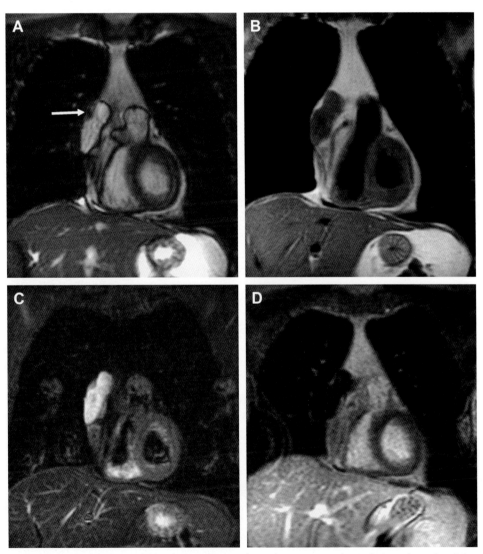

Fig. 14. Pericardial cyst. (*A*) Coronal SSFP image shows a hyperintense mass (*arrow*) that abuts the right atrium. (*B*) This structure is hypointense on T1-weighted images, (*C*) is hyperintense on T2-weighted images, and (*D*) demonstrates no enhancement on DE inversion-recovery images.

parallel the imaging characteristics of simple fluid, usually are hypointense on T1-weighted images (unless they are proteinaceous, in which case they are hyperintense), and are hyperintense on T2-weighted images. They appear hyperintense on SSFP images. They do not enhance after contrast administration.

Thrombus

Thrombus is the most common intracardiac mass and is the most frequent mimic of a cardiac tumor. In the atria, it is located most commonly in the left atrial appendage, especially in patients who have atrial fibrillation. Thrombus also can occur in the right atrium, typically adjacent to central venous lines. Ventricular thrombi occur most commonly in the setting of a cardiomyopathy with diminished left ventricular ejection fraction. The most common site is adjacent to an apical infarction, especially if an apical aneurysm is present. MR imaging is significantly more sensitive than echocardiography in detecting intracardiac thrombus (**Fig. 15**).[89–91] The T1 and T2 properties of thrombus depend on its age. Acute thrombus has high signal intensity on both T1- and T2-weighted images; subacute thrombus has high signal intensity on T1-weighted images but low signal intensity on T2-weighted images; and chronic organized

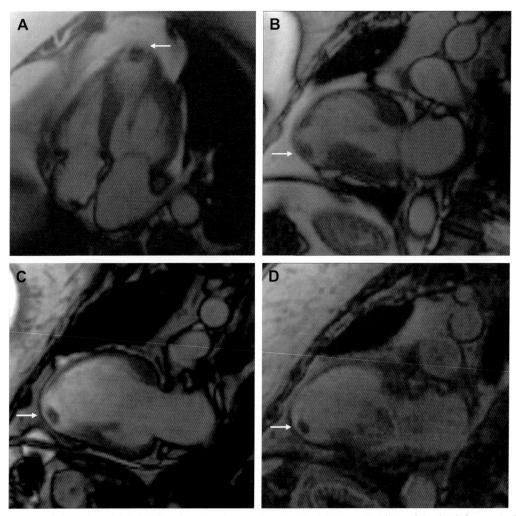

Fig. 15. Apical thrombus. (A) Four-chamber SSFP image shows an isointense mass (arrow) in the left ventricular apex adjacent to a thinned and akinetic apex. This appearance is most consistent with an apical thrombus. Two-chamber SSFP images (B) before and (C) after the administration of contrast demonstrate thinned akinetic myocardium in the anterior wall and apex and an isointense, nonenhancing apical mass (arrow). (D) Two-chamber DE inversion-recovery image shows the thrombus (arrow) to be deeply hypointense and adjacent to hyperenhanced infarcted myocardium.

thrombus usually has low signal intensity on both T1- and T2-weighted images. Thrombus appears dark on SSFP images. Administration of contrast is especially helpful for detecting ventricular thrombi. Thrombus does not enhance after administration of contrast. DE images are very sensitive for detection of thrombus and demonstrate thrombus as a dark, nonenhancing mass that often is adjacent to bright scarred ventricular myocardium (see **Fig. 15D**).[89–91]

SUMMARY

This article has presented the following key points:

- Primary cardiac tumors are rare; 75% of primary tumors are benign, and 25% are malignant.
- Cardiac metastases are 20 to 40 times more common than primary tumors.
- Nontumoral masses and pseudomasses also are a common source of referral for cardiac MR imaging.
- Cardiac MR imaging presently is the modality of choice for evaluation of cardiac masses, providing better tissue characterization than obtained with other modalities.
- A comprehensive cardiac MR imaging examination consists of static morphologic images using fast spin-echo sequences, including single-shot techniques, with T1 and T2 weighting and fat suppression pulses as well as dynamic imaging with cine SSFP techniques. Cardiac flow disturbances can be visualized on SSFP images and quantified with velocity-encoded imaging, and alterations in myocardial contractility can be assessed with tissue-tagging methods. Further tissue characterization is provided with perfusion and DE imaging.
- Specific cardiac tumoral characterization is possible in many cases. When specific tumor characterization is not possible, MR imaging often can demonstrate aggressive versus nonaggressive features that help in differentiating malignant tumors from benign tumors.
- MR imaging is useful in evaluating tumor mimics and is significantly more sensitive than echocardiography in detecting thrombus, which, although not a tumor, is the most common cardiac mass.

REFERENCES

1. Reynen K. Frequency of primary tumors of the heart. Am J Cardiol 1996;77(1):107.
2. Sutsch G, Jenni R, von Segesser L, et al. [Heart tumors: incidence, distribution, diagnosis. Exemplified by 20,305 echocardiographies]. Schweiz Med Wochenschr 1991;121(17):621–9 [in German].
3. Zipes D, Libby P, Bonow R, et al. Braunwald's heart disease. In: A textbook of cardiovascular medicine, vol. 2. Philadelphia: Elsevier Saunders; 2005.
4. Lam KY, Dickens P, Chan AC. Tumors of the heart. A 20-year experience with a review of 12,485 consecutive autopsies. Arch Pathol Lab Med 1993; 117(10):1027–31.
5. McAllister HA Jr, Hall RJ, Cooley DA. Tumors of the heart and pericardium. Curr Probl Cardiol 1999; 24(2):57–116.
6. Abraham KP, Reddy V, Gattuso P. Neoplasms metastatic to the heart: review of 3314 consecutive autopsies. Am J Cardiovasc Pathol 1990;3(3):195–8.
7. Klatt EC, Heitz DR. Cardiac metastases. Cancer 1990;65(6):1456–9.
8. Hoffmann U, Globits S, Schima W, et al. Usefulness of magnetic resonance imaging of cardiac and paracardiac masses. Am J Cardiol 2003;92(7):890–5.
9. Luna A, Ribes R, Caro P, et al. Evaluation of cardiac tumors with magnetic resonance imaging. Eur Radiol 2005;15(7):1446–55.
10. Araoz PA, Eklund HE, Welch TJ, et al. CT and MR imaging of primary cardiac malignancies. Radiographics 1999;19(6):1421–34.
11. Bouton S, Yang A, McCrindle BW, et al. Differentiation of tumor from viable myocardium using cardiac tagging with MR imaging. J Comput Assist Tomogr 1991;15(4):676–8.
12. Reynen K. Cardiac myxomas. N Engl J Med 1995; 333(24):1610–7.
13. Burke A, Virmani R. Tumors of the heart and great vessels. Washington, DC: Armed Forces Institute of Pathology; 1996.
14. Pucci A, Gagliardotto P, Zanini C, et al. Histopathologic and clinical characterization of cardiac myxoma: review of 53 cases from a single institution. Am Heart J 2000;140(1):134–8.
15. Pinede L, Duhaut P, Loire R. Clinical presentation of left atrial cardiac myxoma. A series of 112 consecutive cases. Medicine (Baltimore) 2001;80(3): 159–72.
16. Tazelaar HD, Locke TJ, McGregor CG. Pathology of surgically excised primary cardiac tumors. Mayo Clin Proc 1992;67(10):957–65.
17. Carney JA, Gordon H, Carpenter PC, et al. The complex of myxomas, spotty pigmentation, and endocrine overactivity. Medicine (Baltimore) 1985;64(4): 270–83.
18. Araoz PA, Mulvagh SL, Tazelaar HD, et al. CT and MR imaging of benign primary cardiac neoplasms with echocardiographic correlation. Radiographics 2000;20(5):1303–19.
19. Sparrow PJ, Kurian JB, Jones TR, et al. MR imaging of cardiac tumors. Radiographics 2005;25(5): 1255–76.

20. Masui T, Takahashi M, Miura K, et al. Cardiac myxoma: identification of intratumoral hemorrhage and calcification on MR images. AJR Am J Roentgenol 1995;164(4):850–2.

21. Gowda RM, Khan IA, Nair CK, et al. Cardiac papillary fibroelastoma: a comprehensive analysis of 725 cases. Am Heart J 2003;146(3):404–10.

22. Edwards FH, Hale D, Cohen A, et al. Primary cardiac valve tumors. Ann Thorac Surg 1991;52(5):1127–31.

23. Klarich KW, Enriquez-Sarano M, Gura GM, et al. Papillary fibroelastoma: echocardiographic characteristics for diagnosis and pathologic correlation. J Am Coll Cardiol 1997;30(3):784–90.

24. al-Mohammad A, Pambakian H, Young C. Fibroelastoma: case report and review of the literature. Heart 1998;79(3):301–4.

25. Kondruweit M, Schmid M, Strecker T. Papillary fibroelastoma of the mitral valve: appearance in 64-slice spiral computed tomography, magnetic resonance imaging, and echocardiography. Eur Heart J 2008;29(6):831.

26. Shiraishi J, Tagawa M, Yamada T, et al. Papillary fibroelastoma of the aortic valve: evaluation with transesophageal echocardiography and magnetic resonance imaging. Jpn Heart J 2003;44(5):799–803.

27. Wintersperger BJ, Becker CR, Gulbins H, et al. Tumors of the cardiac valves: imaging findings in magnetic resonance imaging, electron beam computed tomography, and echocardiography. Eur Radiol 2000;10(3):443–9.

28. Lembcke A, Meyer R, Kivelitz D, et al. Images in cardiovascular medicine. Papillary fibroelastoma of the aortic valve: appearance in 64-slice spiral computed tomography, magnetic resonance imaging, and echocardiography. Circulation 2007;115(1):e3–6.

29. Lang-Lazdunski L, Oroudji M, Pansard Y, et al. Successful resection of giant intrapericardial lipoma. Ann Thorac Surg 1994;58(1):238–40 [discussion: 240–31].

30. Hananouchi GI, Goff WB 2nd. Cardiac lipoma: six-year follow-up with MRI characteristics, and a review of the literature. Magn Reson Imaging 1990;8(6):825–8.

31. Matta R, Neelakandhan KS, Sandhyamani S. Right atrial lipoma. Case report. J Cardiovasc Surg (Torino) 1996;37(2):165–8.

32. Doshi S, Halim M, Singh H, et al. Massive intrapericardial lipoma, a rare cause of breathlessness. Investigations and management. Int J Cardiol 1998;66(2):211–5.

33. King SJ, Smallhorn JF, Burrows PE. Epicardial lipoma: imaging findings. AJR Am J Roentgenol 1993;160(2):261–2.

34. Cooper MJ, deLorimier AA, Higgins CB, et al. Atrial flutter-fibrillation resulting from left atrial compression by an intrapericardial lipoma. Am Heart J 1994;127(4 Pt 1):950–1.

35. Friedberg MK, Chang IL, Silverman NH, et al. Images in cardiovascular medicine. Near sudden death from cardiac lipoma in an adolescent. Circulation 2006;113(21):e778–9.

36. Schrepfer S, Deuse T, Detter C, et al. Successful resection of a symptomatic right ventricular lipoma. Ann Thorac Surg 2003;76(4):1305–7.

37. Vanderheyden M, De Sutter J, Wellens F, et al. Left atrial lipoma: case report and review of the literature. Acta Cardiol 1998;53(1):31–2.

38. Burke AP, Rosado-de-Christenson M, Templeton PA, et al. Cardiac fibroma: clinicopathologic correlates and surgical treatment. J Thorac Cardiovasc Surg 1994;108(5):862–70.

39. Cina SJ, Smialek JE, Burke AP, et al. Primary cardiac tumors causing sudden death: a review of the literature. Am J Forensic Med Pathol 1996;17(4):271–81.

40. Walpot J, Shivalkar B, Bogers JP, et al. A patient with cardiac fibroma and a subvalvular aortic stenosis caused by a subvalvular membrane. J Am Soc Echocardiogr 2007;20(7):906e1–906e4.

41. Herman TE, Siegel MJ, McAlister WH. Cardiac tumor in Gorlin syndrome. Nevoid basal cell carcinoma syndrome. Pediatr Radiol 1991;21(3):234–5.

42. Littler BO. Gorlin's syndrome and the heart. Br J Oral Surg 1979;17(2):135–46.

43. Yan AT, Coffey DM, Li Y, et al. Images in cardiovascular medicine. Myocardial fibroma in Gorlin syndrome by cardiac magnetic resonance imaging. Circulation 2006;114(10):e376–9.

44. De Cobelli F, Esposito A, Mellone R, et al. Images in cardiovascular medicine. Late enhancement of a left ventricular cardiac fibroma assessed with gadolinium-enhanced cardiovascular magnetic resonance. Circulation 2005;112(13):e242–3.

45. Grebenc ML, Rosado de Christenson ML, Burke AP, et al. Primary cardiac and pericardial neoplasms: radiologic-pathologic correlation. Radiographics 2000;20(4):1073–103.

46. Kivelitz DE, Muhler M, Rake A, et al. MRI of cardiac rhabdomyoma in the fetus. Eur Radiol 2004;14(8):1513–6.

47. Kaminaga T, Takeshita T, Kimura I. Role of magnetic resonance imaging for evaluation of tumors in the cardiac region. Eur Radiol 2003;13(Suppl 6):L1–L10.

48. Hamilton BH, Francis IR, Gross BH, et al. Intrapericardial paragangliomas (pheochromocytomas): imaging features. AJR Am J Roentgenol 1997;168(1):109–13.

49. Johnson TL, Shapiro B, Beierwaltes WH, et al. Cardiac paragangliomas. A clinicopathologic and immunohistochemical study of four cases. Am J Surg Pathol 1985;9(11):827–34.

50. McGann C, Tazelaar H, Cho SR, et al. In vivo detection of encapsulated intracardiac paraganglioma by delayed gadolinium enhancement magnetic resonance imaging. J Cardiovasc Magn Reson 2005; 7(2):371–5.

51. Orr LA, Pettigrew RI, Churchwell AL, et al. Gadolinium utilization in the MR evaluation of cardiac paraganglioma. Clin Imaging 1997;21(6):404–6.

52. Burke A, Johns JP, Virmani R. Hemangiomas of the heart. A clinicopathologic study of ten cases. Am J Cardiovasc Pathol 1990;3(4):283–90.

53. Oshima H, Hara M, Kono T, et al. Cardiac hemangioma of the left atrial appendage: CT and MR findings. J Thorac Imaging 2003;18(3):204–6.

54. Kiaffas MG, Powell AJ, Geva T. Magnetic resonance imaging evaluation of cardiac tumor characteristics in infants and children. Am J Cardiol 2002;89(10): 1229–33.

55. Lo LJ, Nucho RC, Allen JW, et al. Left atrial cardiac hemangioma associated with shortness of breath and palpitations. Ann Thorac Surg 2002;73(3):979–81.

56. Jougon J, Laborde MN, Parrens M, et al. Cystic lymphangioma of the heart mimicking a mediastinal tumor. Eur J Cardiothorac Surg 2002;22(3):476–8.

57. Kaji T, Takamatsu H, Noguchi H, et al. Cardiac lymphangioma: case report and review of the literature. J Pediatr Surg 2002;37(10):E32.

58. Pennec PY, Blanc JJ. Cardiac lymphangioma: a benign cardiac tumour. Eur Heart J 2006;27(24):2913.

59. Kocaoglu M, Bulakbasi N, Ugurel MS, et al. Value of magnetic resonance imaging in the depiction of intravenous leiomyomatosis extending to the heart. J Comput Assist Tomogr 2003;27(4):630–3.

60. Herrmann MA, Shankerman RA, Edwards WD, et al. Primary cardiac angiosarcoma: a clinicopathologic study of six cases. J Thorac Cardiovasc Surg 1992;103(4):655–64.

61. Janigan DT, Husain A, Robinson NA. Cardiac angiosarcomas. A review and a case report. Cancer 1986; 57(4):852–9.

62. Kakizaki S, Takagi H, Hosaka Y. Cardiac angiosarcoma responding to multidisciplinary treatment. Int J Cardiol 1997;62(3):273–5.

63. Kim EE, Wallace S, Abello R, et al. Malignant cardiac fibrous histiocytomas and angiosarcomas: MR features. J Comput Assist Tomogr 1989;13(4):627–32.

64. Schwab J, Haack G, Wunsch PH, et al. Cardiac angiosarcoma: case report and review of the literature: R.R. Brandt, R. Arnold, R.M. Bohle, T. Dill, C.W. Hamm; Z Kardiol 94:824–828 (2005). Clin Res Cardiol 2006;95(6):351–2 [author reply 352–3].

65. Valeviciene N, Mataciunas M, Tamosiunas A, et al. Primary heart angiosarcoma detected by magnetic resonance imaging. Acta Radiol 2006;47(7):675–9.

66. Deetjen AG, Conradi G, Mollmann S, et al. Cardiac angiosarcoma diagnosed and characterized by cardiac magnetic resonance imaging. Cardiol Rev 2006;14(2):101–3.

67. Yahata S, Endo T, Honma H, et al. Sunray appearance on enhanced magnetic resonance image of cardiac angiosarcoma with pericardial obliteration. Am Heart J 1994;127(2):468–71.

68. Okamoto K, Kato S, Katsuki S, et al. Malignant fibrous histiocytoma of the heart: case report and review of 46 cases in the literature. Intern Med 2001;40(12):1222–6.

69. Burke AP, Cowan D, Virmani R. Primary sarcomas of the heart. Cancer 1992;69(2):387–95.

70. Mader MT, Poulton TB, White RD. Malignant tumors of the heart and great vessels: MR imaging appearance. Radiographics 1997;17(1):145–53.

71. Chung TJ, Cheng L, Yu CY. Left ventricular malignant fibrous histiocytoma. Clin Imaging 2007;31(6): 422–4.

72. Schvartzman PR, White RD. Imaging of cardiac and paracardiac masses. J Thorac Imaging 2000;15(4): 265–73.

73. Villacampa VM, Villarreal M, Ros LH, et al. Cardiac rhabdomyosarcoma: diagnosis by MR imaging. Eur Radiol 1999;9(4):634–7.

74. Vujin B, Benc D, Srdic S, et al. Rhabdomyosarcoma of the heart. Herz 2006;31(8):798–800.

75. Lurito KJ, Martin T, Cordes T. Right atrial primary cardiac osteosarcoma. Pediatr Cardiol 2002;23(4): 462–5.

76. Yamagishi M, Yamada N, Kuribayashi S. Images in cardiology: magnetic resonance imaging of cardiac osteosarcoma. Heart 2001;85(3):311.

77. Durand E, Vanel D, Mousseaux E, et al. A recurrent left atrium leiomyosarcoma. Eur Radiol 1998;8(1): 97–9.

78. Lo FL, Chou YH, Tiu CM, et al. Primary cardiac leiomyosarcoma: imaging with 2-D echocardiography, electron beam CT and 1.5-Tesla MR. Eur J Radiol 1998;27(1):72–6.

79. Clarke NR, Mohiaddin RH, Westaby S, et al. Multifocal cardiac leiomyosarcoma. Diagnosis and surveillance by transoesophageal echocardiography and contrast enhanced cardiovascular magnetic resonance. Postgrad Med J 2002;78(922):492–3.

80. Coskun H, Bozkurt AK, Ozbay G, et al. Primary fibrosarcoma of the heart. Aust N Z J Surg 1995;65(1): 66–8.

81. Hoffstetter P, Djavidani B, Feuerbach S, et al. Myxoid fibrosarcoma of a pulmonary vein with extension into the left atrium. AJR Am J Roentgenol 2006;186(2): 365–7.

82. Itoh A, Okubo S, Nakanishi N, et al. Recurrent epicardial fibrosarcoma which arose 12 years after the first resection. Eur Heart J 1991;12(2):270–2.

83. Ceresoli GL, Ferreri AJ, Bucci E, et al. Primary cardiac lymphoma in immunocompetent patients: diagnostic

and therapeutic management. Cancer 1997;80(8): 1497–506.

84. Butany J, Nair V, Naseemuddin A, et al. Cardiac tumours: diagnosis and management. Lancet Oncol 2005;6(4):219–28.

85. Enochs WS, Petherick P, Bogdanova A, et al. Paramagnetic metal scavenging by melanin: MR imaging. Radiology 1997;204(2):417–23.

86. Mousseaux E, Meunier P, Azancott S, et al. Cardiac metastatic melanoma investigated by magnetic resonance imaging. Magn Reson Imaging 1998;16(1): 91–5.

87. Vogel-Claussen J, Rochitte CE, Wu KC, et al. Delayed enhancement MR imaging: utility in myocardial assessment. Radiographics 2006;26(3):795–810.

88. Pharr JR, Figueredo VM. Lipomatus hypertrophy of the atrial septum and prominent crista terminalis appearing as a right atrial mass. Eur J Echocardiogr 2002;3(2):159–61.

89. Bruder O, Waltering KU, Hunold P, et al. Detection and characterization of left ventricular thrombi by MRI compared to transthoracic echocardiography. Rofo 2005;177(3):344–9 [in German].

90. Mollet NR, Dymarkowski S, Volders W, et al. Visualization of ventricular thrombi with contrast-enhanced magnetic resonance imaging in patients with ischemic heart disease. Circulation 2002;106(23):2873–6.

91. Srichai MB, Junor C, Rodriguez LL, et al. Clinical, imaging, and pathological characteristics of left ventricular thrombus: a comparison of contrast-enhanced magnetic resonance imaging, transthoracic echocardiography, and transesophageal echocardiography with surgical or pathological validation. Am Heart J 2006;152(1):75–84.

Cardiac MR Imaging of Nonischemic Cardiomyopathies

Scott R. Harris, MD[a], James Glockner, MD, PhD[a],
Andrew J. Misselt, MD[a], Imran S. Syed, MD[b], Philip A. Araoz, MD[a],*

KEYWORDS

- Cardiomyopathy • MR imaging
- Delayed enhancements

According to the 1995 World Health Organization (WHO) definition, cardiomyopathy is a disease of the myocardium associated with cardiac dysfunction.[1] The WHO has divided cardiomyopathies into commonly recognized entities, including hypertrophic, restrictive, and dilated forms. This classification system has been criticized for mixing morphologic and functional designations. In 2006, an American Heart Association scientific statement presented an alternative classification scheme, dividing cardiomyopathies into two subgroups: (1) primary cardiomyopathies, which are solely or predominately confined to heart muscle, and (2) secondary cardiomyopathies, which show pathologic involvement of the heart as part of a generalized systemic disorder.[2] Regardless of which classification system is preferred, significant overlap remains in the presentations and appearances of the various cardiomyopathies; thus, defining the underlying form is important for determining clinical course and treatment options for patients (**Table 1**). MR imaging can play a vital role in characterizing the underlying cardiomyopathy and in providing prognostic information of various disease entities.

HYPERTROPHIC CARDIOMYOPATHY

Hypertrophic cardiomyopathy (HCM) is a common genetic disorder affecting 1 in 500 individuals. Characterized histologically by a disarray of myocytes, HCM manifests as hypertrophy of the left ventricular (LV) myocardium. With more than 10 genes affected and variable expression, however, there is a wide range of clinical symptoms and outcomes.[3]

Inherited as an autosomal dominant trait, HCM affects men and women equally. HCM can affect almost any age group, making it unique among cardiovascular diseases. Up to 25% of patients who have HCM achieve normal longevity (75 years or older), but HCM often gains attention as a cause of sudden death among younger affected patients.[3]

HCM is primarily a diastolic disorder, as ventricular hypertrophy results in increased ventricular stiffness. As a result of a noncompliant ventricle, high diastolic filling pressures are required, which eventually may lead to increased atrial size and atrial fibrillation. Systolic function, alternatively, often is hyperdynamic. Eighty percent of the stroke volume is ejected in the first half of systole compared with 57% in normal patients,[4] and obliteration of the ventricular cavity is a classic finding on echocardiography and MR imaging.

Risk for sudden cardiac death is correlated with myocardial thickness and arrhythmias.[3] Dynamic LV outflow obstruction resulting from preferential thickening of the basal segment of the intraventricular septum can lead to a pressure gradient across the outflow tract, producing symptoms such as dyspnea on exertion and exertional syncope. An instantaneous pressure gradient greater than 30 mm Hg also is associated with increased risk

[a] Department of Radiology, Mayo Clinic, 200 First Street SW, Rochester, MN 55905, USA
[b] Department of Cardiology, Mayo Clinic, 200 First Street SW, Rochester, MN 55905, USA
* Corresponding author.
E-mail address: paraoz@mayo.edu (P.A. Araoz).

Magn Reson Imaging Clin N Am 16 (2008) 165–183
doi:10.1016/j.mric.2008.02.010
1064-9689/08/$ – see front matter © 2008 Elsevier Inc. All rights reserved.

Table 1
MR imaging characteristics for nonischemic cardiomyopathies

Cardiomyopathy	Etiology	Findings	Delayed Enhancement
Hypertrophic	Idiopathic/genetic	Wall hypertrophy (>12 mm); diffuse or focal Outflow tract obstruction SAM of the mitral valve ± Delayed enhancement (RV insertion points, wall hypertrophy)	± Delayed enhancement (RV insertion points, wall hypertrophy)
Dilated	Idiopathic/genetic	Dilated LV Global hypokinesis Normal epicardial vessels ⊥ Delayed enhancement (midmyocardial stripe)	60% may show no enhancement ± Delayed enhancement; midmyocardial stripe, subepicardial
Amyloidosis	Mixed (genetic/acquired)	Atrial, ventricular, and valvular thickening Pericardial effusion Diffuse myocardial enhancement, subendocardial enhancement	Diffuse myocardial enhancement, subendocardial predominance, patchy enhancement
ARVD	Genetic/idiopathic	Fatty/fibrofatty changes in RV RV enlargement RV outpouching/aneurysms RV dyskinesis	± Patchy enhancement of RV wall
Noncompaction	Genetic	Hypertrabeculation of inferior and lateral wall of LV Hypokinesis	± Enhancement of the noncompacted trabeculations
Iron-overload	Mixed (genetic/ acquired)	Low signal intensity myocardium T2* time < 20 ms	No evidence of delayed enhancement
Myocarditis	Acquired	Regional wall motion abnormalities	Delayed patchy epicardial enhancement of the lateral wall
Sarcoid	Unknown etiology	Regional wall motion abnormalities not in vascular territory Focal wall thickness Basal wall thinning and aneurysmal formation	Nonvascular territory regional wall motion abnormalities Focal wall thickening or thinning (basal septum and posterior wall) Patchy delayed enhancement
Apical ballooning	Idiopathic	Regional wall motion abnormalities involving all apical segments Hyperdynamic basal segments	No evidence of delayed enhancement
Endomyocardial disease	Idiopathic	Wall thickening primarily involving the apex Decreased LV cavity size	Trilaminar enhancement pattern (thickened wall, inflammatory exudates, thrombus)

for cardiac death. LV outflow tract (LVOT) gradients most often are measured with echocardiography but also can be calculated using phase-contrast MR imaging. The obstructive physiology through the LVOT tract may lead to systolic anterior motion (SAM) of the mitral valve, producing mitral regurgitation (**Fig. 1**). This mitral regurgitation can contribute greatly to patients' symptoms of heart failure.

HCM often is imaged initially with echocardiography. MR imaging, however, provides improved tissue characterization; visualization of anatomic regions, which are sometimes difficult to evaluate with echocardiography (the LV apex, for example); and more accurate and reproducible measurements of LV volume and mass. HCM may manifest as symmetric thickening of the entire LV or as focal asymmetric thickening, which most commonly involves the basal-septal and anterior-basal ventricular segments, or which may involve the entire interventricular septum (**Fig. 2**). Midventricular wall hypertrophy has been seen and this form may result in an apical aneurysm (**Fig. 3**) and eventually apical infarction and thrombus. Apical hypertrophy is a variant more common in Japanese populations (**Fig. 4**). This form is classically associated with large inverted T waves on ECG tracings.

Myocardial wall thickening greater than 12 mm is considered abnormal. These wall measurements should be obtained in the end-diastolic phase of the cardiac cycle using balanced steady-state free precession (b-SSFP) images,

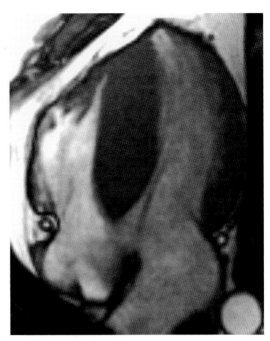

Fig. 2. HCM: b-SSFP four-chamber view demonstrates hypertrophy of the entire ventricular septum.

which provide sharp delineation of the epicardial and endocardial myocardial interfaces. Four-chamber and short-axis views are the best imaging planes for wall measurements (**Fig. 5**). A comparison of the septum and free wall thickness also can be obtained: this ratio is higher in the asymmetric basal form of HCM compared with that of normal patients (1.5 ± 0.8 versus 0.9 ± 0.3).[5]

Angled three-chamber b-SSFP views encompassing the LVOT should be obtained to visualize SAM and mitral regurgitation. In patients who have obstructive physiology, the pressure gradient across the LVOT pulls the anterior mitral leaflet forward. This causes poor coaptation of the mitral valve leaflets, resulting in mitral regurgitation. The mitral regurgitant jet is seen as a signal void on b-SSFP images and usually is directed posteriorly and laterally in the left atrium (**Fig. 6**). Cine phase-contrast sequences can measure peak and average velocities across the LVOT, which can be converted to pressure gradients using the modified Bernoulli equation. Evaluation of pressure gradients provides prognostic information, because a gradient greater than 30 mm Hg is an independent risk factor for sudden cardiac death.[3]

Delayed enhancement sequences provide additional information in patients who have HCM. Two studies have shown that myocardial delayed enhancement (MDE) occurs in the majority (81%) of

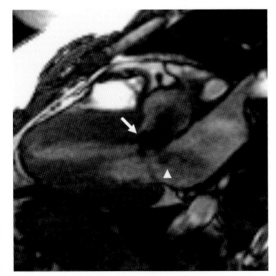

Fig. 1. HCM: b-SSFP three-chamber view shows obstruction of the LVOT (*arrow*) and mitral regurgitation with a posteriorly directed jet (*arrowhead*).

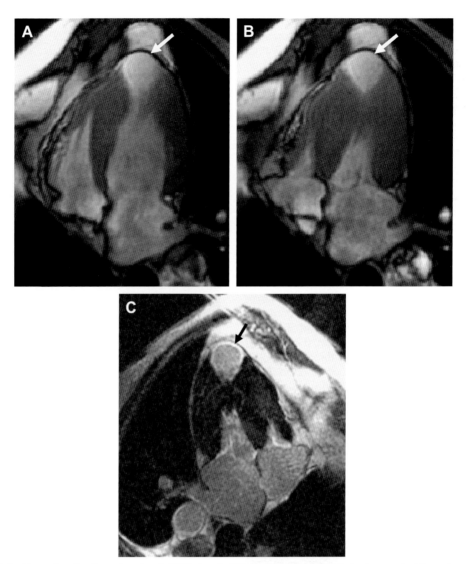

Fig. 3. Apical hypertrophy: four-chamber b-SSFP view in (*A*) diastole and (*B*) systole show apical hypertrophy and a dyskinetic apical pouch (*white arrows*) (*A, B*). (*C*). Four-chamber delayed enhancement image shows transmural delayed enhancement in the apical pouch (*black arrow*), indicating that the pouch is fibrotic and nonviable.

patients who have HCM. Delayed enhancement is not a specific finding, but typical patterns involve the middle third of the myocardium in a patchy distribution in the hypertrophied segment (**Fig. 7**). Approximately one tenth of the myocardium typically is involved. In those patients displaying hyperenhancement, all had involvement at the insertion points of the right ventricle (RV) with the interventricular septum (**Fig. 8**).[6,7] In the authors' institutions, however, MDE has been seen in approximately 50% of patients.

The significance of the delayed gadolinium enhancement is a subject of intense investigation.

Studies have shown that enhancement is seen more commonly in patients who have severe hypertrophy, nonsustained ventricular tachycardia, young age at diagnosis, strong family history, and decreased LV function. These are factors that relate to increased risk for sudden death; however, at this point, enhancement does not support further prognostic information.[7,8]

DILATED CARDIOMYOPATHY

Idiopathic dilated cardiomyopathy (DCM) is defined as biventricular dilation, increased LV

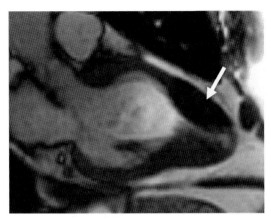

Fig. 4. Apical hypertrophy: b-SSFP two-chamber view of a 65-year-old woman who had marked hypertrophy of the apical segments (*arrow*).

mass secondary to chamber enlargement, and severely depressed systolic function in the setting of normal coronary arteries.[9] Histologically, there is hypertrophy and degeneration of myocytes with alteration of the interstitium resulting from an increase in collagen.[10] Idiopathic DCM typically affects those between ages 20 and 50 and is most common in men. DCM may be familial in 35% to 50% of cases; thus, genetic screening is valuable.[11] Most commonly, patients present with symptoms of severe left-sided heart failure. Systemic and pulmonary emboli and chest pain on exertion are other initial presentations.[9]

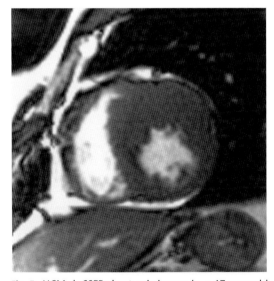

Fig. 5. HCM: b-SSFP short-axis image in a 17-year-old man shows marked hypertrophy involving the anterior and anterior septal segments. The wall thickness measured up to 27 mm.

MR imaging plays an important role in investigating of DCM as it can provide accurate and reproducible measurements of cardiac function and morphology, both predictors of prognosis. In addition, ventricular dilation is a known endpoint for ischemic heart disease and many other entities. Factors, such as ethanol, viruses, and metabolic abnormalities, are linked to cardiac dilation; thus, the underlying cause of dilation must be differentiated clearly, as treatment options differ. Standard b-SSFP four-chamber and short-axis images can be performed to assess ventricular volumes and systolic dysfunction. There may be dilation of all cardiac chambers, although the LV generally demonstrates the most marked changes, including typical increased LV mass. Ventricular walls, however, do not increase in thickness and increased mass is secondary to overall chamber enlargement. Unlike ischemic disease, which demonstrates regional wall motion abnormalities, DCM generally is defined by global hypokinesis resulting in a reduced ejection fraction. The degree of LV dysfunction is a predictor of prognosis.[9] In addition, MR imaging has the ability to visualize secondary complications of the disease, such as intracardiac thrombi and organized plaques, which are present in more than 50% of patients at necropsy.[11]

Morphologic changes may be the only MR imaging features present in DCM as delayed contrast-enhanced sequences show no enhancement in 60% of cases.[10,12,13] A distinctive pattern of delayed enhancement may be seen in a minority of patients. Described by McCrohon and colleagues, a midventricular wall stripe of enhancement has been demonstrated in approximately 30% of patients (**Fig. 9**).[13] This stripe may correlate to midwall fibrosis seen on pathology. It has been suggested, however, that this pattern may be secondary to a previous history of myocarditis; thus, genetic correlation could be beneficial to characterize patients further.[14] This pattern of delayed enhancement recently has been considered an independent prognostic factor for all-cause mortality, sudden cardiac death, and cardiovascular hospitalizations, thus identifying its presence to be of great importance.[15] A third pattern of enhancement has been defined by McCrohon, and colleagues, which is subendocardial in location and indistinguishable from the enhancement pattern of infarction. In this study, patients who had infarction pattern demonstrated normal coronary arteries at diagnosis, but their investigation could not exclude infarction followed by clot lysis as the cause of MDE.

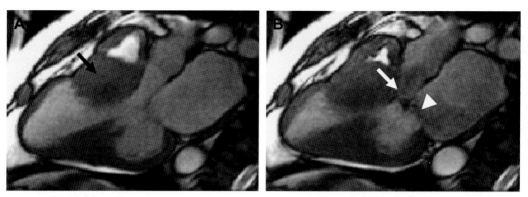

Fig. 6. HCM: b-SSFP three-chamber view in (A) diastole shows marked hypertrophy of the basal septum (arrow). Image in systole (B) shows outflow obstruction (arrow) and mitral regurgitation (arrowhead).

ARRHYTHMOGENIC RIGHT VENTRICULAR DYSPLASIA/CARDIOMYOPATHY

Arrhythmogenic RV dysplasia/cardiomyopathy (ARVD/C) is characterized by arrhythmias and left bundle branch block and patchy fatty/fibrofatty infiltration of the RV free wall.[4] ARVD/C is listed by the WHO as an idiopathic disorder, as it is a progressive myocardial disease with no known underlying cause. Most prevalent in men, it is a common cause of sudden cardiac death in young patients. Some reports state a 30% to 50% genetic association; thus, its diagnosis is of great importance to families.[5]

Two variants of ARVD/C are reported: fatty and fibrofatty.[16] The fatty form is characterized by almost complete replacement of the myocardium without thinning of the ventricular wall. This variant occurs exclusively in the RV. In contrast, the fibrofatty variant is associated with significant thinning of the RV wall. In this case, the LV myocardial wall also may be involved. Other morphologic variations of the RV associated with ARVD/C consist of mild to severe global dilatation of the ventricle, ventricular aneurysms, or outpouchings and segmental hypokinesis. The sites of involvement are found in the so-called "triangle of dysplasia," namely, the RV subtricuspid area, the apex, and the infundibulum.[17]

MR imaging provides information regarding morphologic changes of the RV, an area not easily evaluated with echocardiography. Detection of fat in the RV free wall has long been an component of MR imaging investigation of patients who have suspected ARVD/C, although currently the significance of this finding is uncertain (**Fig. 10**).

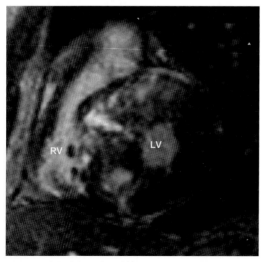

Fig. 7. HCM: delayed enhancement short-axis image demonstrates marked delayed enhancement of hypertrophied LV myocardium suggesting fibrosis.

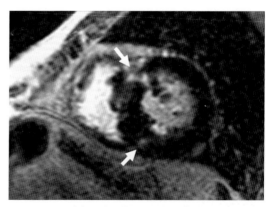

Fig. 8. HCM: delayed enhancement short-axis images demonstrate typical focal hyperenhancement of the RV insertion points (arrows) in a patient who had HCM.

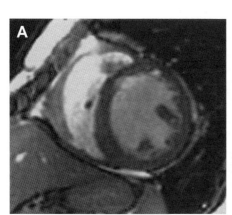
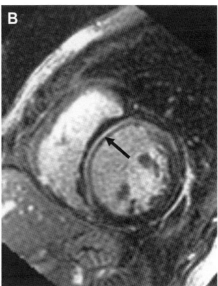

Fig. 9. DCM: (A) short-axis b-SSFP image through the midventricular level demonstrate a dilated LV measuring 64 mm. (B) Delayed enhancement imaging of the same patient displays the distinctive midmyocardial stripe enhancement pattern (arrow).

Because the RV free wall is thin, high–spatial resolution black-blood double inversion recovery sequences typically are used. Some investigators have suggested that these images may be improved by imaging at end systole, when the RV wall thickness is maximal, although this also may result in a higher degree of motion blurring.[18,19] In addition, using fat-suppressed double inversion recovery or triple inversion recovery sequences may provide additional confidence in the presence of fat

by confirming signal dropout in a region of suspected fatty infiltration.

Regional wall motion abnormalities and RV dilatation also are important imaging findings. These features are best evaluated using b-SSFP sequences. Axial and short-axis images should be obtained to adequately assess ventricular morphology and movement and diastolic and systolic function (**Fig. 11**). As discussed previously, mild to severe global dilatation of the

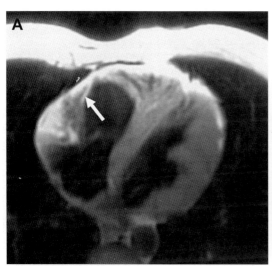
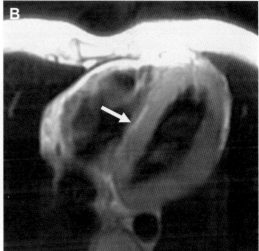

Fig. 10. ARVD: (A) double inversion recovery axial images of the heart demonstrate focal areas of high signal intensity within the RV free wall (arrow). An image slightly more caudal (B) shows fat in the interventricular septum (arrow).

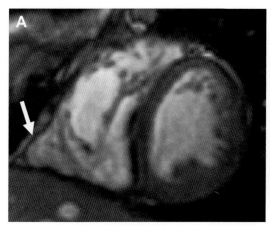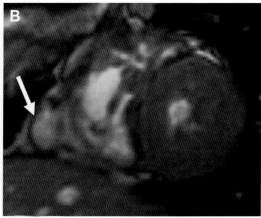

Fig. 11. ARVD: b-SSFP short-axis image in (A) diastole and (B) systole show a small focal dyskinetic segment of the free wall of the RV (arrow).

ventricle, ventricular aneurysms, and segmental hypokinesia are objective findings associated with the disorder. Reports also have demonstrated a reduced RV ejection fraction in some patients.[20]

Diagnosis of ARVD/C cannot be based solely on the presence of fat in the RV wall. Several studies have shown the presence of fat within the myocardium without the clinical disorder of ARVD/C.[21] A study by Bomma and colleagues demonstrated that expert readers had difficulty distinguishing patients who had ARVD from normal controls based on MR imaging findings alone and noted that the one of the most important errors was the strong tendency of readers to associate the identification of RV fat with ARVD/C.[22] The diagnosis of ARVD/C is based on a 1994 Task Force of the Working Group Myocardial and Pericardial Disease of the European Society of Cardiology and of the Scientific Council on Cardiomyopathies of the International Society and Federation of Cardiology report by McKenna and colleagues, which defines major and minor criteria for the disorder (Table 2).[23] Many, if not most, of these criteria involve clinical and laboratory information; therefore, the diagnosis of ARVD/C never should be based solely on imaging findings.

In one postmortem study, focal myocarditis and inflammation secondary to cell death was found in 67% of cases of ARVD.[24] Tandri and colleagues demonstrated a good agreement between the presence of fibrosis on histology and the delayed enhancement with contrast-enhanced–inversion recovery sequences.[25] As a result, delayed hyperenhancement may be evident in patients who have ARVD. The use of MDE in diagnosis of patients who have ARVD is an exciting development;

however, the sensitivity and specificity of this finding have yet to be determined in large studies, and it is true that ARVD is not the only cause of RV delayed enhancement.

VENTRICULAR NONCOMPACTION

LV noncompaction is a rare cardiomyopathy that is poorly described in the literature. According to the WHO, ventricular noncompaction is categorized as an unclassified cardiomyopathy. Between 5 and 8 weeks of embryonic life, a spongy meshwork of fibers undergoes "compaction" from the epicardium to the endocardium from the base to the apex.[26] An arrest of this normal development is believed the underlying factor of this cardiomyopathy. As a result of this developmental anomaly, multiple prominent trabeculations and intertrabecular recesses can be seen on imaging.

Originally described as a congenital disease in young patients, this disorder recently has been described in adults.[27] The incidence of ventricular noncompaction was 0.014% in one series of patients. These patients, however, originally were referred for an abnormal echocardiogram; thus, the true incidence may be lower.[26] Others have reported rates as high as 0.05%.[27] Noncompaction is more prevalent in men and generally isolated to the LV, although RV involvement also is described (Fig. 12). In addition to the morphologic changes of hypertrabeculation or noncompaction, patients may develop thromboembolic events, experience malignant arrhythmias, and progress to worsening heart failure.

In more than 80% of patients, the apical and midventricular inferior and lateral segments are affected (Fig. 13). The anterior wall and the septum

Table 2
Criteria for diagnosis of arrhythmogenic right ventricular dysplasia/cardiomyopathy

Factor	Major Criteria	Minor Criteria
Global or regional dysfunction and structural alterations	Severe dilatation of the RV and reduced RV ejection fraction, severe segmental dilatation of the RV, localized RV aneurysms (akinetic or dyskinetic areas with diastolic bulging)	Mild dilatation of the RV or reduced RV ejection, mild segmental dilatation of the RV, regional RV hypokinesia
Tissue characterization	Fibrofatty replacement of RV myocardium at endocardial biopsy	—
Repolarization abnormalities	—	Inverted T waves (V2-V3)
Depolarization or conduction abnormalities	Epsilon waves prolonged QRS complex (>110 ms) in V1-V3	Late potentials
Arrhythmias	—	VT with LBBB, frequent VES
Family history	Familial disease confirmed at necropsy or surgery	Familial history of premature sudden death due to suspected ARVD, family history (clinical diagnosis based on present

Data from McKenna WJ, Thiene G, Nava A, et al. Diagnosis of arrhythmogenic right ventricular dysplasia/cardiomyopathy. Task Force of the Working Group Myocardial and Pericardial Disease of the European Society of Cardiology and of the Scientific Council on Cardiomyopathies of the International Society and Federation of Cardiology. Br Heart J 1994;71(3):215–8.

are much less frequently involved. The location of involvement is useful in differentiating normal variants of hypertrabeculation, which commonly course from the free wall to the septum in normal patients.[28] In addition to location, magnetic resonance and echocardiographic criteria have been established for the compacted to noncompacted myocardium. A noncompacted to compacted ratio greater than 2.3 in end diastole is

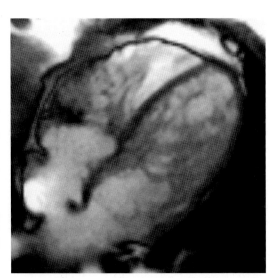

Fig. 12. Noncompaction: b-SSFP four-chamber view of the heart shows marked increased trabeculation of the LV.

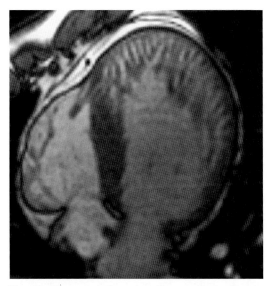

Fig. 13. Noncompaction: another patient demonstrates increased noncompacted to compacted myocardium toward the apex on this b-SSFP four-chamber view.

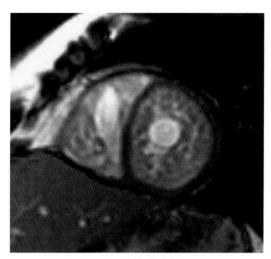

Fig. 14. Noncompaction: short-axis b-SSFP images in end diastole clearly demonstrate marked circumferential LV trabeculation. On cine imaging there was mild global decrease in systolic function with an ejection fraction of 50%.

considered diagnostic by MR imaging criteria (**Fig. 14**).[29] This differs from echocardiography criteria, in which an end-systolic myocardial thickness ratio between the compacted epicardial to the noncompacted endocardial layer greater than or equal to 2 is diagnostic of the disorder.[30] As stated previously, hypertrabeculation may be seen in normal variants and in patients who have hypertrophied hearts secondary to dilation, hypertension, or valvular disease. In such patients, the ratio of the trabeculated heart to normal myocardium by definition never reaches 2.[30] Some argue that this definition of thickness may be too strict. Less florid cases are described that do not meet magnetic resonance or echocardiographic criteria but have the characteristic patterns of increased trabeculation and myocardial recesses. In a study by Oechslin and colleagues, all noncompacted segments demonstrated hypokinesia.[30] Even the normally compacted myocardium occasionally demonstrated hypokinesia with approximately 90% of the cases studied displaying ejection fractions less than 50%.

A recent study examined a group of patients referred for heart failure and demonstrated that 24% of these patients fulfilled criteria for noncompaction based on the three current echocardiography definitions in the literature.[31] Alternatively, 8% of patients within the control or normal group also met the criteria for noncompaction based on current definitions. In several studies, large subsets of patients are asymptomatic. Certain clinical characteristics are found significantly more common in nonsurvivors than in long-term survivors of noncompaction: higher LV end-diastolic diameter at presentation, New York Heart Association class III/IV, chronic atrial fibrillation, and bundle branch block.[32] The greater recognition of ventricular noncompaction as cardiac imaging techniques improve raises the possibility that noncompaction may exist over a broad spectrum, essentially a normal variant in some patients and a disabling cardiomyopathy in others.

SARCOID

Sarcoid is a multisystem disease of unknown etiology characterized by noncaseating granulomas. Sarcoid affects people of all races, both genders, and all ages. It is most common in adults under the age of 40. The incidence in the United States is 35.5 cases per 100,000 blacks and 10.9 cases per 100,000 whites; thus, thousands of patients are affected each year.[33] Pulmonary involvement is the most common presentation; however, clinical manifestations depend on the location and extent of granulomatous inflammation.

Cardiac sarcoid is common but rarely clinically identified. Autopsy studies have shown cardiac involvement in nearly 50% of sarcoid patients; however, clinically significant cardiac sarcoid affects only 5%.[34] This is a small but significant percentage, because symptoms range from benign arrhythmias to heart block, intractable heart failure, intense chest pain, and fatal ventricular fibrillation.

Cardiac involvement may precede, follow, or occur concurrently with involvement of the lungs or other organs. If cardiac manifestations occur in patients who have multisystem sarcoidosis, the diagnosis is relatively clear. When cardiac dysfunction is the sole manifestation of sarcoidosis, however, the diagnosis often is never contemplated and usually not confirmed because of the lack of specific diagnostic tests. Endomyocardial biopsy may be entertained; however, this procedure has a low sensitivity of only 20% and is invasive.[35] Early corticosteroid intervention once myocardial involvement is detected is the mainstay of treatment.

Diagnostic evaluation for cardiac sarcoidosis has involved ECG, echocardiography, and thalium[201] scanning. Smedema and colleagues, however, demonstrated that 11% of patients who had cardiac sarcoid were diagnosed only through cardiac MR imaging.[36] These patients had a shorter clinical course and there was limited myocardial involvement compared with those diagnosed by traditional methods. Therefore, cardiac MR imaging may be beneficial for the diagnosis and subsequent treatment early in the disease process.

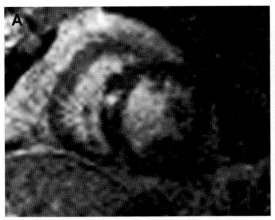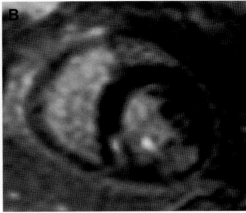

Fig. 15. Sarcoidosis: two patients who had known sarcoidosis. (*A*) Short-axis delayed enhancement images show patchy areas of hyperenhancement in the interventricular septum. (*B*) Similar findings are seen in the lateral free wall of a second patient.

Findings of cardiac involvement are not specific but do allow for differentiating other disease processes. On T2-weighted sequences, active disease may demonstrate areas of high signal intensity and myocardial swelling. The focal increased wall thickness may mimic HCM. Sarcoid granulomas can demonstrate a central fibrotic area with peripheral hyperenhancement representing edema.[37] Later in the disease course, myocardial thinning and aneurysmal formation may develop. A posterior basal aneurysm is the most common location. In addition, regional wall motion abnormalities may be identified that do not correspond to vascular distributions. MDE images typically demonstrate patchy areas of hyperenhancement that do not correspond to a vascular territory (**Fig. 15**). These findings are nonspecific and can mimic other processes. The basal septal myocardium is affected most commonly, but any region can be affected, and the appearance is similar to the subepicardial enhancement of myocarditis. The subendocardium usually is spared allowing distinction from ischemic disease.

Cardiac MR imaging likely is beneficial in the follow-up of patients who have known sarcoid. In one study, serial MR imaging scans demonstrated clearing of cardiac involvement and improved cardiac function patients treated with steroids. In patients who had not received steroids there was progression of disease.[34]

IRON OVERLOAD CARDIOMYOPATHY

The body has no means of excreting iron; therefore, patients requiring transfusion therapy often have elevated levels of iron throughout the body. After stores within the liver are filled, iron is deposited in other organs, such as the pancreas, spleen, and heart (**Fig. 16**). Iron initially is stored as a component of transferrin. After the transferrin binding sites are exhausted, free iron exists as non–transferrin-bound iron, which has a higher toxicity compared with bound iron as it may cause free radical formation and peroxidase damage to membrane lipids and proteins.

Myocardial iron deposition occurs initially without symptoms. When symptoms develop, myocardial iron levels generally are high and there is rapid deterioration in cardiac function. Nonspecific findings on routine b-SSFP sequences may be seen, including LV dilation and reduced systolic

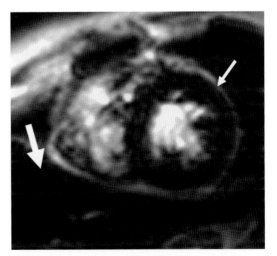

Fig. 16. Iron-overload cardiomyopathy: short axis b-SSFP image. Notice relative low signal intensity of the myocardium (*small arrow*) and the liver (*large arrow*) and spleen in a patient who had thalassemia.

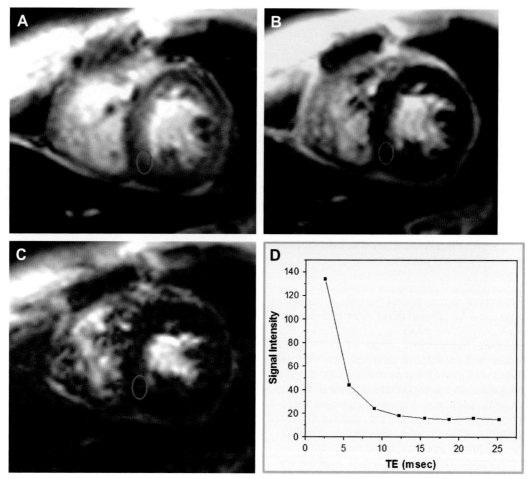

Fig. 17. Iron-overload cardiomyopathy: (*A*) short-axis b-SSFP image with a small region of interest on the interventricular septum. Imaging this region at multiple inversion times (*B, C*) allows for plotting of signal versus echo time (*D*), which allows for calculation calculation of T2*.

and diastolic function. As iron levels increase, signal dropout on b-SSFP and other pulse sequences may be noted.

Global reduction in myocardial T2* is a relatively specific finding for iron deposition. Iron particles cause local variations in the magnetic field, resulting in rapid loss of phase coherence in the transverse plane and reduced T2*. This signal loss can be quantified, typically using multiecho gradient-echo sequences: the signal intensity of each pixel is plotted versus echo time and the resulting curve fit to the expected exponential decay function to generate parametric images of T2* or R2* (relaxivity, or the inverse of T2*) (**Fig. 17**).

Normal values for myocardial T2* at 1.5 T are 33 ± 7.8 ms. In symptomatic patients who have iron overload, myocardial T2* values typically are below 20 ms, associated with declining LV function and increasing LV end-diastolic dimension and mass.[38,39] This technique may be important for identifying and monitoring therapy, as myocardial involvement is not well correlated with serum ferritin or hepatic liver iron load measurements.

AMYLOIDOSIS

Amyloidosis is a deposition disorder that easily may be confused with other cardiomyopathies. Amyloidosis results in the deposition of twisted β-pleated sheet fibrils (amyloid) and is classified by the composition of the amyloid fibril. Within the heart, deposition can occur within the myocardium of the ventricle and atria, valve leaflets, and within the coronary arteries. This pattern of deposition disrupts contractile function and conduction and influences coronary artery flow, producing clinical symptoms.

The most common form of amyloidosis accounting for 85% of all new cases is immunoglobulin amyloidosis. The building block of this form is an immunoglobulin light chain protein and includes primary amyloidosis, multiple myeloma, and other plasma cell dyscrasias, such as B-cell lymphoma and Waldenström's macroglobulinemia. Primary amyloidosis is a plasma cell disorder in which approximately 5% to 10% of bone marrow plasma cells have clonal dominance of a light chain isotype. This is manifested by a predominance of lambda versus kappa free light chains in a 3:1 ratio. In comparison, plasma cell dyscrasias, such as multiple myeloma, usually have a lambda-to-kappa ratio of 1:2.[40] Primary amyloidosis is a rare but devastating disorder with a median survival of 4 months if untreated. Immunoglobulin amyloidosis involves the heart in 60% of patients and ultimately leads to patient death from associated heart failure or arrhythmia.[41]

Several less common forms of amyloidosis also exist. Familial or hereditary amyloidosis is an autosomal dominant disorder caused most commonly by a mutation in a transthyretin gene—a gene in which more than 70 mutations have been identified. Senile systemic amyloidosis affects approximately 25% of patients over age 80 and is derived from normal transthyretin protein. Senile amyloid usually is isolated to the heart and most commonly involves the atria. Secondary amyloidosis is characterized by reactive amyloid fibrils. These fibrils are acute-phase reactants produced in response to systemic inflammation, such as tuberculosis, leprosy, rheumatoid arthritis, familial Mediterranean fever, inflammatory bowel syndrome, chronic lung diseases, and chronic infections.

Although cardiac biopsy is the gold standard for diagnosis, less invasive techniques are available. At echocardiography, diffuse ventricular thickening with a granular sparkle may be suggestive of the diagnosis.[11] MR imaging also shows promise in this area. On standard b-SSFP cine sequences, symmetric thickening of the ventricles and atria with enlarged chamber size may be noted. Valve leaflets and the papillary muscles may demonstrate thickening. Pericardial and pleural effusions are common (**Fig. 18**).

Histologically, cardiac amyloidosis is characterized by interstitial expansion with amyloid protein. Amyloid shows an asymmetric distribution, with greater involvement of the subendocardium with respect to the subepicardium.[42] On delayed enhancement imaging, the increased myocardial interstitial volume results in delayed washout of gadolinium and diffuse myocardial enhancement. This also commonly results in difficulty nulling

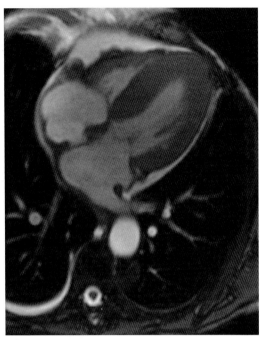

Fig. 18. Amyloidosis: four-chamber b-SSFP image shows biventricular myocardial thickening. Thickening of the atrial walls also is evident. Ancillary findings consistent with amyloid are the small pericardial and pleural effusions.

myocardium for delayed enhancement images, as shown in a study by Maceira and colleagues.[43] The diagnosis of amyloid should be entertained when the nulling inversion time of myocardium is less than that of the ventricular cavity or blood pool (**Fig. 19**).[43]

In the same study by Maceira and colleagues, it was established that gadolinium washes out of the blood pool faster in patients who have amyloid compared with normal patients. This effect was amplified with decreased renal function, which is believed linked to a greater total body amyloid load. Because of this increased clearance, the blood pool is darker in amyloid patients than normal patients at standard inversion times of 200 to 300 ms.[42]

MYOCARDITIS

Myocarditis is an acute injury to the cardiac muscle, which often is the sequela of viral infection. Patients may present with vague symptoms, such as lethargy, palpitations, and chest pain. Abnormal laboratory findings often are seen, including ECG changes and elevated cardiac enzymes. The clinical presentation can mimic acute

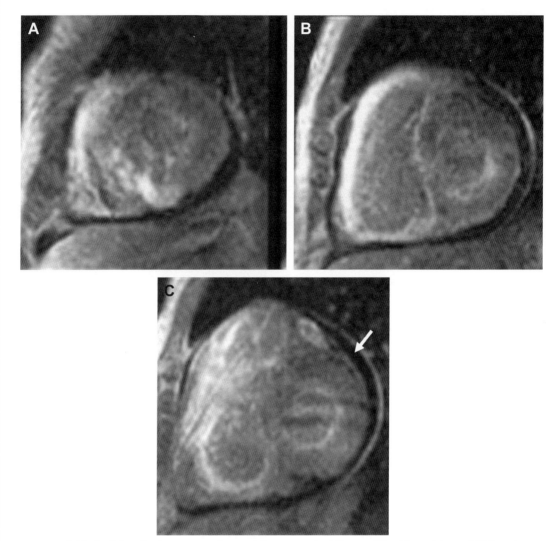

Fig.19. Amyloidosis: delayed enhancement short-axis images at the (*A*) apex, (*B*) midventricle, and (*C*) base in a patient who had cardiac amyloidosis show diffuse abnormal enhancement of the myocardium. Note the markedly abnormal enhancement of the RV myocardium. A pericardial effusion also is visible (*arrow*) (*C*).

coronary syndrome and this should be excluded before the diagnosis of myocarditis is assured. Most patients who have myocarditis spontaneously recover; however, some experience severe complications, and myocarditis is a leading cause of sudden death in adults less than 40 years of age.[44]

Myocarditis traditionally has been a diagnosis of exclusion or a presumed diagnosis in patients who have acute coronary syndrome but normal coronary arteries. Endomyocardial biopsy is considered the gold standard for diagnosis but has a high risk/benefit ratio and a sensitivity of only 50% to 63%.[45] MR imaging provides a noninvasive method of diagnosis and therapeutic monitoring.

Segmental wall motion abnormalities and associated pericardial effusions may be seen with myocarditis; however, these are nonspecific findings that also are common in patients who have acute myocardial infarction. In active myocarditis, there is disruption of myocyte cell membranes and subsequently an increase in free water within the myocardium. This results in increased T2 signal or hyperintensity on fluid sensitive sequences, also a nonspecific finding.[46]

Key imaging features that allow discrimination between myocarditis and myocardial infarction are myocardial perfusion and MDE sequences. In early studies, acute myocarditis was shown to rarely have first-pass perfusion abnormalities

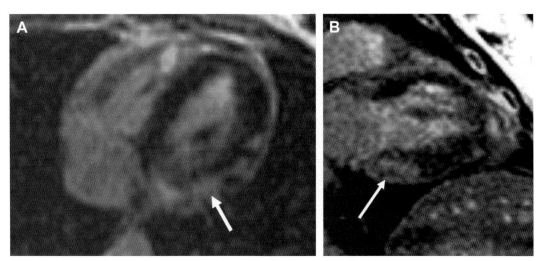

Fig. 20. Myocarditis: (*A*) axial and (*B*) two-chamber delayed enhancement images demonstrate patchy subepicardial hyperenhancement of the inferolateral and inferior wall of the left ventricle (*arrows*) in keeping with the questioned history of myocarditis in this 18-year-old female patient.

(4%), which are seen more commonly in acute myocardial infarction.[47] In a study evaluating delayed enhancement patterns in patients who had acute myocarditis, 88% of patients displayed abnormal enhancement. This enhancement typically involves the lateral LV free wall located in the subepicardium (**Fig. 20**).[14] This location is an important discriminator as the subendocardium is spared, the typical location in myocardial infarction (**Fig. 21**). Follow-up imaging in recovering

from myocarditis has demonstrated decreasing enhancement and improved LV function.

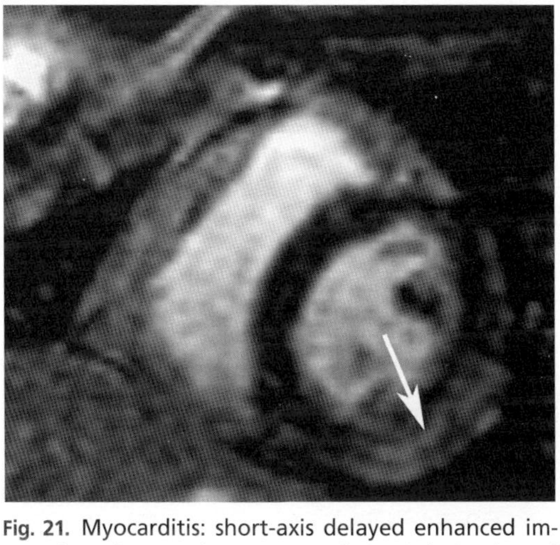

OTHER CARDIOMYOPATHIES

Many other cardiomyopathies exist that occur much less frequently than the aforementioned disease entities. Often, the clinical history must be put into context and subsequent imaging may provide additional information. Cardiomyopathy may be secondary to tachyarrhythmias and those associated with pregnancy. Peripartum cardiomyopathy demonstrates LV dysfunction (LVEF < 45%) in the absence of another identifiable disease process within 1 month ante partum to 5 months' post partum.[48] The exact cause of this disease process is unknown, but MR imaging is able to provide additional clinical information, such as LV function and the presence of myocardial damage/fibrosis. MR imaging may be useful in evaluating cardiac dysfunction related to infectious agents or Lyme disease and Chagas' disease or may be used to evaluate underlying metabolic disorders. Two further diseases that often have interesting imaging features despite their infrequent occurrence are endomyocardial disease and apical ballooning (or takotsubo) syndrome.

Endomyocardial Disease

Endomyocardial disease is a rare restrictive cardiomyopathy that may be secondary to idiopathic hypereosinophilia syndrome or endomyocardial fibrosis. Although these two entities often are

Fig. 21. Myocarditis: short-axis delayed enhanced image show hyperenhancement of the inferior lateral wall in a subepicardial location (*arrow*) in keeping with myocarditis.

described interchangeably, they possess distinct variations, including geographic variations, the presence of eosinophilia, and differing clinical courses.[11] Three phases of hypereosinophilia are described, including necrosis, thrombosis, and fibrosis.[49] This may cause significant subendocardial fibrotic wall thickening of either ventricle, which is most common at the apex. This wall thickening results in a decreased cavity size and restricted filling. Cine imaging allows visualization of diastolic dysfunction whereas delayed enhanced imaging classically demonstrates a trilaminar appearance consisting of normal myocardium, thickened fibrotic endocardium with inflammatory exudate, and overlying thrombus (**Fig. 22**).[50]

Apical Ballooning (Takotsubo) Syndrome

This unique cardiomyopathy often is confused with myocardial ischemia. Apical ballooning syndrome shows severe cardiac dysfunction, typically involving the apex, in the presence of normal coronary arteries. This entity most commonly affects postmenopausal women after emotional or physical stress. The pathogenesis of the disease is unknown but is speculated to involve the release of catecholamines with subsequent cardiac toxicity. Named for its resemblance to a Japanese fishing pot, the syndrome involves hypokinesis or akinesis of the apical cardiac segments with hypercontractility of the basal segments. This finding can be demonstrated easily with cine MR imaging (**Fig. 23**). Furthermore, with the addition of postcontrast imaging, the finding can be differentiated from myocardial infarction with the lack of delayed myocardial hyperenhancement. Apical ballooning syndrome is frequently referred to as transient LV cardiomyopathy as patients generally have a good prognosis and recovery of the cardiac dysfunction can occur within weeks of the primary event.

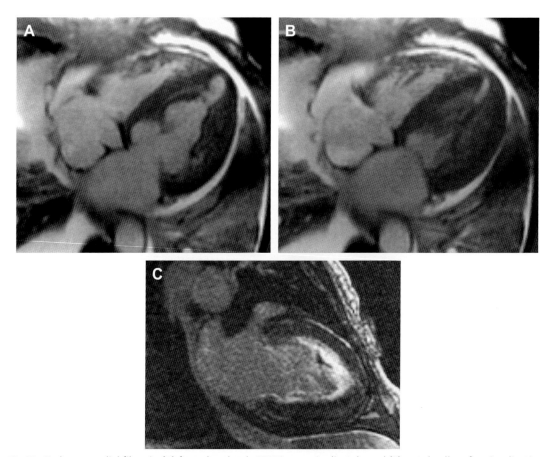

Fig. 22. Endomyocardial fibrosis: (*A*) four-chamber b-SSFP images in diastole and (*B*) systole allow for visualization of thrombus within the apex of the of the LV. (*C*) Delayed enhancement two-chamber view of the LV demonstrates the trilaminar appearance consistent with endomyocardial fibrosis.

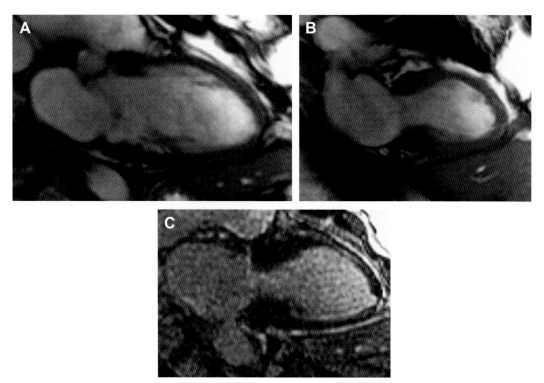

Fig. 23. Apical ballooning: (*A*) diastolic b-SSFP two-chamber view with normal-appearing ventricle. (*B*) The same view in systole shows hyperdynamic function of the base of the heart whereas the apex is akinetic. (*C*) Delayed enhancement imaging does not show any hyperenhancement of the myocardium. Epicardial coronary arteries were normal. Findings were consistent with apical ballooning syndrome.

SUMMARY

- There is a varied and extensive group of diseases that may affect the myocardium and its subsequent function, collectively referred to as cardiomyopathies.
- Many of these cardiomyopathies have similar clinical presentations, but the underlying condition determines which of the variety of prognoses and treatment options are selected.
- Cardiac MR imaging plays a vital role in characterizing the range of entities, thus is crucial for patient evaluation and management.
- In addition to the exquisite morphologic and functional imaging provided by routine cardiac MR imaging sequences, delayed enhanced imaging can allow for differentiation between diseases and can provide prognostic information. As the speed and technical ease of cardiac imaging improve, MR imaging will assume an ever-increasing role in the care of patients who have cardiomyopathy.

REFERENCES

1. Richardson P, McKenna W, Bristow M, et al. Report of the 1995 World Health Organization/International Society and Federation of Cardiology Task Force on the Definition and Classification of Cardiomyopathies. Circulation 1996;93(5):841–2.
2. Maron BJ, Towbin JA, Thiene G, et al. Contemporary definitions and classification of the cardiomyopathies: an American Heart Association scientific statement from the Council on Clinical Cardiology, Heart Failure and Transplantation Committee; quality of care and outcomes research and functional genomics and translational biology interdisciplinary working groups; and Council on Epidemiology and Prevention. Circulation 2006;113(14):1807–16.
3. Maron BJ, McKenna WJ, Danielson GK, et al. American College of Cardiology/European Society of Cardiology clinical expert consensus document on hypertrophic cardiomyopathy. A report of the American College of Cardiology Foundation Task Force on Clinical Expert Consensus Documents and the European Society of Cardiology Committee for Practice Guidelines. J Am Coll Cardiol 2003;42(9):1687–713.
4. Nathan AW, SID. Essential cardiology. 3rd edition. London: Blackwell; 1997.
5. Bogaert J, Taylor AM. Nonischemic myocardial disease. In: Bogaert J, Dymarkowski S, Taylor AM, editors. Clinical cardiac MRI. New York (NY): Springer Verlag Inc.; 2005. p. 285–304.

6. Choudhury L, Mahrholdt H, Wagner A, et al. Myocardial scarring in asymptomatic or mildly symptomatic patients with hypertrophic cardiomyopathy. J Am Coll Cardiol 2002;40(12):2156–64.

7. Moon JC, McKenna WJ, McCrohon JA, et al. Toward clinical risk assessment in hypertrophic cardiomyopathy with gadolinium cardiovascular magnetic resonance. J Am Coll Cardiol 2003;41(9):1561–7.

8. Dumont CA, Monserrat L, Soler R, et al. Clinical significance of late gadolinium enhancement on cardiovascular magnetic resonance in patients with hypertrophic cardiomyopathy. Rev Esp Cardiol 2007;60(1):15–23 [in Spanish].

9. Dec GW, Fuster V. Idiopathic dilated cardiomyopathy. N Engl J Med 1994;331(23):1564–75.

10. Knaapen P, Gotte MJ, Paulus WJ, et al. Does myocardial fibrosis hinder contractile function and perfusion in idiopathic dilated cardiomyopathy? PET and MR imaging study. Radiology 2006;240(2):380–8.

11. Hare JM. The dilated, restrictive, and infiltrative cardiomyopathies. Braunwald's heart disease: a textbook of cardiovascular medicine. 8th edition. St. Louis (MO): Saunders; 2007. p. 1739–60.

12. Wu E, Judd RM, Vargas JD, et al. Visualisation of presence, location, and transmural extent of healed Q-wave and non-Q-wave myocardial infarction. Lancet 2001;357(9249):21–8.

13. McCrohon JA, Moon JC, Prasad SK, et al. Differentiation of heart failure related to dilated cardiomyopathy and coronary artery disease using gadolinium-enhanced cardiovascular magnetic resonance. Circulation 2003;108(1):54–9.

14. Mahrholdt H, Goedecke C, Wagner A, et al. Cardiovascular magnetic resonance assessment of human myocarditis: a comparison to histology and molecular pathology. Circulation 2004;109(10):1250–8.

15. Assomull RG, Prasad SK, Lyne J, et al. Cardiovascular magnetic resonance, fibrosis, and prognosis in dilated cardiomyopathy. J Am Coll Cardiol 2006; 48(10):1977–85.

16. Corrado D, Basso C, Thiene G. Arrhythmogenic right ventricular cardiomyopathy: diagnosis, prognosis, and treatment. Heart 2000;83(5):588–95.

17. Fontaine G, Fontaliran F, Frank R. Arrhythmogenic right ventricular cardiomyopathies: clinical forms and main differential diagnoses. Circulation 1998;97(16):1532–5.

18. Kayser HW, van der Wall EE, Sivananthan MU, et al. Diagnosis of arrhythmogenic right ventricular dysplasia: a review. Radiographics 2002;22(3):639–48 [discussion: 649–50].

19. Castillo E, Tandri H, Rodriguez ER, et al. Arrhythmogenic right ventricular dysplasia: ex vivo and in vivo fat detection with black-blood MR imaging. Radiology 2004;232(1):38–48.

20. Ferrari VA, Scott CH. Arrhythmogenic right ventricular cardiomyopathy: time for a new look. J Cardiovasc Electrophysiol 2003;14(5):483–4.

21. Sen-Chowdhry S, Lowe MD, Sporton SC, et al. Arrhythmogenic right ventricular cardiomyopathy: clinical presentation, diagnosis, and management. Am J Med 2004;117(9):685–95.

22. Bomma C, Rutberg J, Tandri H, et al. Misdiagnosis of arrhythmogenic right ventricular dysplasia/cardiomyopathy. J Cardiovasc Electrophysiol 2004;15(3): 300–6.

23. McKenna WJ, Thiene G, Nava A, et al. Diagnosis of arrhythmogenic right ventricular dysplasia/cardiomyopathy. Task force of the working group myocardial and pericardial disease of the European society of cardiology and of the scientific council on cardiomyopathies of the international society and federation of cardiology. Br Heart J 1994; 71(3):215–8.

24. Basso C, Thiene G, Corrado D, et al. Arrhythmogenic right ventricular cardiomyopathy. Dysplasia, dystrophy, or myocarditis? Circulation 1996;94(5): 983–91.

25. Tandri H, Saranathan M, Rodriguez ER, et al. Noninvasive detection of myocardial fibrosis in arrhythmogenic right ventricular cardiomyopathy using delayed-enhancement magnetic resonance imaging. J Am Coll Cardiol 2005;45(1):98–103.

26. Weiford BC, Subbarao VD, Mulhern KM. Noncompaction of the ventricular myocardium. Circulation 2004;109(24):2965–71.

27. Ritter M, Oechslin E, Sutsch G, et al. Isolated noncompaction of the myocardium in adults. Mayo Clin Proc 1997;72(1):26–31.

28. Boyd MT, Seward JB, Tajik AJ, et al. Frequency and location of prominent left ventricular trabeculations at autopsy in 474 normal human hearts: implications for evaluation of mural thrombi by two-dimensional echocardiography. J Am Coll Cardiol 1987;9(2):323–6.

29. Petersen SE, Selvanayagam JB, Wiesmann F, et al. Left ventricular non-compaction: insights from cardiovascular magnetic resonance imaging. J Am Coll Cardiol 2005;46(1):101–5.

30. Oechslin EN, Attenhofer Jost CH, Rojas JR, et al. Long-term follow-up of 34 adults with isolated left ventricular noncompaction: a distinct cardiomyopathy with poor prognosis. J Am Coll Cardiol 2000; 36(2):493–500.

31. Kohli SK, Pantazis AA, Shah JS, et al. Diagnosis of left-ventricular non-compaction in patients with left-ventricular systolic dysfunction: time for a reappraisal of diagnostic criteria? Eur Heart J 2008; 29(1):89–95.

32. Jenni R, Oechslin EN, van der Loo B. Isolated ventricular non-compaction of the myocardium in adults. Heart 2007;93(1):11–5.

33. Henke CE, Henke G, Elveback LR, et al. The epidemiology of sarcoidosis in Rochester, Minnesota: a population-based study of incidence and survival. Am J Epidemiol 1986;123(5):840–5.

34. Vignaux O, Dhote R, Duboc D, et al. Clinical significance of myocardial magnetic resonance abnormalities in patients with sarcoidosis: a 1-year follow-up study. Chest 2002;122(6):1895–901.

35. Uemura A, Morimoto S, Hiramitsu S, et al. Histologic diagnostic rate of cardiac sarcoidosis: evaluation of endomyocardial biopsies. Am Heart J 1999;138 (2 Pt 1):299–302.

36. Smedema JP, Snoep G, van Kroonenburgh MP, et al. The additional value of gadolinium-enhanced MRI to standard assessment for cardiac involvement in patients with pulmonary sarcoidosis. Chest 2005; 128(3):1629–37.

37. Vignaux O. Cardiac sarcoidosis: spectrum of MRI features. AJR Am J Roentgenol 2005;184(1):249–54.

38. Anderson LJ, Holden S, Davis B, et al. Cardiovascular T2-star (T2*) magnetic resonance for the early diagnosis of myocardial iron overload. Eur Heart J 2001;22(23):2171–9.

39. Cheong B, Huber S, Muthupillai R, et al. Evaluation of myocardial iron overload by T2* cardiovascular magnetic resonance imaging. Tex Heart Inst J 2005;32(3):448–9.

40. Hassan W, Al-Sergani H, Mourad W, et al. Amyloid heart disease. New frontiers and insights in pathophysiology, diagnosis, and management. Tex Heart Inst J 2005;32(2):178–84.

41. Shah KB, Inoue Y, Mehra MR. Amyloidosis and the heart: a comprehensive review. Arch Intern Med 2006;166(17):1805–13.

42. Maceira AM, Joshi J, Prasad SK, et al. Cardiovascular magnetic resonance in cardiac amyloidosis. Circulation 2005;111(2):186–93.

43. Mahrholdt H, Wagner A, Judd RM, et al. Delayed enhancement cardiovascular magnetic resonance assessment of non-ischaemic cardiomyopathies. Eur Heart J 2005;26(15):1461–74.

44. Feldman AM, McNamara D. Myocarditis. N Engl J Med 2000;343(19):1388–98.

45. Laissy JP, Messin B, Varenne O, et al. MRI of acute myocarditis: a comprehensive approach based on various imaging sequences. Chest 2002;122(5):1638–48.

46. Gagliardi MG, Bevilacqua M, Di Renzi P, et al. Usefulness of magnetic resonance imaging for diagnosis of acute myocarditis in infants and children, and comparison with endomyocardial biopsy. Am J Cardiol 1991;68(10):1089–91.

47. Laissy JP, Hyafil F, Feldman LJ, et al. Differentiating acute myocardial infarction from myocarditis: diagnostic value of early- and delayed-perfusion cardiac MR imaging. Radiology 2005;237(1):75–82.

48. Gilles A, Antoine M, Vincent JL, et al. Peripartum cardiomyopathy. Rev Med Brux 2001;22(5):436–8 [in French].

49. Ogbogu PU, Rosing DR, Horne MK III. Cardiovascular manifestations of hypereosinophilic syndromes. Immunol Allergy Clin North Am 2007;27(3):457–75.

50. Syed IS, Martinez MW, Feng DL, et al. Cardiac magnetic resonance imaging of eosinophilic endomyocardial disease. Int J Cardiol 2007;29.

MR Imaging of the Pericardium

Andrew J. Misselt, MD[a], Scott R. Harris, MD[a],
James Glockner, MD, PhD[a], DaLi Feng, MD[b],
Imran S. Syed, MD[b], Philip A. Araoz, MD[a],*

KEYWORDS

- MR imaging • Pericardium • Mesothelioma
- Constrictive • Pericardial effusion

The heart is separated from the remaining mediastinal structures by the pericardium, a thin covering that provides structural support and barrier protection for the heart. It also improves the mechanics of the heart by coupling the right and left chambers to each other and by lubricating the heart's motion in the chest.

Despite the apparent usefulness of the pericardium, it is not an essential structure, and normal cardiac function can be sustained in its absence.[1] Although the pericardium provides a supportive role, it is the diseased pericardium that is of primary interest.

The pericardium can be developmentally malformed or absent. Other states of pericardial abnormality, such as pericarditis (thickening and inflammation), pericardial effusion (retained fluid within the pericardial layers), and pericardial masses, arise as a response to various diseases.

IMAGING

Echocardiography is often the first-line modality for imaging the pericardium. In most situations, this highly portable tool with outstanding spatial and temporal resolution provides sufficient diagnostic information. Echocardiography is not optimal, however, for every patient or situation. Obesity and chronic obstructive pulmonary disease may limit the acoustic window, and even in optimal patients small pericardial effusions may be difficult to visualize and pericardial thickening is frequently not detectable. Also,

echocardiography provides only a limited opportunity for tissue characterization.

The pericardium can also be imaged using MR imaging or CT. There is substantial overlap in the capabilities of these two modalities, with both offering multiplanar imaging and multigated cine reconstructions. Presently, CT offers a faster examination with superior anatomic detail. MR imaging, however, is more useful for soft tissue characterization.[2,3] Furthermore, if the patient has a regular heart rhythm, MR imaging can provide better display of cardiac motion.[4] Ultimately, the best choice of modality depends on the specific patient, clinical question, and operator preference.

A successful MR imaging protocol for imaging the pericardium starts with an effective basic cardiac examination. In addition to routine short axis stack, four-chamber, and three-chamber cine sequences (SSFP), axial black-blood, perfusion, and postcontrast delayed enhancement images should be included. To differentiate definitively between fluid and fat it may be useful to obtain selective double inversion recovery (IR) and triple IR images in the same plane. Additional techniques include myocardial tagging and inspiratory and expiratory real-time cine acquisition.[5,6]

PERICARDIAL ANATOMY

The pericardium is a bilayered sac into which the heart and origins of the great vessels have been invaginated (**Fig. 1**). A commonly used analogy for the embryologic development of the pericardium is inserting one's hand into a balloon and then

[a] Department of Radiology, Mayo Clinic, 200 First Street SW, Rochester, MN 55905, USA
[b] Department of Cardiology, Mayo Clinic, 200 First Street SW, Rochester, MN 55905, USA
* Corresponding author.
E-mail address: paraoz@mayo.edu (P.A. Araoz).

Magn Reson Imaging Clin N Am 16 (2008) 185–199
doi:10.1016/j.mric.2008.02.011
1064-9689/08/$ – see front matter © 2008 Elsevier Inc. All rights reserved.

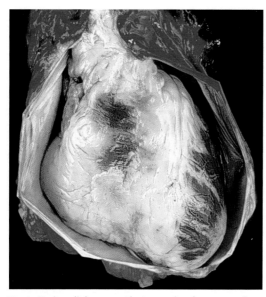

Fig. 1. Pericardial space. Photograph of gross pericardial specimen with fibrous pericardium incised and reflected revealing the pericardial space.

deflating it. This analogy creates a useful image of the heart (hand) contained within the cavity of the bilayered pericardium (the balloon). In addition to the heart and great vessels, the pericardium contains small blood vessels, the lymphatics draining the mediastinal lymph nodes, and branches of the phrenic and vagal nerves.[1]

Structurally, the pericardium is composed of two layers. The outside layer is a tough fibrous structure called the "fibrous pericardium." The fibrous pericardium is thicker than the inner layer and it provides mechanical support by attaching to the surrounding mediastinal structures.[1,7] The inner layer of the pericardium, called the "serosal pericardium" (also known as the "visceral pericardium"), forms a continuous sac by investing both the epicardium and the interior surface of the surrounding fibrous pericardium. The serosal pericardium is made of a thin layer of mesothelial cells, which produce the lubricating serous fluid of the pericardial sac.[8] In the physiologic state the pericardial sac contains between 15 and 50 mL of fluid.[9] The combined thickness of both layers of pericardium should measure less than 2 mm.

Normally, the fibrous pericardium is the only visualized portion of the pericardium because the visceral pericardium adds an imperceptibly thin contribution. The normal pericardium is seen as a less than 2-mm thin band of low signal between the epicardial and mediastinal fat layers (**Fig. 2**).[10] Occasionally, a small amount of

physiologic fluid derived from the serosal pericardium collects within the pericardium and can be seen on cross-sectional imaging as it pools within the potential spaces of the pericardial sac (**Fig. 3**).

The reflections of the serosal pericardium form two complex tubes. One tube surrounds the origins of the aorta and pulmonary trunk. The second tube surrounds the origins of the superior vena cava, inferior vena cava, and pulmonary veins. A passage way called the "transverse sinus" connects the two serosal pericardial tubes. The transverse sinus is divided into several recesses including the superior and inferior aortic recesses and the right and left pulmonic recesses. The oblique sinus is the second pericardial sinus and it is located in a cul-de-sac behind the left atrium. Recesses of the oblique sinus include the postcaval recess, the right pulmonary venous recess, and the left pulmonary venous recess (**Fig. 4**).[8,11,12]

PERICARDITIS

Clinically, pericarditis presents as chest pain, which is often sharp and may worsen with changes in position. In most cases the cause of pericarditis is thought to be a viral infection. Often the precise viral agent is not identified. These cases remain idiopathic in origin. Other etiologies include radiation; injury, such as trauma or myocardial infarction; bacterial, fungal, or tuberculous infections; metabolic causes, such as uremia, rheumatic, autoimmune-related; and malignancy. Commonly, the diagnosis of pericarditis is made on clinical grounds. Causes of chest pain including myocardial infarction, myocarditis, pericarditis, pulmonary embolism, and musculoskeletal pain can have wide and overlapping spectrum of presentation. In complex cases imaging may be used to arrive at a definitive diagnosis. Generally, an MR imaging examination occurs well down the path of the diagnostic work-up after causes of chest pain, such as myocardial infarction or pulmonary embolism, have been excluded on the basis of biomarkers or other imaging tests.

As the name implies, pericarditis is inflammation of the pericardium. Acutely, the pericardium may develop a small effusion and become slightly thickened (**Fig. 5**). Most cases resolve in a short time and are treated primarily with nonsteroidal anti-inflammatory medicines. If imaged in this acute setting one is likely to see a minimally thickened and enhancing pericardium, perhaps with a small pericardial effusion (**Fig. 6**). The imaging findings of pericarditis generally abate in concert with the clinical manifestations. This is not

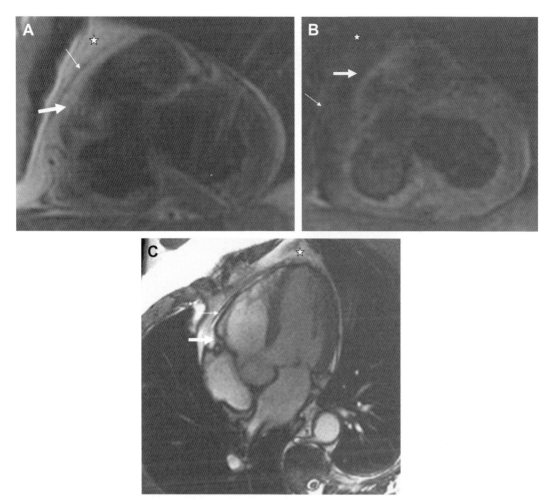

Fig. 2. Normal pericardium. (*A*) Short axis black blood (double inversion recovery) image in a 55-year-old man showing normal pericardium (*thin arrow*), which is superficial to the epicardial fat layer (*thick arrow*) and deep to the mediastinal fat (*star*). (*B*) Short axis black blood at the same level with nulling of fat signal (triple inversion recovery) shows the signal drop-out of the mediastinal and epicardial fat. (*C*) Four-chamber SSFP in the same patient. Note the T2/T1 weighting of the image with both fat and fluid yielding bright signal.

universally true, however, and patients may maintain a degree of pericardial enhancement well after clinical resolution of the disease, perhaps caused by secondary fibrosis of the pericardium.[13] Occasionally, a patient may progress to a scenario called "chronic relapsing pericarditis" in which the clinical course is characterized by episodic recurrence despite treatment. Often steroids are used to manage this more persistent inflammation. Over time, if the pericarditis does not resolve, the pericardial effusion may increase, or the pericardium may become more thickened and perhaps fibrotic or calcified.[14] Chronic pericarditis is identified based on patient history, and by demonstrating a thicker pericardium, and possibly areas of calcification.[14]

PERICARDIAL EFFUSION

Pericardial effusion refers to excessive fluid within the pericardial sac (>50 mL). In addition to occurring as a response to pericarditis, pericardial effusion can often result from fluid overload states, such as heart or renal failure. Alternatively, pericardial effusions may develop as a result of disruption of cardiac lymphatic drainage caused by infection or neoplasm, or in response to injuries, such as infarction, blunt or penetrating trauma, and radiation.[15]

The size of a pericardial effusion may be semi-quantitatively assessed by measuring the thickness of the fluid anterior to the right ventricle. Using criteria established by echocardiography,

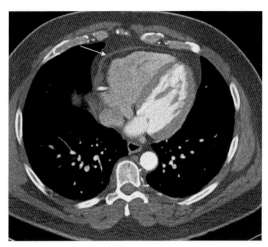

Fig. 3. Normal amount of pericardial fluid. Axial CT of a 50-year-old man showing normal fluid (*arrow*) within the pericardial space.

a pericardial effusion may be quantified as small (<5 mm); moderate (5–10 mm); or large (>10 mm). A small effusion may be difficult to detect using any modality, although MR imaging has been reported to be more sensitive than echocardiography.[16] Generally, it is the differentiation of fluid from pericardial fat or pericardial thickening that proves challenging. When the pericardial space appears thickened with bright signal on SSFP imaging, the signal intensity may be caused by either fat or fluid contribution because of the T2/T1 weighting of the image. In this situation, double and triple IR sequences can aid in the differentiation. Double IR images null the signal contribution of fluid, whereas tripple IR images null the signal contribution of fat. Using these complementary techniques one can usually differentiate between fluid and fat with confidence.

In addition to quantifying the amount of fluid, MR imaging may characterize the pericardial effusion as simple or proteinaceous based on the signal characteristics.[17] Specific types of pericardial effusion, such as hydropericardium, hemopericardium, chylopericardium, or pneumopericardium, may be deduced by their respective signal characteristics. Simple effusions show decreased signal on T1-weighted images and increased signal with T2 weighting (**Fig. 7**). Hemopericardium has signal that varies with the degradation of the blood, although complex or infected fluid has heterogeneous signal and may have some increased intensity on T1-weighted images (**Fig. 8**). Air in the pericardial space is evident as a signal void.

PERICARDIAL TAMPONADE

From a physiologic standpoint, it is not the cause or even the volume of pericardial fluid that is most important. Rather, it is the time course of fluid accumulation that is most physiologically significant.[18] Indeed, if a pericardial effusion from any cause develops slowly enough, adaptive expansion of the pericardium may ultimately accommodate a pericardial fluid volume of up to 3 L with little consequence.[8] Conversely, if a pericardial effusion develops without time for adaptive enlargement of the pericardium, the increase in pressure within the pericardial sac impacts the function of the heart.

Pericardial tamponade (also referred to as "cardiac tamponade") is a physiologic state in which pericardial pressure derived from a rapid increase in pericardial fluid impairs cardiac function.[19] When pericardial fluid accumulates quickly, before adaptive enlargement of the pericardium can occur, the increased volume of fluid within a contained space increases the pericardial pressure. Because the heart is surrounded by the pericardium the increased pericardial pressure is transmitted to all four cardiac chambers.

During tamponade, increased pericardial pressure exerts its collapsing force on the outer surface of the heart throughout the cardiac cycle. The effects of tamponade can be predicted by comparing a given pericardial pressure with the normal intracardiac pressures (**Table 1**). As the pericardial pressure rises, it becomes more difficult to fill the heart. The cavae and hepatic veins, which are exterior to the pericardial pressure, dilate to accommodate the back pooling of blood. Further increases in pericardial pressure can lead to a reduction of ventricular filling. This reduction in preload results in a reduction in cardiac output as expected from the Frank-Starling mechanism. Eventually, if the pericardial pressure exceeds the ability of the circulation to fill the heart, the cardiac chambers, especially the right atrium and right ventricle, collapse.[20]

Imaging

MR imaging is seldom used in the setting of pericardial tamponade because of the hemodynamic instability of the patient; however, patients with pericardial effusions frequently undergo MR imaging evaluations. By understanding the physiology of tamponade, the examiner can differentiate a well-compensated pericardial effusion from tamponade. Changes in intrathoracic pressure caused by respiration play an exaggerated role (**Table 2**), although these findings are presently best demonstrated with real-time imaging with

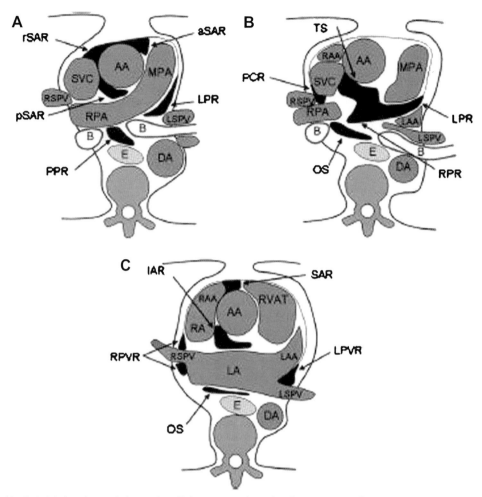

Fig. 4. (A–C) Axial drawings of the pericardial spaces at three levels. Drawings of the pericardial sinuses and recesses at three closely adjacent slice levels in the axial plane above the heart base. AA, ascending aorta; B, bronchus intermedius; DA, descending aorta; E, esophagus; IAR, inferior aortic recess; LA, left atrium; LAA, left atrial appendage; LPR, left pulmonic recess; LPVR, left pulmonic vein recess; LSPV, left superior pulmonary vein; MPA, main pulmonary artery; OS, oblique sinus; PCR, postcaval sinus; pSAR, posterior superior aortic recess; PRP, posterior pericardial recess; RA, right atrium; RAA, right atrial appendage; RPA, right pulmonary artery; RPR, right pulmonic recess; RPVR, right pulmonic vein recess; rSAR, right superior aortic recess; RSPV, right superior pulmonary vein; RVAT, right ventricular outflow tract; SAR, superior aortic recess; SVC, superior vena cava. (From Rienmuller R, Groll R, Lipton MJ. CT and MR imaging of pericardial disease. Radiol Clin North Am 2004;42:587–601; with permission.)

echocardiography or cardiac catheterization. A patient with tamponade may demonstrate enlarged vena cavae and hepatic veins. The heart size, however, excluding the pericardial space, is normal or decreased. This is contrary to restrictive cardiomyopathy and partial pericardial constriction in which the atria are typically enlarged. Throughout the cardiac cycle there is enhanced intraventricular coupling from the taut pericardial space. This most often manifests as abnormal motion of the intraventricular septum. If the pericardial pressures are particularly high, or if the patient is imaged in expiration (which decreases

right ventricular filling), there may be partial collapse of the right ventricle during diastole. There may also be the associated clinical findings of Kussmaul's sign or pulsus paradoxus (Table 3).

CONSTRICTIVE PERICARDITIS

Constrictive pericarditis is a physiologic condition in which a thickened, rigid, and often calcified pericardium impairs cardiac function (Fig. 9).[21] The findings of constrictive pericarditis are similar to restrictive cardiomyopathy, which broadly refers to an intrinsic myocardial process in which

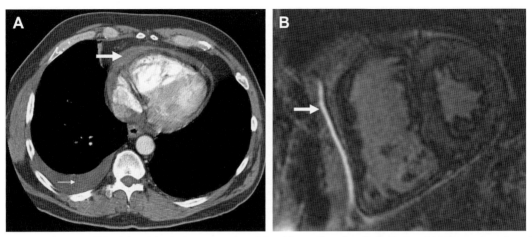

Fig. 5. Acute pericarditis. (*A*) Axial CT of acute pericarditis with small pericardial effusion (*thick arrow*) and small pleural effusion (*thin arrow*) in a 64-year-old man. (*B*) Follow-up short axis, delayed enhancement MR image 1 week later shows brightly enhancing pericardium (*arrow*) with signal intensity higher than subcutaneous fat. The pericardial effusion has resolved.

the heart muscle itself is thickened and stiff.[22] Clinically separating constrictive pericarditis from restrictive cardiomyopathy can be difficult.[23] Amyloid cardiomyopathy is a specific example of a restrictive process. In amyloid cardiomyopathy protein deposition thickens and stiffens the muscle and limits the heart's function. Treatments for restrictive cardiomyopathy have limited efficacy and the prognosis is dismal. The heart failure caused by constrictive pericarditis can be cured, however, by surgical resection of the pericardium (**Fig. 9C**). The distinction between the two entities is critical and imaging is often used to identify appropriate surgical candidates.

Most commonly, constrictive pericarditis occurs after open heart surgery. Other leading causes

include prior radiation, infection, noninfectious inflammation, or idiopathic etiologies.[21] In most cases the pericardium is thick, and in about a quarter of patients the pericardium is calcified.[24] The entire pericardium can be affected or the constriction may be caused by just a portion of the pericardium. In a small minority of cases, perhaps less than 5%, constrictive physiology may be present in the setting of pericardium with normal thickness at imaging, but demonstrable fibrosis at pathology.[25]

Imaging

Typically, a patient with constrictive pericarditis has a thickened pericardium, measuring greater

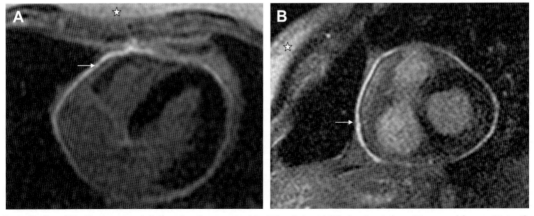

Fig. 6. Pericarditis. Postcontrast delayed enhancement in (*A*) axial and (*B*) short axis in a 46-year-old man. Note the brightly enhancing pericardium (*arrow*) with signal intensity higher than subcutaneous fat (*star*).

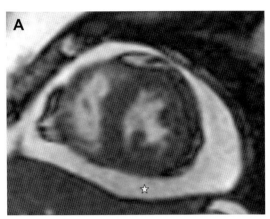
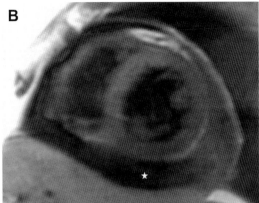

Fig. 7. Simple pericardial effusion. Short axis SSFP (A) and double inversion recovery (B) images in a 43-year-old woman. The fluid (star) demonstrates bright signal with T2/T1 weighting of SSFP image and dark signal on the double inversion recovery image.

than 4 mm.[26] It is possible the pericardium enhances, although this is not a necessary feature. There may be a small pericardial effusion. The ventricles may be narrowed at the apical aspect with a tubular appearance. The inferior vena cava is usually dilated. The atria may or may not be dilated because atrial dilatation depends on whether the entire pericardium is abnormal or just the anterior portion. Of note, most patients with restrictive cardiomyopathy have atrial dilation, so this is a relatively insensitive finding. The most sensitive and specific finding is the septal bounce (Fig. 10).[23] In one series the septal bounce was present in 85% of patients with constrictive pericarditis, and in no patients without constriction.[27]

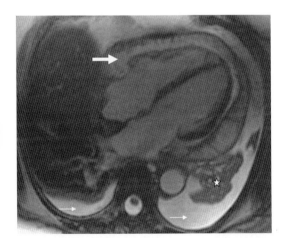

Fig. 8. Complex pericardial effusion. Axial SSFP image shows a complex pericardial effusion in a 68-year-old woman. Note stranded appearance of the complex fluid in the pericardial space (thick arrow). Pleural effusions (thin arrows) and atelectatic lung (star) are also present.

Constrictive Physiology

In the setting of pericardial constriction, initial ventricular filling is normal. As the intracardiac volume approaches the constraining limit of the rigid pericardium, the intraventricular pressures rise sharply and equalize and diastolic filling terminates abruptly (Fig. 11).[28] Because the heart fills poorly, preload is reduced and there is an overall decrease in cardiac performance.

The abnormal hemodynamic forces of constrictive pericarditis are best explained in the context of intrathoracic pressure changes during respiration.[29] The heart is isolated from the chest by the rigid and noncompliant pericardium and so the heart effectively behaves as an extrathoracic structure. At the same time the confining space of the rigid pericardium couples the ventricles to each other so that a pressure change in one ventricle is transmitted to the other.[30] This results in an exaggerated response to changes in intrathoracic pressure.[22]

Inspiration, Constrictive Pericarditis

The main imaging feature of constrictive physiology during inspiration is the septal bounce. The septal bounce is a transient leftward shift of the interventricular septum (which normally bows into the right ventricle). During inspiration the negative intrathoracic pressure gradient draws blood into the intrathoracic systemic veins (innominate veins and superior and inferior vena cavae) causing the right heart to fill more rapidly than the left. In early diastole the right ventricular pressure is transiently higher than the left, causing the septum to bow leftward. This increased right ventricular pressure is only in early diastole and only temporary. In mid diastole the left ventricular pressure once

Table 1
Normal chamber pressures

Chamber/Vessel	Diastolic (mm Hg)	Systolic (mm Hg)	Mean (mm Hg)
Right atrium	4	4	3–4
Right ventricle	2	15	—
Pulmonary artery	7	15	12
Left atrium	10	7	8
Left ventricle	8	120	—
Aorta	80	120	100

again becomes higher, pushing the septum rightward, and in late diastole the pressures equalize. The result is that the ventricular septum shivers, or vibrates, as it expends its kinetic energy between two chambers of equal pressure (see **Fig. 11**; **Fig. 12**).

If the capacity for right ventricular expansion is sufficiently reduced, paradoxical elevation of the jugular venous pressure with inspiration (clinically manifest as jugular venous distention) may be appreciated (Kussmaul's sign). This happens because the increased pressure in the small fixed ventricular volume is transmitted backward to the systemic veins, resulting in elevation of the jugular venous pressure.

In the left heart, the rigid pericardium isolates the left atrium and ventricle from the decrease in intrathoracic pressures experienced in the chest during inspiration. The pressure gradient derived from the discrepancy in pressure exaggerates the normal physiologic pattern and blood pools within the low-pressure pulmonary venous circulation with greater tenacity at the expense of left heart filling.

Expiration, Constrictive Pericarditis

The opposite is true in expiration, in which the increase in intrathoracic pressure normally slows the systemic venous return to the right heart while simultaneously increasing pulmonary venous return to the left heart (**Table 4**). Because the heart is isolated from the chest by the rigid pericardium,

however, the normal differences between the right and left ventricles are exaggerated. The right heart filling is further decreased and the increase in left heart filling is exaggerated (up until the point of pericardial constriction). This scenario can be observed by measuring differences in mitral inflow velocities during respiration, which are increased during expiration and decreased during inspiration. Flattening of the ventricular septum may occur in late diastole when the ventricular pressures equalize, but because the ventricle normally bows rightward, the septal bounce is less prominent.

Effusive Constrictive Pericarditis

Effusive constrictive pericarditis combines the findings of pericardial tamponade and constrictive pericarditis. This entity is seen most often following treatment with radiation. Typically, symptoms of heart failure prompt an imaging evaluation, at which time a pericardial effusion is identified. After the pericardial effusion has been drained, however, the abnormal physiology persists.[31] This is best demonstrated with cardiac catheterization obtained with pre-pericardial and post-pericardial drainage pressure measurements or with echocardiography.[32] Similar findings (persistent constriction after pericardial effusion drainage) could also likely be appreciated with CT or MR imaging, although these modalities are rarely used in this setting.

Table 2
Alterations in cardiac filling with respiratory variation, normal physiology

	Inspiration	Expiration
Venus return to right atrium (right heart filling)	Increased	Decreased
Venus return to left atrium (left heart filling)	Slightly decreased	Slightly increased

Table 3
Alterations in cardiac filling with respiratory variation, tamponade physiology

	Inspiration	Expiration
Right heart filling	Decreased (Kussmauls sign)[a]	Severely decreased
Left heart filling	Severely decreased (pulsus paradoxus)[b]	Decreased

[a] Kussumaul's sign is the paradoxical elevation of the jugular venous distention with inspiration. Normally with inspiration the jugular venous distention is decreased.
[b] Pulsus paradoxus is classically the absence of radial pulse during inspiration.

DEVELOPMENTALLY ABNORMAL OR ABSENT PERICARDIUM

Embryologically, the pericardium is formed by the medial migration of the two pleuropericardial folds. As these two structures progress and ultimately fuse, the thorax is divided into the pericardial cavity and pleural cavities. If a pleuropericardial fold is redundant, it may pinch off and form a pericardial cyst or diverticulum. Conversely, if a pleuropericardial fold is diminutive,

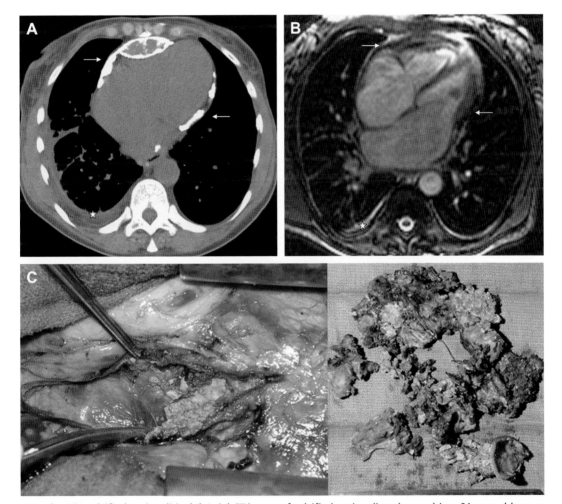

Fig. 9. Chronic, calcified pericarditis. (*A*) Axial CT image of calcified pericardium (*arrows*) in a 64-year-old woman with constrictive pericarditis. A pleural effusion is also present (*star*). (*B*) Axial SSFP image of same patient. The calcified pericardium shows decreased signal on MR imaging (*arrows*). (*C*) Intraoperative photos from same patient during pericardial stripping for constrictive pericarditis shows the thickened, calcified pericardium.

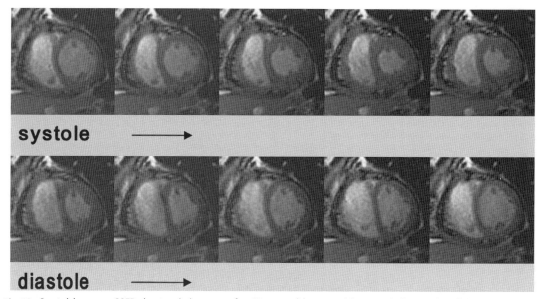

systole ⟶

diastole ⟶

Fig. 10. Septal bounce. SSFP short axis images of a 69-year-old man with constrictive pericarditis. Images were acquired during inspiration. The top row shows the ventricles contracting during systole. The bottom row shows the ventricles relax during diastole. Note the mild bowing of intraventricular septum to the left during early diastole and the undulating septum during mid to late diastole (septal bounce).

a partially or completely absent pericardium may ensue.

Complete absence of the pericardium is rare and is manifest by levopostion of the heart with no directly associated cardiac abnormality.[33] Congenital abnormalities often occur in concert, however, and anomalies of the chest wall, lungs, heart, or diaphragm may also be present.[34] Partial absence of the pericardium is also infrequent,

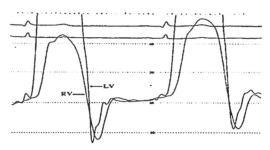

Fig. 11. Ventricular pressure tracing of patient with constrictive pericarditis. Cardiac catheterization pressure tracing of the right ventricle (RV) and left ventricle (LV) throughout the cardiac cycle in a patient with constrictive pericarditis. Right ventricular pressure transiently exceeds left ventricular pressure in early diastole. Later in diastole, the ventricular pressures equalize. (*From* Goldstein JA. Cardiac tamponade, constrictive pericarditis, and restrictive cardiomyopathy. Curr Probl Cardiol 2004;29:503–67; with permission.)

but more common than complete absence.[35] In normal conditions the pericardium acts as a barrier, preventing the invagination of the lung tissue into the space between the aorta and pulmonary artery. If the pericardial deficit overlies the great vessels, lung tissue is seen between the aorta and pulmonary artery. If the pericardium along the posterolateral wall of the left ventricle is absent, the left ventricle is posteriorly displaced (**Fig. 13**).[36] A focally deficient pericardium may also allow a part of the heart to herniate through the hole. When this type of trans-pericardial cardiac herniation occurs, it most often involves the left atrial appendage. In such situations, surgical closure may be performed.[37]

Pericardial Cysts and Masses

Pericardial cysts or diverticula are fluid-containing structures that abut the pericardium (**Fig. 14**). They are often found in the cardiophrenic space, but they can occur along any surface of the pericardium.[9] Pericardial cysts are usually unilocular and they do not enhance with contrast.[38] Additionally, a pericardial cyst should not exert mass effect on the myocardium. If there is mass effect or enhancement, an alternative diagnosis should be sought.

Coronary artery aneurysms are sometimes mistaken for pericardial masses. They may arise as a result of infection, surgical anastomosis,

Table 4
Alterations in cardiac filling with respiratory variation, constrictive physiology

	Inspiration	Expiration
Right heart filling	Relatively normal early in diastole, but abruptly terminates because of the constraining pericardium (Kussmauls sign)	Slightly decreased
Left heart filling	Severely decreased (pulsus paradoxus)	Rapid in early diastole, but abruptly terminates because of the constraining pericardium
Septal bowing	Transient leftward in early diastole, may shiver or vibrate in mid to late diastole	Rightward in early diastole (the normal finding), may flatten in late diastole

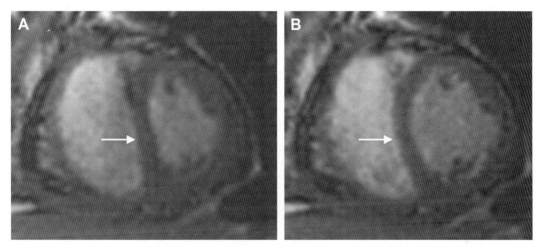

Fig. 12. Septal motion of constrictive pericarditis. Short axis SSFP images during (*A*) early and (*B*) late diastole in the same patient. Note the leftward bowing of the intraventricular septum (*arrow*) during early diastole.

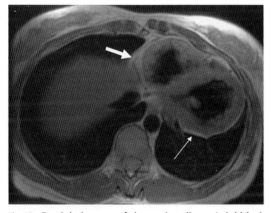

Fig. 13. Partial absence of the pericardium. Axial black blood MR image of a 44-year-old woman demonstrating partial absence of the pericardium. The thick arrow shows a portion of normal pericardium. There is partial absence over the left ventricular free wall (*thin arrow*) with posterior displacement of the left ventricle.

vasculitis, or atherosclerosis. A coronary artery aneurysm should be suspected when a smoothly marginated, enhancing mass is seen along the expected course of a coronary artery (**Fig. 15**).

In general, solid pericardial masses are rare. The most common solid pericardial masses are metastases, which in autopsy series have been identified in 10% to 12% of patients with known malignancies.[39] About 25% of patients with known pericardial metastasis have impaired cardiac function, most often caused by pericardial effusion with tamponade physiology.[34] Other tumors involving the pericardium arise as extensions from structures in the adjacent mediastinum. Primary tumors of the pericardium include mesothelioma, fibrosarcoma, angiosarcoma, and malignant teratoma.[40] Benign tumors include fibromas, hemangiomas, lipomas, and benign teratomas. The most common primary malignant tumor of the pericardium is mesothelioma

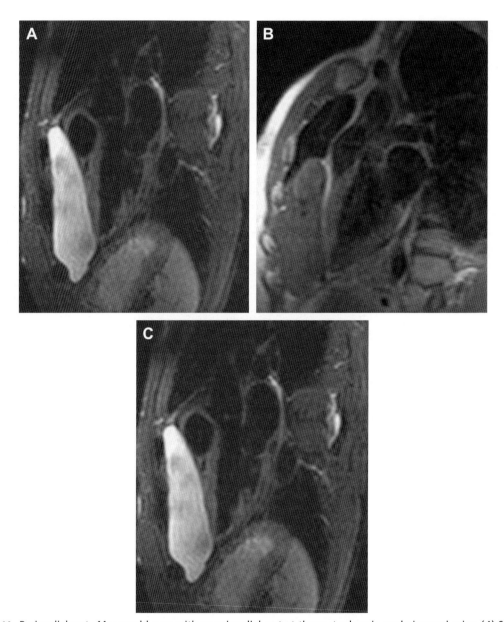

Fig. 14. Pericardial cyst. 44-year-old man with a pericardial cyst at the costophrenic angle imaged using (*A*) SSFP, (*B*) double inversion recovery, and (*C*) triple inversion recovery MR imaging sequences. The cyst behaves like fluid: bright on SSFP and triple inversion recovery and dark on double inversion recovery.

(Fig. 16). Like mesothelioma of the pleura, pericardial mesothelioma is associated with prior asbestos exposure.[41] Angiomyosarcoma heterogenously enhances and tends to occur in the right atrium and involve the pericardium.[42]

Imaging

The best starting place for imaging masses or congenital heart findings is with axial black blood images. One successful approach is to use double IR black blood images followed by triple IR images in the same plane (usually axial). The double IR images are T1 weighted and provide a detailed overview of the anatomy. The triple IR images are T2 weighted with nulled signal from fat, and are useful for identify cysts and differentiating fluid from fat. It follows then that a pericardial cyst or diverticulum should have a high signal intensity on T2-weighted images and low signal intensity on T1-weighted

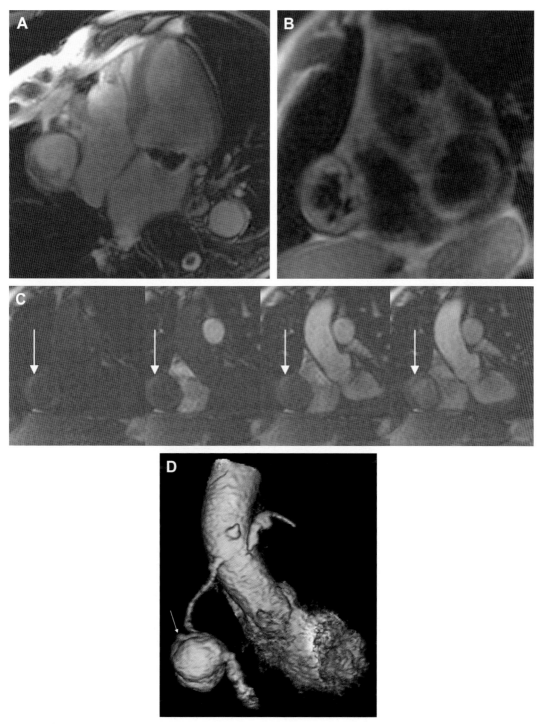

Fig. 15. Right coronary artery aneurysm. An 80-year-old man with a right coronary artery aneurysm (*arrow*). (*A*) Four-chamber SSFP, (*B*) short axis black blood, (*C*) short axis perfusion, and (*D*) three-dimensional rendered MR images. Note the position within the right atrioventricular groove (*A*), mass effect on the right heart (*B*), and progressive enhancement of the aneurysm concomitant with the aorta (*C*).

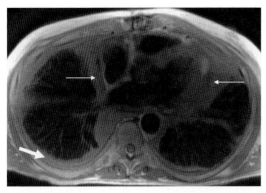

Fig. 16. Pericardial mesothelioma. Axial double inversion recovery MR image of a 63-year-old man with mesothelioma involving the pericardium (*thin arrows*) and pleura (*thick arrow*).

images. If the cyst in question contains proteinaceous debris, however, relatively increased signal intensity may be appreciated on T1-weighted images.[33] Pericardial cysts do not enhance or have mass effect. Coronary artery aneurysms should follow the arterial distribution. If an enhancing mass extends beyond the expected coronary artery distribution and exerts mass effect, malignancy should be strongly considered.

SUMMARY

Imaging of the pericardium requires understanding of anatomy, normal and abnormal physiology, tissue characterization, and the evaluation of masses. MR imaging is well-suited for answering clinical questions regarding the pericardium. Short axis, four-chamber, and three-chamber cine sequences (SSFP), axial black-blood, perfusion, and postcontrast delayed enhancement images should be included in the evaluation of suspected pericardial disease. To differentiate definitively between fluid and fat in patients with pericardial disease, it may be useful to obtain selective double IR and triple IR images in the same plane. Additional techniques include myocardial tagging and inspiratory and expiratory real-time cine acquisition.

Pericardial diseases that may be effectively imaged with MR imaging include pericarditis, pericardial effusion, cardiac and pericardial tamponade, constrictive pericarditis, pericardial cysts, absence of the pericardium, and pericardial masses. Although benign and malignant primary tumors of the pericardium may be occasionally encountered, the most common etiology of a pericardial mass is metastatic disease.

REFERENCES

1. Axel L. Assessment of pericardial disease by magnetic resonance and computed tomography. J Magn Reson Imaging 2004;19(6):816–26.
2. Gulati G, Sharma S, Kothari SS, et al. Comparison of echo and MRI in the imaging evaluation of intracardiac masses. Cardiovasc Intervent Radiol 2004; 27(5):459–69.
3. Semelka RC, Shoenut JP, Wilson ME, et al. Cardiac masses: signal intensity features on spin-echo, gradient-echo, gadolinium-enhanced spin-echo, and TurboFLASH images. J Magn Reson Imaging 1992;2(4):415–20.
4. Pereles FS, Kapoor V, Carr JC, et al. Usefulness of segmented trueFISP cardiac pulse sequence in evaluation of congenital and acquired adult cardiac abnormalities. AJR Am J Roentgenol 2001;177(5): 1155–60.
5. Kuhl HP, Spuentrup E, Wall A, et al. Assessment of myocardial function with interactive non-breath-hold real-time MR imaging: comparison with echocardiography and breath-hold Cine MR imaging. Radiology 2004;231(1):198–207.
6. Reichek N. MRI myocardial tagging. J Magn Reson Imaging 1999;10(5):609–16.
7. Fuster V, Alexander RW, O'Rourke RA. Diseases of the pericardium. In: Fuster V, Alexander RW, O'Rourke RA, editors. 11th edition, Hurst's the heart, vol. 2. York (PA): The McGraw-Hill Companies, Inc.; 2004.
8. Rienmuller R, Groll R, Lipton MJ. CT and MR imaging of pericardial disease. Radiol Clin North Am 2004; 42(3):587–601.
9. Breen JF. Imaging of the pericardium. J Thorac Imaging 2001;16(1):47–54.
10. Sechtem U, Tscholakoff D, Higgins CB. MRI of the normal pericardium. AJR Am J Roentgenol 1986; 147(2):239–44.
11. Groell R, Schaffler GJ, Rienmueller R. Pericardial sinuses and recesses: findings at electrocardiographically triggered electron-beam CT. Radiology 1999;212(1):69–73.
12. Broderick LS, Brooks GN, Kuhlman JE. Anatomic pitfalls of the heart and pericardium. Radiographics 2005;25(2):441–53.
13. Teraoka K, Hirano M, Yannbe M, et al. Delayed contrast enhancement in a patient with perimyocarditis on contrast-enhanced cardiac MRI: case report. Int J Cardiovasc Imaging 2005;21(2–3): 325–9.
14. Sechtem U, Tscholakoff D, Higgins CB. MRI of the abnormal pericardium. AJR Am J Roentgenol 1986;147(2):245–52.
15. Oyama N, Oyama N, Komuro K, et al. Computed tomography and magnetic resonance imaging of the pericardium: anatomy and pathology. Magn Reson Med Sci 2004;3(3):145–52.

16. White CS. MR evaluation of the pericardium. Top Magn Reson Imaging 1995;7(4):258–66.

17. Glockner JF. Imaging of pericardial disease. Magn Reson Imaging Clin N Am 2003;11(1):149–62.

18. Refsum H, Junemann M, Lipton MJ, et al. Ventricular diastolic pressure-volume relations and the pericardium: effects of changes in blood volume and pericardial effusion in dogs. Circulation 1981;64(5):997–1004.

19. Tsang TS, Oh JK, Seward JB. Diagnosis and management of cardiac tamponade in the era of echocardiography. Clin Cardiol 1999;22(7):446–52.

20. Singh S, Wann LS, Schuchard GH, et al. Right ventricular and right atrial collapse in patients with cardiac tamponade: a combined echocardiographic and hemodynamic study. Circulation 1984;70(6):966–71.

21. Myers RB, Spodick DH. Constrictive pericarditis: clinical and pathophysiologic characteristics. Am Heart J 1999;138(2 Pt 1):219–32.

22. Nishimura RA. Constrictive pericarditis in the modern era: a diagnostic dilemma. Heart 2001;86(6):619–23.

23. Giorgi B, Mollet NR, Dymarkowski S, et al. Clinically suspected constrictive pericarditis: MR imaging assessment of ventricular septal motion and configuration in patients and healthy subjects. Radiology 2003;228(2):417–24.

24. Ling LH, Oh JK, Breen JF, et al. Calcific constrictive pericarditis: is it still with us? Ann Intern Med 2000;132(6):444–50.

25. Talreja DR, Edwards WD, Danielson GK, et al. Constrictive pericarditis in 26 patients with histologically normal pericardial thickness. Circulation 2003;108(15):1852–7.

26. Masui T, Finck S, Higgins CB. Constrictive pericarditis and restrictive cardiomyopathy: evaluation with MR imaging. Radiology 1992;182(2):369–73.

27. Francone M, Dymarkowski S, Kalantzi M, et al. Real-time cine MRI of ventricular septal motion: a novel approach to assess ventricular coupling. J Magn Reson Imaging 2005;21(3):305–9.

28. Goldstein JA. Cardiac tamponade, constrictive pericarditis, and restrictive cardiomyopathy. Curr Probl Cardiol 2004;29(9):503–67.

29. Hurrell DG, Nishimura RA, Higano ST, et al. Value of dynamic respiratory changes in left and right ventricular pressures for the diagnosis of constrictive pericarditis. Circulation 1996;93(11):2007–13.

30. Santamore WP, Bartlett R, Van Buren SJ, et al. Ventricular coupling in constrictive pericarditis. Circulation 1986;74(3):597–602.

31. Hancock EW. A clearer view of effusive-constrictive pericarditis. N Engl J Med 2004;350(5):435–7.

32. Sagrista-Sauleda J, Angel J, Sanchez A, et al. Effusive-constrictive pericarditis. N Engl J Med 2004;350(5):469–75.

33. Maksimovic R, Dill T, Seferovic PM, et al. Magnetic resonance imaging in pericardial diseases: indications and diagnostic value. Herz 2006;31(7):708–14.

34. Van Son JA, Danielson GK, Schaff HV, et al. Congenital partial and complete absence of the pericardium. Mayo Clin Proc 1993;68(8):743–7.

35. Abbas AE, Appleton CP, Liu PT, et al. Congenital absence of the pericardium: case presentation and review of literature. Int J Cardiol 2005;98(1):21–5.

36. Yamano T, Sawada T, Sakamoto K, et al. Magnetic resonance imaging differentiated partial from complete absence of the left pericardium in a case of leftward displacement of the heart. Circ J 2004;68(4):385–8.

37. Wang ZJ, Reddy GP, Gotway MB, et al. CT and MR imaging of pericardial disease. Radiographics 2003;23(Spec issue):S167–80.

38. Grizzard JD, Ang GB. Magnetic resonance imaging of pericardial disease and cardiac masses. Magn Reson Imaging Clin N Am 2007;15(4):579–607.

39. Chiles C, Woodard PK, Gutierrez FR, et al. Metastatic involvement of the heart and pericardium: CT and MR imaging. Radiographics 2001;21(2):439–49.

40. Maisch B, Seferovic PM, Ristic AD, et al. Guidelines on the diagnosis and management of pericardial diseases executive summary. The Task Force on the Diagnosis and Management of Pericardial Diseases of the European Society of Cardiology. Eur Heart J 2004;25(7):587–610.

41. Kim JS, Kim HH, Yoon Y. Imaging of pericardial diseases. Clin Radiol 2007;62(7):626–31.

42. Araoz PA, Eklund HE, Welch TJ, et al. CT and MR imaging of primary cardiac malignancies. Radiographics 1999;19(6):1421–34.

MR Imaging of Ischemic Heart Disease

Gautham P. Reddy, MD, MPH[a],*, Sandra Pujadas, MD[b],
Karen G. Ordovas, MD[a], Charles B. Higgins, MD[a]

KEYWORDS

- Heart disease • Coronary artery disease
- Atherosclerosis • MR imaging

Ischemic heart disease (IHD) is the leading cause of morbidity and mortality in the United States and other industrialized countries,[1] and the diagnosis and therapy of IHD is a significant issue. The complex pathophysiology of IHD represents a substantial difficulty in the diagnostic evaluation of IHD. The ischemic cascade consists of several components leading up to the syndrome of angina pectoris (**Fig. 1**).[2] The first result of coronary obstruction is myocardial hypoperfusion. Decreased perfusion leads to diastolic dysfunction of the left ventricle, followed by systolic dysfunction. Persistence of blood flow impairment can lead to electrocardiographic changes and, ultimately, angina.

When IHD is suspected or confirmed, the primary imaging modality is echocardiography. When appropriate, complementary examinations can be performed. These include stress perfusion scintigraphy, cardiac catheterization, coronary angiography, and CT. MR imaging techniques have developed rapidly over the past several years, and MR imaging has the ability to delineate myocardial perfusion, ventricular function, and myocardial viability in a single examination. Although coronary MR angiography is promising, in recent years it has been supplanted as a noninvasive imaging modality by coronary CT angiography. The other capabilities of MR imaging suggest that it will be performed more and more frequently for the assessment of IHD.

EVALUATION OF MYOCARDIAL ISCHEMIA WITH PHARMACOLOGIC STRESS

The goal of imaging in IHD is to detect disease before symptoms occur, to confirm disease in the symptomatic patient, or to monitor disease progression over time. Referring to the ischemic cascade,[2] it is evident that myocardial ischemia can be identified with one of two broad approaches: assessing either myocardial perfusion or left ventricular wall motion and contractility. Examinations are performed under stress. Stress perfusion scintigraphy and stress echocardiography are most commonly performed with exercise stress, but for these examinations an alternative is pharmacologic stress. It is not feasible for a patient to exercise while undergoing an MR imaging examination unless an expensive and somewhat cumbersome customized exercise system is installed. Most institutions therefore apply pharmacologic stress for the MR imaging evaluation of myocardial ischemia. The two main categories of pharmacologic stress agents are: (1) vasodilators, such as adenosine or dipyridamole, and (2) beta agonists, such as dobutamine.

Vasodilators cause heterogeneity of coronary blood flow, which results in myocardial ischemia. Dipyridamole blocks the cellular uptake and metabolism of adenosine and thereby causes an increase in the concentration of interstitial adenosine. Adenosine produces an increase in intracellular cyclic adenosine monophosphate (c-AMP) by acting directly on surface adenosine receptors in the vascular wall smooth muscle. Through several mechanisms, the increased level of c-AMP causes relaxation of the vascular smooth muscle, leading to vasodilation. Both of these stress agents, dipyridamole and adenosine, decrease vascular resistance and thereby increase coronary blood flow by a factor of four to five times that of

[a] Department of Radiology, University of California, San Francisco, 505 Parnassus Avenue, Box 0628, San Francisco, CA 94143, USA
[b] Unidad de Imagen Cardiaca, Hospital de la Santa Creu i Sant Pau, Barcelona, Spain
* Corresponding author. Department of Radiology, Suite M396, 505 Parnassus Avenue, Box 0628, University of California, San Francisco, San Francisco, CA 94143-0628.
E-mail address: gautham.reddy@radiology.ucsf.edu (G.P. Reddy).

Magn Reson Imaging Clin N Am 16 (2008) 201–212
doi:10.1016/j.mric.2008.03.002
1064-9689/08/$ – see front matter © 2008 Elsevier Inc. All rights reserved.

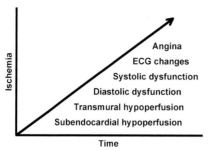

Fig. 1. The ischemic cascade. The sequence of events in the progression of ischemia. (*Reprinted from* Pujadas S, Reddy GP, Lee JJ, et al. Magnetic resonance imaging in ischemic heart disease. Semin Roentgenol 2003;38: 320–9; with permission.)

the resting level. If no coronary stenosis is present, the flow in the coronary system dilates uniformly, but if there is a flow-limiting stenosis, the portion of the distal vessel is fully dilated even during rest, and there is no increase in blood flow in the affected territory, resulting in flow heterogeneity. Moreover, vasodilatation in the normally perfused myocardium worsens the ischemia in the ischemic region by reducing perfusion pressure to the affected area, a phenomenon known as "coronary steal."

At many centers, the standard regimen for dipyridamole stress is the slow intravenous infusion of 0.56 mg/kg over a period of 4 minutes. MR imaging can begin 2 minutes after the beginning of the infusion. Alternatively, if dipyridamole is administered while the patient is on the detachable MR imaging table in the holding area outside of the scanner room, the patient can be closely monitored during administration of the drug, and a 12-lead ECG can be performed immediately after completion of the infusion. MR imaging can be performed immediately after the ECG is checked. Adenosine is typically administered intravenously at a rate of

140 μg/kg/min, and imaging can begin after 3 minutes. Because of its relatively short half-life, adenosine is administered when the patient is on the MR imaging table in the scanner room.

Contraindications for these pharmacologic stress agents include asthma and high-grade atrioventricular block. See **Table 1** for a more complete list of contraindications. During infusion of the stress agent, patients may develop symptoms, such as flushing, dizziness, nausea, and chest discomfort. Infusion of the stress agent should be halted and the study terminated if the patient develops bronchospasm, ventricular arrhythmia, or high-grade atrioventricular block.

An important difference between dipyridamole and adenosine is that dipyridamole has a longer half-life and therefore a slower onset and longer duration of action, approximately 30 minutes. This longer duration of action usually necessitates the use of aminophylline, an antagonist, to reverse the effect of dipyridamole after the MR imaging examination. Vasodilation increase in myocardial blood flow with dipyridamole is comparable to that of adenosine, although it may be more variable.[3] In contrast, the vasodilation produced by adenosine is of a shorter duration because of its relatively short half-life, which is less than 10 seconds. The effects of adenosine can therefore be reversed simply by discontinuing its administration. Nevertheless, it is important to keep aminophylline close at hand for emergency administration as an antidote to either adenosine or dipyridamole. It is important that patients avoid medication or food containing aminophylline, theophylline, or xanthines (including coffee, tea, cocoa products, and cola) for at least 24 hours before the stress examination.

Dobutamine is the most commonly used pharmacologic agent for stress wall motion studies. It is ideal for such examination because it is an

Table 1 Contraindications to pharmacologic stress	
Dobutamine	Unstable angina pectoris Severe arterial hypertension ($\geq$220/120 mm Hg) Hemodynamically significant aortic stenosis Complex cardiac arrhythmias Hypertrophic obstructive cardiomyopathy Myocarditis, pericarditis, or endocarditis Other major diseases
Adenosine/dipyridamole	Unstable angina pectoris Severe arterial hypertension ($\geq$220/120 mm Hg) Asthma/severe obstructive pulmonary disease Atrioventricular block $\geq$IIa Carotid artery stenosis

inotropic drug whose effect is similar to that of exercise. Dobutamine produces tachycardia and an increase in contractility, leading to an increase in oxygen demand, and ultimately regional ischemia in territories perfused by stenotic or occluded coronary arteries. The vasodilator effect of dobutamine is not as profound as that of adenosine or dipyridamole. The stress protocol for dobutamine MR imaging is the same as that for stress echocardiography: the drug is administered intravenously in increments of 10 μg/kg/min every 3 minutes, up to a maximal dose of 40 μg/kg/min. It is important to monitor the patient carefully for symptoms and blood pressure changes and to assess the examination for wall motion abnormalities (**Fig. 2**B). The examination should be terminated if the patient develops symptoms (such as chest pain), wall motion abnormalities, arrhythmia, severe hypotension or hypertension, or ECG changes that suggest ischemia (such as ST depression or T wave inversion). Contraindications to dobutamine are listed in **Table 1**. A defibrillator and medications needed for emergency treatment should be kept at hand and readily available.

EVALUATION OF MYOCARDIAL PERFUSION

The functional significance of a coronary stenosis depends several factors, including the severity of stenosis, presence of collateral blood flow, microcirculation, and coronary artery autoregulation. A functional test is necessary for the evaluation of the hemodynamic severity of a coronary stenosis. The first consequence of a flow-limiting coronary stenosis is the diminishment of myocardial perfusion,[2,4] and several noninvasive techniques have been applied to the assessment of myocardial perfusion.

Positron Emission Tomography

Positron emission tomography (PET) is the standard of reference (gold standard) for the evaluation of myocardial perfusion.[5] PET allows for the absolute quantification of regional myocardial perfusion. Although it is a tomographic technique, its spatial resolution is not high enough to delineate subendocardial perfusion defects. PET has other drawbacks: it is relatively expensive, and its availability is relatively limited.

Radionuclide Scintigraphy

For clinical purposes, the primary method for assessment of myocardial perfusion is single photon emission computed tomography (SPECT). SPECT myocardial perfusion imaging uses the radioisotopes thallium-201 or technetium-99m. SPECT

has demonstrated good sensitivity (80%–90%) and specificity (75%–85%) for myocardial perfusion defects.[6–8] This technique has disadvantages, including relatively poor spatial resolution and artifacts, such as attenuation of tracer signal in the inferior wall because of overlying soft tissue. Such artifacts can be common, especially in women, although they can be overcome with attenuation correction.[9]

MR Perfusion Imaging

Contrast agent
First-pass MR imaging with gadolinium-chelate contrast agent has been shown to be a feasible technique for the assessment of myocardial perfusion.[10–13] Gadolinium chelates are paramagnetic agents that quickly diffuse across the capillary membrane into the extracellular space but cannot enter cells that have intact membranes. Approximately 30%–50% of the bolus of contrast agent enters the myocardial interstitium on the first pass, and myocardial gadolinium concentration and enhancement is closely related to myocardial blood flow.[10] By assessing the pattern of myocardial signal intensity over time after intravenous contrast administration, it is possible to identify differences in myocardial perfusion (**Fig. 3**). In the clinical setting, images are usually interpreted qualitatively, although semiquantitative analysis can also be performed. Qualitative image interpretation can be done by visual inspection. Perfusion defects can be categorized as reversible, in which the defect is seen only on stress imaging, or fixed, in which the defect is identified on both the stress and rest images. Semiquantitative methods can be used to estimate coronary flow reserve or myocardial perfusion reserve.[14–16] For semiquantitative analysis, a contrast agent dose of 0.02 to 0.025 mmol/kg is optimal for ensuring a relatively linear relationship between gadolinium concentration and myocardial signal intensity. If qualitative evaluation is desired, it is preferable to use a higher dose of contrast agent (0.05 mmol/kg). In both situations, gadolinium chelate is administered as an intravenous bolus at a typical injection rate of 2 mL/sec, which is best achieved with use of a mechanical injector.

Imaging pulse sequences
Myocardial blood flow is the primary determinant of gadolinium concentration in the myocardium within 5 minutes of a bolus contrast administration. After 5 minutes of the injection, concentration of the contrast agent is determined primarily by diffusion and eventually by recirculation. Rapid imaging sequences are therefore necessary to allow the

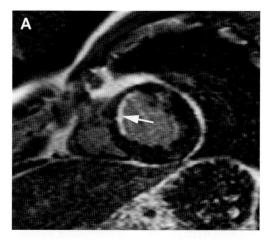

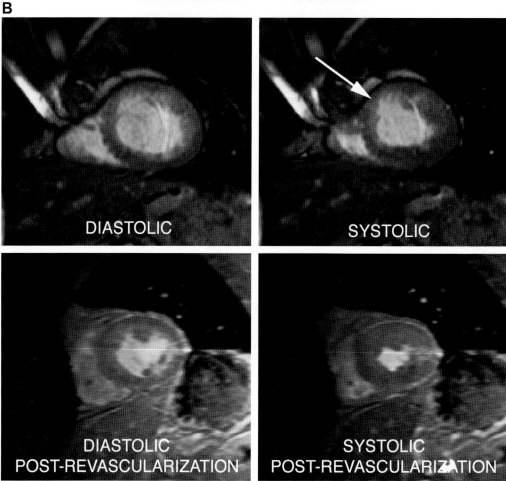

Fig. 2. MR imaging of a patient who had a nontransmural myocardial infarction and left ventricular dysfunction. (A) Viability study. Short-axis view of the left ventricle showing nontransmural hyperenhancement (*arrow*) of the anteroseptal wall. (B) Cine MR imaging study in the short-axis view at the level of the infarction showing diastolic (*left*) and systolic (*right*) images before revascularization (*upper images*) and 4 months after revascularization (*lower images*). Before revascularization there is akinesis of the anteroseptal wall (absence of systolic thickening). Because the viability study shows a limited extent (<50% of the myocardial wall) of the hyperenhancing area, we would expect functional recovery after revascularization. As expected, the study performed 4 months after revascularization shows normal left ventricular function (concentric wall thickening during systole). (*Reprinted from* Pujadas S, Reddy GP, Lee JJ, et al. Magnetic resonance imaging in ischemic heart disease. Semin Roentgenol 2003;38:320–9; with permission.)

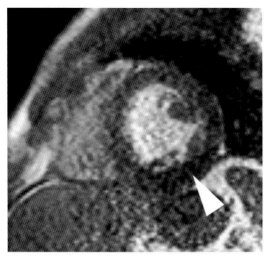

Fig. 3. Perfusion MR imaging study. Short-axis view at the mid-ventricular level demonstrates a perfusion defect in the inferior wall (*arrowhead*) corresponding to a stenosis of the right coronary artery in a right-dominant system.

identification of regional myocardial perfusion defects during the first pass of the contrast agent and to provide adequate spatial resolution. For clinical purposes it is vital to obtain myocardial perfusion MR images at several (three or more) anatomic levels in multiple imaging planes: the short-axis and vertical and horizontal long-axis planes. Several sequences can be used for MR perfusion imaging; each of these pulse sequences involves a tradeoff among several parameters: temporal resolution, spatial resolution, and image acquisition time.

Fast gradient-echo sequences are T1-weighted pulse sequences that yield a high signal-to-noise ratio and excellent image contrast. The primary drawback of this technique is its limited temporal resolution.

Echoplanar imaging makes multislice imaging possible without loss of temporal resolution because of its extremely fast acquisition time, typically 50 to 100 milliseconds. It should be noted that this type of sequence has not been widely used in the clinical setting because the images can be suboptimal because they are highly susceptible to artifacts. Moreover, this sequence yields a relatively poor combination of spatial resolution and signal-to-noise ratio.

Hybrid echoplanar imaging is a compromise between single-shot echoplanar imaging and fast gradient-echo sequences and has some features of both. Excellent results have been obtained using this sequence in conjunction with the sensitivity encoding technique.[17] This combination can

lead to excellent signal-to-noise ratio and spatial and temporal resolution.

Image postprocessing and validation studies
It has been shown that first-pass MR imaging techniques can be used to quantify myocardial perfusion reserve by analyzing signal intensity (SI) time changes.[14] Because gadolinium is an extravascular contrast agent, it rapidly diffuses to the extracellular space. Myocardial perfusion and contrast agent diffusion, which are related to blood flow, contribute to the SI-time curve.[18] The early portion of this SI-time curve is influenced primarily by myocardial perfusion, whereas the later portions are more significantly influenced by diffusion of the contrast agent.

Myocardial perfusion reserve is calculated as a ratio: the impulse response amplitude for hyperemic flow divided by the impulse response amplitude for basal flow.[14] Using this definition, Al-Saadi and colleagues[15] reported a sensitivity of 90% and a specificity of 85% for the detection of coronary stenosis with first-pass perfusion MR imaging in patients, using a threshold value of 1.5 for myocardial perfusion reserve. The primary limitation of this study was the incomplete coverage of the myocardium because the image acquisition was limited to a single slice through the heart. Another study used hybrid echoplanar imaging to compare multislice first-pass MR imaging to PET and quantitative coronary angiography.[16] That study reported a high correlation between MR imaging and PET for the identification of myocardial ischemia, and good sensitivity (87%) and specificity (85%) in comparison to quantitative coronary angiography, the standard of reference.

MR perfusion imaging: approach
The resting sequence is acquired with multiple simultaneous slices using the hybrid echoplanar technique. Images are performed in the short-axis plane to encompass the entire heart, and at least one slice should be obtained in the horizontal and vertical long axes. Gadolinium chelate contrast agent is infused as a compact intravenous bolus as imaging begins. After the resting sequence is performed, it takes approximately 10 minutes for the contrast agent to wash out from the myocardium. After 10 minutes, the pharmacologic stress agent (adenosine or dipyridamole) is administered intravenously, and the stress first-pass MR imaging study is performed. The stress study is compared visually to the resting study for qualitative assessment, and when needed, the images can be analyzed on a computer workstation for quantitative evaluation of perfusion.

ASSESSMENT OF VENTRICULAR FUNCTION (WALL MOTION)
Dobutamine Stress MR Imaging

Several studies of stress function MR imaging have used dipyridamole to detect regional wall motion abnormalities. These studies have reported reasonable specificity but relatively low sensitivity, in the 62% to 85% range, for the detection of significant coronary artery stenosis.[19–21] Dobutamine is the ideal choice for wall motion studies. Clinical studies have demonstrated good results for dobutamine stress MR imaging for the identification of significant obstructive coronary artery disease, with sensitivities in the 80% to 90% range and specificities in the 80% to 100% range.[22–28]

In current clinical practice, dobutamine stress echocardiography is the technique that is most frequently used to assess wall motion under pharmacologic stress. Comparing dobutamine MR imaging to dobutamine echocardiography, Nagel and colleagues[22] reported that there was superior sensitivity and specificity with dobutamine MR imaging. The results demonstrated sensitivity of 86% for dobutamine MR imaging versus 74% for echocardiography, and a specificity of 86% for MR imaging and 70% for echocardiography. Accuracy was shown to be higher (86%) for MR imaging than for dobutamine echocardiography (73%). In a subgroup of patients who had echocardiography that was of moderate or low quality, dobutamine MR imaging performed markedly better than did dobutamine echocardiography.[23,29]

Dobutamine MR imaging has several advantages over dobutamine echocardiography for wall motion assessment. The outstanding image quality and high spatial resolution permit highly accurate evaluation of the ventricular wall thickness and wall thickening because the endocardial border is more clearly depicted than on echocardiography. The results of MR imaging examinations are more reliably reproducible than those of echocardiography, and they are not as dependent on the operator.

Dobutamine MR imaging does have some limitations. Specifically, claustrophobia is a relative contraindication, and the presence of certain metallic objects and implanted devices in the body may be absolute contraindications. Perhaps more importantly, it is relatively difficult to monitor the patient for adverse effects. A 12-lead ECG cannot be obtained, and this limits the ability to detect ischemic ST changes. Wall motion abnormalities sometimes can be detected before such ST changes occur, but cine imaging is not typically acquired in real time, and there is usually a delay of a few minutes before wall motion can be assessed by visual inspection. In addition, if a patient has significant adverse effects or complications related to dobutamine administration, access to the patient may be impaired or delayed in the MR imaging environment. Because of these limitations, dobutamine MR imaging most typically serves as an adjunct to dobutamine echocardiography for the detection of coronary obstructive disease in patients whose echocardiograms are nondiagnostic or are of suboptimal image quality. It should be noted, however, that severe complications are unusual, occurring in only 0.25% of patients,[30,31] a rate similar to that of dobutamine stress echocardiography.

Image acquisition
For the detection of wall motion abnormalities, cine MR imaging is performed. Most commonly, steady-state free precession imaging is used because of the fast imaging time and improvement in image quality. Alternative cine MR imaging techniques are the gradient-echo and segmented k-space turbo gradient-echo sequences. Most commonly, images encompassing the entire heart are acquired in the short-axis view. Acquisitions in the horizontal and vertical long-axis planes are optional, but they can be useful.

Image interpretation
It is ideal to interpret dobutamine MR imaging studies using a multiple cine loop display, which allows different anatomic levels and different levels of stress (with progressive doses of dobutamine) to be evaluated simultaneously. The left ventricle should be analyzed at 17 segments per level of stress, in line with the standards outlined by the American Society of Echocardiography[32] and the American Heart Association (**Fig. 4**). Wall motion of each left ventricular segment is assessed visually and assigned 1 to 4 points, with 1 point for normokinetic segments, 2 for hypokinetic, 3 for akinetic, and 4 for dyskinetic. The points are totaled for all segments and then divided by the number of segments to generate a wall motion score. Normal contraction yields a wall motion score of 1, whereas wall motion abnormalities produce a higher score. During stress with escalating doses of dobutamine, abnormalities include a lack of increase in systolic wall thickening and reduced wall thickening compared with a lower level of stress.

ASSESSMENT OF MYOCARDIAL VIABILITY

Left ventricular function is one of the primary determining factors of long-term survival in patients

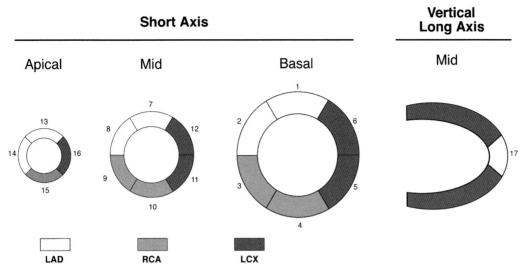

Fig. 4. Seventeen-segment model suggested by the American Heart Association. The coronary territories are shown. (*Reprinted from* Pujadas S, Reddy GP, Lee JJ, et al. Magnetic resonance imaging in ischemic heart disease. Semin Roentgenol 2003;38:320–9; with permission.)

who have IHD. Severe dysfunction of the left ventricle indicates a poor prognosis.[33–35] In many cases ventricular dysfunction can be reversible, however. Reversible myocardial dysfunction in patients who have IHD can be present in the setting of "hibernating" myocardium, which is myocardium with impaired function at rest because of chronic ischemia. Reversible dysfunction also occurs in patients who have "stunned" myocardium, which is tissue with reduced contractility that persists after severe or repetitive hypoperfusion, even after restoration of coronary blood flow.

Numerous studies have shown that in patients who have IHD left ventricular function can improve after revascularization procedures—percutaneous transluminal coronary angioplasty and stent placement or coronary artery bypass graft (CABG) surgery.[36–38] It may be especially important to ascertain viability in regions with severe segmental dysfunction in patients who have multivessel coronary artery disease when CABG is under consideration. It has been reported that the extent of viability before CABG surgery is an indicator of long-term prognosis.[39,40]

Furthermore, the diagnosis of a prior myocardial infarction is clinically important whether or not a revascularization procedure is necessary; such a diagnosis has implications for patient outcome.[41–43] It can be difficult to substantiate the diagnosis of a prior myocardial infarction if it was not diagnosed at the time of the acute infarction. Viability imaging can readily demonstrate infarcted tissue.

Myocardial Viability: Techniques

Various noninvasive techniques can be used to discern myocardial viability (**Table 2**). PET scanning, SPECT thallium or technetium scintigraphy, and dobutamine stress echocardiography are examinations that can identify the presence of viable myocardium. Although they may be clinically useful, these techniques have significant drawbacks. The disadvantages of PET include its relatively high cost and limited availability. SPECT

Table 2 Noninvasive methods of viability assessment	
Technique	Viability Marker
PET	Glucose metabolism
SPECT	Sarcolemma functional integrity
Dobutamine echo/MR imaging	Contractile reserve
Delayed-enhancement MR imaging	Myocardial scar/infarct

Abbreviation: Echo, echocardiography.

imaging has poor spatial resolution and problems with signal attenuation. In addition, it has been demonstrated that PET and SPECT can overestimate tissue viability when compared with the standard of functional recovery after revascularization; the specificity of these techniques is lower than modalities that evaluate contractile reserve.[44] Moreover, PET and SPECT scanning often cannot distinguish transmural nonviability from subendocardial nonviability. Dobutamine stress echocardiography has relatively poor spatial resolution. Up to 15% of studies are suboptimal because of poor image quality, and quality of the examinations is also substantially influenced by the experience of the operator and interpreting physician.

Assessment of Viability by Delayed-Enhancement MR Imaging

Twenty years ago, it was reported that ECG-gating spin-echo MR imaging following intravenous contrast administration demonstrated high signal intensity in infarcted myocardium. This phenomenon has come to be known as "hyperenhancement."[45,46]

The cellular mechanisms that cause hyperenhancement have not been completely elucidated. In acute myocardial infarction, hyperenhancement seems to occur because of the increased volume of distribution of contrast agent resulting from myocardial interstitial edema and myocyte membrane disruption.[10,47,48] Chronic infarction also demonstrates hyperenhancement. Regions of chronic infarction are characterized by a dense collagenous tissue, and interstitial space between collagen fibers in the scar tissue may be much greater than the interstitial space between myocytes in viable myocardium. After administration of contrast agent, the larger interstitial space of infarcted regions can lead to a greater concentration of contrast agent in these areas.[49] It has also been reported that there are abnormal kinetics of the contrast agent molecules, resulting in delayed washout of contrast agent in infarcted and reperfused regions compared with normal myocardium.[50]

Simonetti and colleagues[51] reported a segmented inversion recovery sequence that has led to a substantial improvement in image quality, improving the potential of MR imaging to evaluate myocardial viability. The technique uses a segmented inversion recovery pulse sequence. The inversion time is set to null the signal from viable myocardium and thereby increase the contrast between the hyperenhanced tissue (corresponding to infarction) and the null region (corresponding to viable myocardium) (**Fig. 5**). The imaging sequence is acquired approximately 10 to 15 minutes after the administration of gadolinium chelate contrast medium, hence the term "delayed hyperenhancement," or simply, "delayed enhancement."

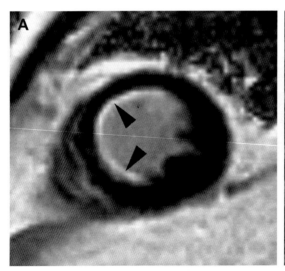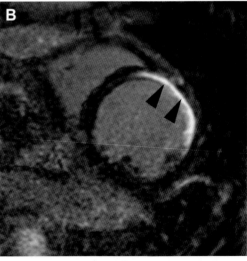

Fig. 5. Viability imaging. Vertical long-axis MR images of the left ventricle in two different patients. Studies were performed approximately 10 minutes after intravenous administration of gadolinium chelate contrast agent. (*A*) Patient who had subendocardial infarction, manifest as high signal intensity (*arrowheads*) in the septal wall. Given that the transmural extent of infarction is less than 50%, functional recovery after revascularization would be predicted. (*B*) Patient who had transmural infarction of the apex (*arrowheads*), indicated by high signal intensity of the full thickness of the myocardial wall. The areas of enhancement delineate nonviable myocardium. Functional recovery after revascularization would not be predicted. Medical management is therefore indicated in this patient.

In the segmented inversion recovery acquisition, the magnetization of the myocardium is prepared with a nonselective 180-degree inversion pulse that increases T1 weighting. The inversion time (TI) is the period between the application of the 180-degree pulse and the center of acquisition of the segmented k-space. To null the myocardium, the TI is selected such that the magnetization of the viable myocardium is near zero, resulting in dark signal of the myocardium. Delayed enhancement leads to T1 lowering, causing the infarcted myocardium to appear bright. This bright signal intensity of the enhancing infarct stands in stark contrast to the dark signal intensity of viable myocardium and allows the precise demarcation of the location and extent of the infarcted region.[51,52]

It is crucial to remember that areas that are at risk yet viable do not demonstrate delayed enhancement.[52–54] In myocardium that is viable but subject to reversible ischemia, the distribution volume of the gadolinium chelate is similar to that of normal myocardium and does not manifest delayed enhancement. Cellular membranes remain intact in the setting of severe but reversible ischemia, and contrast agent is therefore excluded from the intracellular space.

Contrast-enhanced MR imaging permits the depiction of the "no-reflow" phenomenon, which is characterized by significantly impaired myocardial perfusion even though there is patency of the artery supplying the infarcted territory. After arterial occlusion and on reperfusion, microvascular occlusion results from microvascular damage, which causes local activation and adhesion of neutrophils. Areas subject to the no-reflow phenomenon can be distinguished on delayed-enhancement MR imaging as a dark region toward the endocardial core of the infarct, completely surrounded by hyperenhancing tissue. Because the no-reflow area is surrounded by infarcted tissue, it can be differentiated from viable myocardium (**Fig. 6**).

Validation studies in humans

Studies in humans have validated the delayed-enhancement technique for the diagnosis of both acute and chronic myocardial infarction.[51,55–58] Klein and colleagues[56] reported that delayed-enhancement MR imaging can delineate the location and size of nonviable myocardium in close correlation with PET scanning. Moreover, delayed-enhancement MR imaging detected infarcted tissue with a greater sensitivity than that of PET, because of the higher spatial resolution of MR imaging. Other studies have confirmed the accuracy of delayed-enhancement MR imaging to detect and to identify location, size, and transmural

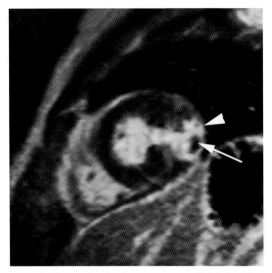

Fig. 6. Patient who had acute myocardial infarction. Short-axis view at midventricular level showing transmural hyperenhancement (*arrowhead*) of the posterolateral wall with a dark area (*arrow*) in the core corresponding to a no-reflow area. (*Reprinted from* Pujadas S, Reddy GP, Lee JJ, et al. Magnetic resonance imaging in ischemic heart disease. Semin Roentgenol 2003;38:320–9; with permission.)

extent of Q-wave and non–Q-wave myocardial infarction (see **Fig. 5**).[58]

The most important application of delayed-enhancement MR imaging for assessment of myocardial viability is the potential to predict functional recovery after revascularization with PTCA or CABG. In the seminal study on this topic, Kim and colleagues[59] showed that delayed-enhancement MR imaging could detect reversible myocardial dysfunction and suggest whether a coronary revascularization procedure would be effective in restoring function. Poor regional function did not improve in segments with substantial delayed enhancement, whereas there was functional recovery of dysfunctional myocardium that did not demonstrate delayed enhancement. Importantly, the transmural extent of delayed enhancement was an important factor in the prediction of recovery of regional function. If the transmural extent of delayed enhancement was more than 50%, the myocardium was unlikely to regain function after revascularization. But delayed enhancement involving less than 50% of the wall thickness was likely to improve function after a revascularization procedure. Knowledge of the transmural extent of viability can therefore improve accuracy in the prediction of functional recovery after revascularization (see **Fig. 2**).[60] A major advantage of MR imaging over PET is the superior spatial resolution of MR imaging, which can be used to distinguish transmural infarct from subendocardial infarct involving less than 50% of the wall thickness.

Imaging approach

To perform a delayed-enhancement sequence, gadolinium-chelate contrast medium is infused intravenously at a dose of 0.15 to 0.2 mmol/kg. The inversion recovery acquisition is obtained approximately 10 to 15 minutes later in the short-axis and long-axis planes. The TI is selected to null the signal in viable myocardium (typically 200–300 milliseconds), giving it a dark appearance. The greater the delay after contrast agent administration, the higher TI should be to null the viable myocardium. Myocardial perfusion or stress function sequences can be obtained and correlated with the viability images.

SUMMARY/KEY POINTS

- Although echocardiography remains the mainstay of imaging for patients who have known or suspected heart disease, MR imaging has become more frequently used in recent years and is now poised to become even more widespread.
- MR imaging is highly accurate for the assessment of myocardial perfusion, and can be used as an adjunct to stress perfusion scintigraphy.
- The accuracy of dobutamine stress function MR imaging is greater than that of stress echocardiography. Although dobutamine MR imaging has some limitations, it is a useful alternative study when stress echocardiography is suboptimal.
- MR viability imaging with the delayed-enhancement technique is useful for the accurate prediction of the recovery of regional function in ischemic myocardium. Its high spatial resolution gives it an advantage over PET scanning in the setting of subendocardial infarction. Viability MR imaging can be combined with perfusion or functional sequences to provide global, accurate evaluation of IHD.

REFERENCES

1. Murray CJ, Lopez AD. Alternative visions of the future: projecting mortality and disability, 1990–2020. Boston: Harvard University Press; 1996. p. 325–95.
2. Nesto RW, Kowalchuk GJ. The ischemic cascade: temporal sequence of hemodynamic, electrocardiographic and symptomatic expressions of ischemia. Am J Cardiol 1987;59:23C–30C.
3. Chan SY, Brunken RC, Czernin J, et al. Comparison of maximal myocardial blood flow during adenosine infusion with that of intravenous dipyridamole in normal men. J Am Coll Cardiol 1992;20:979–85.
4. Leong-Poi H, Rim SJ, Le DE, et al. Perfusion versus function: the ischemic cascade in demand ischemia: implications of single-vessel versus multivessel stenosis. Circulation 2002;105:987–92.
5. Muzik O, Duvernoy C, Beanlands RS, et al. Assessment of diagnostic performance of quantitative flow measurements in normal subjects and patients with angiographically documented coronary artery disease by means of nitrogen-13 ammonia and positron emission tomography. J Am Coll Cardiol 1998;31:534–40.
6. Maddahi J, Van Train K, Prigent F, et al. Quantitative single photon emission computed thallium-201 tomography for detection and localization of coronary artery disease: optimization and prospective validation of a new technique. J Am Coll Cardiol 1989;14:1689–99.
7. Tamaki N, Takahashi N, Kawamoto M, et al. Myocardial tomography using technetium-99m-tetrofosmin to evaluate coronary artery disease. J Nucl Med 1994;35:594–600.
8. Zaret BL, Rigo P, Wackers FJ, et al. Myocardial perfusion imaging with 99m-Tc tetrofosmin. Comparison to 201-Tl imaging and coronary angiography in a phase III multicenter trial. Circulation 1985;91:313–9.
9. Perault C, Loboguerrero A, Liehn JC, et al. Quantitative comparison of prone and supine myocardial SPECT MIBI images. Clin Nucl Med 1995;20:678–84.
10. Diesbourg LD, Prato FS, Wisenberg G, et al. Quantification of myocardial blood flow and extracellular volumes using a bolus injection of Gd-DTPA: kinetic modeling in canine ischemic disease. Magn Reson Med 1992;23:239–53.
11. Manning WJ, Atkinson DJ, Grossman W, et al. First-pass nuclear magnetic resonance imaging studies using gadolinium-DTPA in patients with coronary artery disease. J Am Coll Cardiol 1991;18:959–65.
12. Wendland MF, Saeed M, Masui T, et al. Echo-planar MR imaging of normal and ischemic myocardium with gadodiamide injection. Radiology 1993;186:535–42.
13. Edelman RR, Li W. Contrast-enhanced echo-planar MR imaging of myocardial perfusion: preliminary study in humans. Radiology 1994;190:771–7.
14. Wilke N, Jerosch-Herold M, Wang Y, et al. Myocardial perfusion reserve: assessment with multisection, quantitative, first-pass MR imaging. Radiology 1997;204:373–84.
15. Al-Saadi N, Nagel E, Gross M, et al. Noninvasive detection of myocardial ischemia from perfusion reserve based on cardiovascular magnetic resonance. Circulation 2000;101:1379–83.

16. Schwitter J, Nanz D, Kneifel S, et al. Assessment of myocardial perfusion in coronary artery disease by magnetic resonance: a comparison with positron emission tomography and coronary angiography. Circulation 2001;103:2230–5.

17. Plein S, Ryf S, Schwitter J, et al. Dynamic contrast-enhanced myocardial perfusion MRI accelerated with k-t sense. Magn Reson Med 2007;58:777–85.

18. Tong CY, Prato FS, Wisenberg G, et al. Techniques for the measurement of the local myocardial extraction efficiency for inert diffusible contrast agents such as gadopentate dimeglumine. Magn Reson Med 1993;30:332–6.

19. Pennell DJ, Underwood SR, Longmore DB. Detection of coronary artery disease using MR imaging with dipyridamole infusion. J Comput Assist Tomogr 1990;14:167–70.

20. Baer FM, Smolarz K, Jungehulsing M, et al. Feasibility of high dose dipyridamole-magnetic resonance imaging for detection of coronary artery disease and comparison with coronary angiography. Am J Cardiol 1992;69:51–6.

21. Baer FM, Smolarz K, Theissen P, et al. Identification of hemodynamically significant coronary stenoses by dipyridamole magnetic resonance imaging and 99mTc methoxyisobutyl-isonitrile SPECT. Int J Card Imaging 1993;9:133–45.

22. Nagel E, Lehmkuhl HB, Bocksch W, et al. Noninvasive diagnosis of ischemia-induced wall motion abnormalities with the use of high-dose dobutamine stress MRI: comparison with dobutamine stress echocardiography. Circulation 1999;99:763–70.

23. Hundley WG, Hamilton CA, Thomas MS, et al. Utility of fast cine magnetic resonance imaging and display for the detection of myocardial ischemia in patients not well suited for second harmonic stress echocardiography. Circulation 1999;100:1697–702.

24. Pennell DJ, Underwood SB, Manzara CC, et al. Magnetic resonance imaging during dobutamine stress in coronary artery disease. Am J Cardiol 1992;70:34–40.

25. van Rugge FP, Holman ER, van der Wall EE, et al. Quantification of global and regional left ventricular function by cine magnetic resonance imaging during dobutamine stress in normal human subjects. Eur Heart J 1993;14:456–63.

26. van Rugge FP, van der Wall EE, Spanjersberg SJ, et al. Magnetic resonance imaging during dobutamine stress for detection and localization of coronary artery disease. Quantitative wall motion analysis using a modification of the centerline method. Circulation 1994;90:127–38.

27. Baer FM, Voth E, Theissen P, et al. Gradient echo magnetic resonance imaging during incremental dobutamine infusion for the localization of coronary artery stenosis. Eur Heart J 1994;15:218–25.

28. Baer FM, Voth E, Theissen P, et al. Coronary artery disease: findings with GRE MR imaging and Tc-99mm-methosysobutyl-isonitrile SPECT during simultaneous dobutamine stress. Radiology 1994;193:203–9.

29. Nagel E, Lehmkuhl HB, Klein C, et al. Influence of image quality on the diagnostic accuracy of dobutamine stress magnetic resonance imaging in comparison with dobutamine stress echocardiography for the noninvasive detection of myocardial ischemia. Z Kardiol 1999;88:622–30.

30. Picano E, Mathias W, Pingitore A, et al. Safety and tolerability of dobutamine-atropine stress echocardiography: a prospective, multicenter study. Echo Dobutamine International Cooperative Study Group. Lancet 1994;344:1190–2.

31. Mertes H, Sawada RG, Ryan T, et al. Symptoms, adverse effects, and complications associated with dobutamine stress echocardiography. Experience in 1118 patients. Circulation 1993;88:15–9.

32. Pina IL, Balady GJ, Hanson P, et al. Guidelines for clinical exercise testing laboratories. Circulation 1995;91:912–21.

33. Harris PJ, Harrell FE, Lee KL, et al. Survival in medically treated coronary artery disease. Circulation 1979;60:1259–69.

34. Hammermeister KE, DeRouen TA, Dodge HT. Evidence from a nonrandomized study that coronary surgery prolongs survival in patients with two-vessel coronary disease. Circulation 1979;59:430–5.

35. Mock MB, Ringqvist I, Fisher LD, et al. Survival of medically treated patients in the coronary artery surgery study (CASS) registry. Circulation 1982;66:562–8.

36. Braunwald E, Rutherford JD. Reversible ischemic left ventricular dysfunction: evidence for the "hibernating myocardium." J Am Coll Cardiol 1986;8:1467–70.

37. Ragosta M, Beller GA, Watson DD, et al. Quantitative planar rest-redistribution 201Tl imaging in detection of myocardial viability and prediction of improvement in left ventricular function after coronary bypass surgery in patients with severely depressed left ventricular function. Circulation 1993;87:1630–41.

38. Elefteriades JA, Tolis G, Levi E, et al. Coronary artery bypass grafting in severe left ventricular dysfunction: excellent survival with improved ejection fraction and functional state. J Am Coll Cardiol 1993;22:1411–7.

39. Pagley PR, Beller GA, Watson DD, et al. Improved outcome after coronary bypass surgery in patients with ischemic cardiomyopathy and residual myocardial viability. Circulation 1997;96:793–800.

40. Chaudhry FA, Tauke JT, Alessandrini RS, et al. Prognostic implications of myocardial contractile reserve in patients with coronary artery disease and left

ventricular dysfunction. J Am Coll Cardiol 1999;34: 730–8.

41. Kannel WB, Sorlie P, McNamara PM. Prognosis after initial myocardial infarction: the Framingham study. Am J Cardiol 1979;44:53–9.

42. Nicod P, Gilpin E, Dittrich H, et al. Short- and long-term clinical outcome after Q wave and non-Q wave myocardial infarction in a large patient population. Circulation 1989;79:528–36.

43. Coll S, Castaner A, Sanz G, et al. Prevalence and prognosis after a first nontransmural myocardial infarction. Am J Cardiol 1983;51:1584–8.

44. Bax JJ, Wijns W, Cornel JH, et al. Accuracy of currently available techniques for prediction of functional recovery after revascularization in patients with left ventricular dysfunction due to chronic coronary artery disease: comparison of pooled data. J Am Coll Cardiol 1997;30:1451–60.

45. Rehr RB, Peshock RM, Malloy CR, et al. Improved in vivo magnetic resonance imaging of acute myocardial infarction after intravenous paramagnetic contrast agent administration. Am J Cardiol 1986; 57:864–8.

46. de Roos A, van Rossum AC, van der Wall E, et al. Reperfused and nonreperfused myocardial infarction: diagnostic potential of Gd-DTPA–enhanced MR imaging. Radiology 1989;172:717–20.

47. Saeed M, Wendland MF, Masui T, et al. Reperfused myocardial infarctions on T1- and susceptibility-enhanced MRI: evidence for loss of compartmentalization of contrast media. Magn Reson Med 1994; 31:31–9.

48. Schwitter J, Saeed M, Wendland MF, et al. Influence of severity of myocardial injury on distribution of macromolecules: extravascular versus intravascular gadolinium-based magnetic resonance contrast agents. J Am Coll Cardiol 1997;30:1086–94.

49. Kim RJ, Choi KM, Judd RM. Assessment of myocardial viability by contrast enhancement. In: Higgins CB, De Roos A, editors. Cardiovascular MRI and MRA. Philadelphia: Lippincott Williams & Wilkins; 2002. p. 209–37.

50. Kim RJ, Chen EL, Lima JA, et al. Myocardial Gd-DTPA kinetics determine MRI contrast enhancement and reflect the extent and severity of myocardial injury after acute reperfused infarction. Circulation 1996;94:3318–26.

51. Simonetti OP, Kim RJ, Fieno DS, et al. An improved MR imaging technique for the visualization of myocardial infarction. Radiology 2001;218:215–23.

52. Kim RJ, Fieno DS, Parrish TB, et al. Relationship of MRI delayed contrast enhancement to irreversible injury, infarct age, and contractile function. Circulation 1999;100:1992–2002.

53. Fieno DS, Kim RJ, Chen EL, et al. Contrast-enhanced magnetic resonance imaging of myocardium at risk: distinction between reversible and irreversible injury throughout infarct healing. J Am Coll Cardiol 2000;36:1985–91.

54. Hillenbrand HB, Kim RJ, Parker MA, et al. Early assessment of myocardial salvage by contrast-enhanced magnetic resonance imaging. Circulation 2000;102:1678–83.

55. Gerber BL, Rochitte CE, Bluemke DA, et al. Relationship between Gd-DTPA contrast enhancement and regional inotropic response in the periphery and center of myocardial infarction. Circulation 2001; 104:998–1004.

56. Klein C, Nekolla SG, Bengel FM, et al. Assessment of myocardial viability with contrast-enhanced magnetic resonance imaging. Comparison with positron emission tomography. Circulation 2002;105:162–7.

57. Mahrholdt H, Wagner A, Holly TA, et al. Reproducibility of chronic infarct size measurement by contrast-enhanced magnetic resonance imaging. Circulation 2002;106:2322–7.

58. Wu E, Judd RM, Vargas JD, et al. Visualisation of presence, location and transmural extent of healed Q-wave and non-Q-wave myocardial infarction. Lancet 2001;357:21–8.

59. Kim RJ, Wu E, Rafael A, et al. The use of contrast-enhanced magnetic resonance imaging to identify reversible myocardial dysfunction. N Engl J Med 2000;343:1445–53.

60. Choi KM, Kim RJ, Gubernikoff G, et al. Transmural extent of acute myocardial infarction predicts long-term improvement in contractile function. Circulation 2001;104:1101–7.

MR Imaging of the Thoracic Aorta

Derek G. Lohan, MD*, Mayil Krishnam, MD, Roya Saleh, MD, Anderanik Tomasian, MD, J. Paul Finn, MD

KEYWORDS

- Aorta • MR • Aortography • Dissection • Aortitis • Imaging

Contemporary vascular physicians practice in an environment very different from their predecessors', in which a wide spectrum of morphologic and functional imaging techniques is available. Echocardiography, transthoracic (TTE) or transesophageal (TEE); conventional catheter angiography; and multidetector CT (MDCT) until recently have been the cornerstones of thoracic aortic interrogation. The decision regarding optimal modality has rested on several key factors, including patient age and suspected pathology. Furthermore, 18-fluorodeoxyglucose positron emission tomography has been applied to aortic imaging, particularly in the presence of suspected inflammatory aortitis.[1]

Recently, however, dramatic advances have been realized in MR imaging and, in particular, magnetic resonance angiography (MRA), allowing for detailed and comprehensive large field-of-view (FOV) evaluation of the aorta and great vessels, without exposure to ionizing radiation or iodinated contrast agents. This article describes the current role of MR imaging in the assessment of the thoracic aorta, considers available imaging techniques, and illustrates the application of these techniques to a range of relevant pathologies.

MR IMAGING TECHNIQUES

A potentially confounding variety of MR techniques currently is available for the purpose of vascular interrogation. Many advanced practices are converging, however, toward a subset of techniques that are fast, reliable, and reproducible, including

- Spin-echo imaging, usually focused on the vessel wall and surrounding soft tissues and producing black-blood images of the patent lumen. These images contain little or no information about flow direction or pattern.
- Contrast-enhanced MRA (CE-MRA), highly time resolved or highly spatially resolved, which produces detailed images of 3-D or 4-D vascular lumen anatomy.
- Complementary techniques, which provide some information about flow and vascular anatomy, including steady-state free precession (SSFP) (in single-shot[2] and gated cine forms[3]), fat-suppressed gradient-echo imaging, and phase-contrast flow quantification.

Intuitively, it seems that a comprehensive examination of the thoracic aorta involves using at least two approaches. The following section discusses a variety of MR imaging techniques that the authors believe should be included in the armamentarium of diagnostic imagers for optimal vascular imaging.

Spin-Echo Techniques

Often referred to as "black-blood techniques" in relation to vascular imaging, because of the lack of signal seen in flowing blood, spin-echo (SE) techniques allow depiction of the vessel wall while highlighting contrast between mural morphology and the luminal signal-void.[4] ECG gating usually is used. Currently, most implementations of SE imaging use echo-trains for fast acquisition, usually in a breath-hold.[5]

Conventional spin echo

Using repetition times (TR) governed by the R-R interval, conventional SE can be used to image the thoracic aorta with modest T1 weighting. This

Department of Radiology, David Geffen School of Medicine at the University of California, 10945 Le Conte Avenue, Suite 3371, Peter V. Ueberroth Building, Los Angeles, CA 90095 7206, USA
* Corresponding author.
E-mail address: derek.lohan@gmail.com (D.G. Lohan).

Magn Reson Imaging Clin N Am 16 (2008) 213–234
doi:10.1016/j.mric.2008.02.016
1064-9689/08/$ – see front matter © 2008 Elsevier Inc. All rights reserved.

mri.theclinics.com

may be useful in the presence of suspected mural pathology, such as intimal flaps, plaque ulceration, or intramural hematoma. As individual sections are obtained at various intervals of the cardiac cycle during conventional multislice SE imaging, however, the effects of flow can be confounding. Slow flow during diastole, within aortic aneurysms, or the false lumen of a dissection and entry or exit slice phenomena may give rise to intermittent artifactual high intraluminal signal.[6] SE techniques should be interpreted with caution when signal is seen within the vascular lumen and correlation should be performed with more predictable techniques, such as CE-MRA or SSFP imaging.

Spin-echo train imaging

Offering the advantages of rapid data acquisition and improved image resolution, SE train techniques represent an improvement over conventional SE for vascular imaging. These often use double inversion pulses to null the blood signal.[7,8] The first of these 180° RF pulses is nonslice selective, which is followed by a slice-selective "reversion" radiofrequency (RF) pulse, which restores signal to the section being imaged, into which the nulled blood flows at time TI (**Fig. 1**).

An extreme version of SE train imaging is half-Fourier single-shot turbo spin-echo (HASTE), a T2-weighted, rapid technique in which the data for a complete image are acquired within a single heartbeat.[9,10] This approach has advantages in patients in whom breath-holding poses a problem for alternative imaging sequences. In many cases, SE imaging of the aorta can be limited to black-blood HASTE, combined with some of the following techniques.

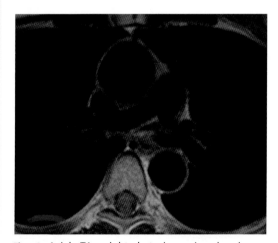

Fig. 1. Axial T1-weighted turbo spin-echo image through the upper mediastinum. There is homogeneous suppression of intraluminal signal (black-blood technique), increasing the conspicuity of the aortic wall.

Gradient-Recalled Echo Techniques

Fat-saturated postcontrast T1-weighted spoiled gradient-echo (SPGR) imaging, in 2-D or 3-D implementations, allows evaluation of the aortic wall in a variety of clinical scenarios, such as suspected inflammatory aortitis or dissection.[11,12] When preceded by precontrast SPGR imaging, T1 hyperintensity may be evident with intramural hematoma. The extent of mural enhancement in the presence of inflammation can be assessed on postcontrast images (**Fig. 2**).[13] This approach combines excellent spatial and contrast resolution with rapid data acquisition, such that entire thoracic coverage may be achieved during a single breath-hold.

Steady-State Free Precession Techniques

SSFP is a steady-state gradient-echo technique that exploits the coherent transverse magnetization remaining when the TR used is shorter than the T1 and T2 of the tissue. Signal on SSFP is dependent on the T2/T1 ratio, rather than on blood flow. Providing rapid bright-blood images with high-contrast resolution, SSFP techniques allow complete thoracic evaluation within seconds, facilitating diagnostic image quality even when breath-holding is suboptimal.[14] SSFP, however, is sensitive to off-resonance artifacts, which may manifest as dark bands or hyperintense foci and must be interpreted in context. Off-resonance effects with SSFP are more problematic at 3 tesla.[15]

3-D versions of SSFP recently have been applied to aortic and coronary arterial imaging in breath-hold[16] and free-breathing formats (**Fig. 3**).[17] The use of navigator gating makes free-breathing SSFP an alternative to CE-MRA, although at present this approach is limited by long data acquisition times in patients who have erratic respiratory patterns or irregular cardiac rhythms.

Phase-Contrast Flow Mapping

Application of bipolar velocity-encoding gradient pulses to flowing spins results in a phase shift of these spins, which is proportional to the velocity at which they are traveling in the direction of the gradient.[18] Conversely, stationary tissues undergo zero net phase shift change and thus have zero phase. As phase can have values only between +180° and −180°, the positive or negative halves of this spectrum are assigned to flow in one direction, whereas the remaining half denotes flow in the opposing direction. The flow sensitivity of the gradient pulses is defined by the velocity-encoding value (VENC), which is the velocity that

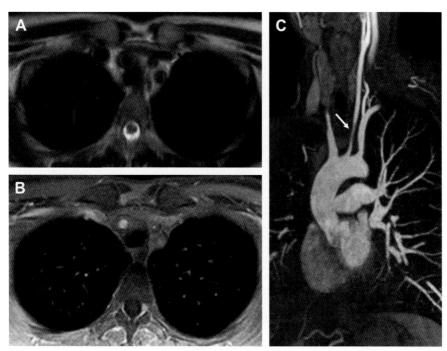

Fig. 2. A 42-year-old woman who had Takayasu's arteritis, currently on medical treatment. Pre- (*A*) and postcontrast (*B*) axial GRE acquisitions through the supra-aortic vessels shows circumferential thickening of the innominate, left common carotid, and left subclavian artery walls, without mural enhancement. Corresponding luminal compromise is seen on sagittal oblique CE-MRA MIP reconstruction (*C*), the greatest degree of stenosis occurring in the left common carotid artery (*arrow*).

produces exactly 180° of phase shift. Depending on the flow present within a vessel, the flow sensitivity may be erroneously chosen such that phase exceeds 180° phase shift, mimicking (incrementally) fast flow in the opposite direction, slow flow in the opposite direction, or slow flow in the same direction. For normal aortic flow, a VENC of 150 cm per second is appropriate, but if higher velocities are anticipated (as in aortic stenosis), values of 250 cm per second or more should be used (**Fig. 4**).

Accurate flow quantification using phase-contrast flow mapping requires that several criteria are fulfilled, including stable hardware with minimization or control of eddy currents. Also, the orientation of the imaging plane should be perpendicular to the vessel in question for through-plane flow, the VENC should be appropriate, reliable ECG gating should be used, and care should be taken in regions prone to susceptibility artifact (such as adjacent to metallic prostheses or air-filled structures, such as the lungs or paranasal sinuses). Provided all these criteria are fulfilled, phase-contrast flow mapping allows derivation of several accurate flow parameters, including time-flow and time-velocity curves. Although extensively and successfully applied in a 2-D capacity

in past years, more recently this technique has been adapted to allow 3-D flow depiction, facilitating a more comprehensive assessment of global and local blood-flow characteristics.[19,20]

Cardiac-Gated Cine Imaging

Although in the past, spoiled fast low-angle shot (FLASH) sequences commonly were used for the purpose of cardiac and aortic cine imaging,[20] more recently steady-state techniques (SSFP) have become the cornerstone of such imaging, offering the advantages of higher SNR, shorter imaging duration, and freedom from the reliance on inflow effects for signal generation (**Fig. 5**).[3] This ECG-gated, k-space segmented pulse sequence has benefited from the application of parallel imaging techniques, allowing high temporal resolution, large FOV imaging of the thoracic aorta, and left ventricular outflow during acceptable breath-holds as low as 5 to 6 seconds. The inherently high blood tissue contrast achieved using SSFP imaging repeatedly is shown to aid evaluation of aortic mural and valvular characteristics, allowing exclusion of the presence of aortic dissection, for example, with a high level of diagnostic confidence.[21,22] A candy cane sagittal

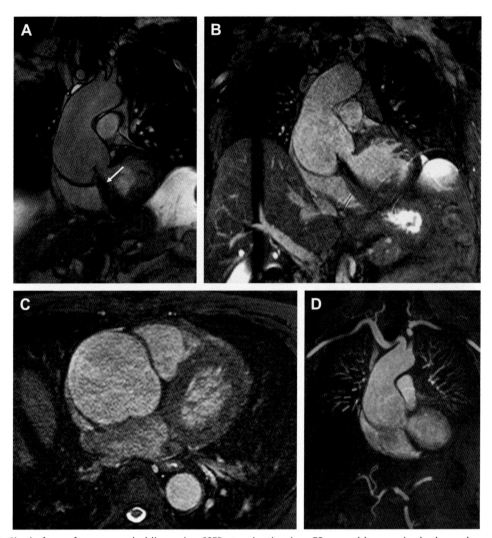

Fig. 3. Single frame from coronal oblique cine-SSFP examination in a 53-year-old man who had annular ectasia (*A*). Noted is the presence of fusiform aortic root dilatation and secondary aortic valvular regurgitation (*arrow*). The morphologic root dilatation and functional valvular insufficiency are evident on coronal 3-D free-breathing SSFP (*B*). Given the 3-D nature of this free-breathing sequence, multiplanar reconstruction is then possible in any desired plane, as shown in (*C*). As this approach is respiratory and cardiac-gated, the aortic annulus and sinuses are seen to greater effect than on the corresponding non–ECG-gated CE-MRA reconstruction (*D*).

oblique view, oriented along the plane of the ascending and descending aortas, is of particular usefulness in such aortic evaluation. Furthermore, this approach allows concurrent assessment of the effect of such pathology on the aortic root and valve complex, of paramount importance in the case of ascending aortic pathology.[23]

Time-Resolved Magnetic Resonance Angiography

Time-resolved MRA (TR-MRA) represents a powerful complement to conventional 3-D CE-MRA, allowing dynamic evaluation of circulatory patency,

confident separation of the arterial and venous phases of luminal enhancement by a compact bolus of gadolinium (Gd) contrast, and facilitation of qualitative and quantitative measures of parenchymal perfusion, such as time-to-peak signal intensity, maximal upslope of the curve, maximal signal intensity, and mean transit time.[24] This technique generates rapid sequential T1-weighted imaging using a 3-D SPGR sequence with ultrashort TR (<2 ms) and echo times (TE) (<1 ms).[25] The use of parallel imaging and temporal echo sharing has improved the performance of TR-MRA.[26] TR-MRA may be of particular value in the evaluation of inhomogeneous aortic flow and dissections, where

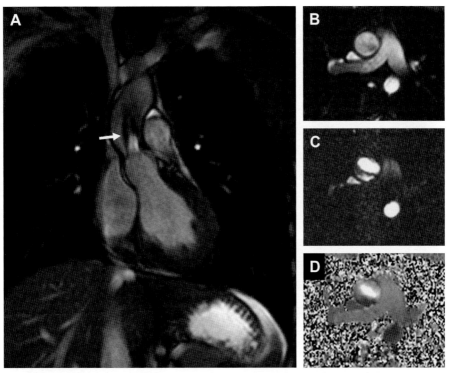

Fig. 4. Williams syndrome and supravalvular aortic stenosis. A flame-shaped area of signal dephasing results from turbulence beyond the affected level in *A (arrow)*. *(B–D)* Magnitude and phase-sensitive images at the level of the stenosis. An elevated peak velocity of 281 cm/s was confirmed on flow quantification.

opacification of multiple phases of enhancement of true and false lumens, respectively, may be beyond the scope of conventional CE-MRA (**Fig. 6**).[27] An alternative approach to TR-MRA involves the use of highly undersampled radial or spherical k-space trajectories where the center of k-space is sampled frequently and the periphery is undersampled. Full k-space 3-D images are calculated with a moving temporal window and data sharing. These approaches are intriguing but require intensive data manipulation before image calculation and are sensitive to off-resonance artifacts.

Contrast-Enhanced Magnetic Resonance Angiography

Many of the most significant advances in vascular MR imaging have involved CE- MRA. This technique exploits the T1-shortening effect of Gd with marked increase of intraluminal signal intensity during the first pass of the contrast bolus. CE-MRA also has benefited significantly from the introduction of parallel imaging techniques and concomitant advances in radiofrequency technology.[28] Although invoking a penalty with regard to SNR, a compromise that may be mitigated by imaging at 3 tesla, the benefits of parallel acquisition

outweigh its disadvantages. CE-MRA with parallel imaging can be used to increase speed, coverage and spatial resolution in any combination.[29]

As is the case with TR-MRA, conventional CE-MRA involves the application of a 3-D SPGR sequence with ultrashort TR and TE. Again, the TR is maintained as low as is practicable, such that k-space filling may be achieved during first-pass passage of the Gd bolus (**Fig. 7**).

Imaging Planes

Comprehensive thoracic aortic evaluation necessitates that images are acquired in several complementary planes, such that the entire hairpin course is fully evaluated. Direct coronal and sagittal images may address the shortcomings of true axial views to a limited extent; however, a sagittal oblique, left anterior oblique candy cane view, traversing the planes of the ascending, transverse, and descending aorta, is recommended such that subtle abnormalities of the arch may be confidently excluded (**Fig. 8**). This imaging plane also is of considerable benefit in demonstrating the extent intimal dissection flaps and their relationship to the origins of the supra-aortic branch vessels. Ectasia, resulting from long-standing hypertension, atherosclerosis, or advanced patient

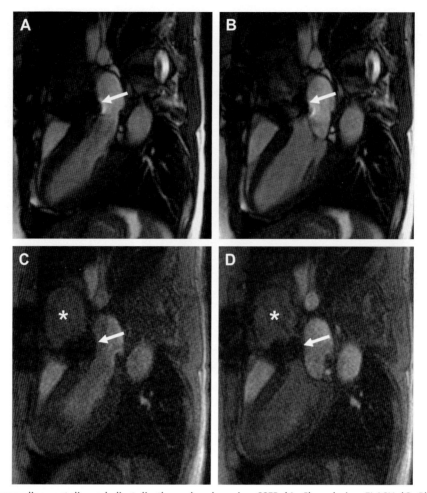

Fig. 5. Corresponding systolic and diastolic three-chamber cine SSFP (*A*, *B*) and cine FLASH (*C*, *D*) images in a 52-year-old female patient who had aortic valve prosthesis (*arrows*). Although FLASH images are of lower spatial and contrast resolution than the SSFP acquisitions, note that magnetic susceptibility has less detrimental effect on image quality with the former, where visualization of the ascending aorta (*) remains possible.

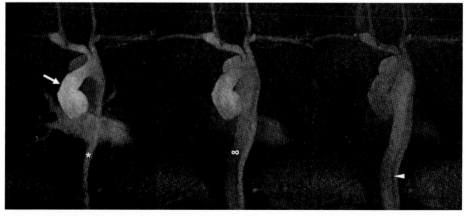

Fig. 6. Sequential TR-MRA images from 49-year-old man who had previous type A aortic dissection and subsequent aortic root graft replacement (*arrow*). An intimal flap remains (*arrowhead*). There is rapid opacification of the true lumen (*) with respect to the false lumen (∞).

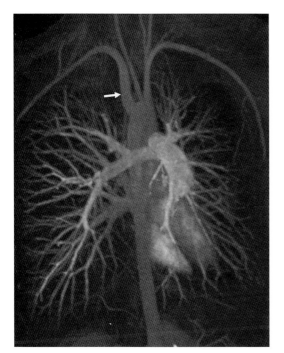

Fig. 7. Frontal full-thickness subtracted MIP image from CE-MRA examination in a 27-year-old man who had aberrant origin of the right subclavian artery (*arrow*), arising separate and distal to the other supra-aortic branch vessels.

age, may render selection of a single sagittal oblique plane, on which the entire thoracic aorta is included, impossible, necessitating piecemeal aortic evaluation on successive images.

In the presence of aortic dissection or aneurysmal dilatation, particularly when involving the ascending portion of the thoracic aorta, cine imaging of the left ventricular outflow tract represents an essential component to the evaluation of the effect of such pathology on ventricular function. Although complementary cardiac functional evaluation, including the right heart and cardiac valves, is necessary only for those who have concomitant heart disease, the authors normally perform cine imaging of the aortic valve, in transverse and vertical long-axis projections, with phase-contrast flow-quantification immediately above the valvular level to quantify the degree of aortic regurgitation/stenosis, when detected.

SPECIFIC PATHOLOGY
Aortic Dissection and Intramural Hematoma

Aortic dissection is a life-threatening condition resulting from disruption of the intimal layer of the aorta, with propagation of a false passage located within the media, and elevation of an intimal flap.[30] The DeBakey[31] and Stanford[32] classifications have become synonymous with this condition, reflecting the therapeutic and prognostic differences between dissections involving the ascending aorta (DeBakey types I and II and Stanford type A) and those sparing this vascular segment (DeBakey Type III and Stanford Type B). The significance of such ascending aortic involvement rests in its potential for proximal migration of the dissection flap to involve the coronary arterial

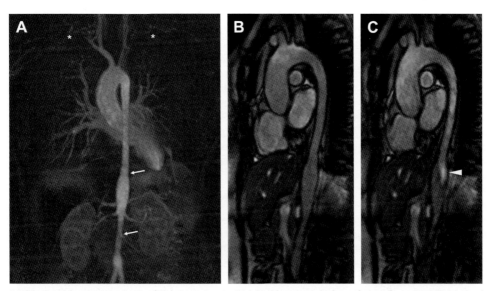

Fig. 8. A 37-year-old woman who had Takayasu's arteritis. Single arterial phase frame from TR-MRA examination (*A*) shows distal thoracic and abdominal aortic luminal stenosis (*arrows*). Also noted are bilateral subclavian artery occlusions (*). Diastolic (*B*) and systolic (*C*) candy cane SSFP cine views show the presence of hemodynamic turbulence at the level of the proximal aortic stenosis (*arrowhead*).

ostia or aortic valve, with potentially catastrophic consequences.

Intramural hematoma represents thrombus within the medial layer of the aorta with an intact intima. Spontaneous rupture of the vasa vasorum of the aortic media is considered an initiating process. Often discussed separately, aortic dissection and intramural hematoma may be considered as variants of the same spectrum, thus are considered in unison here. The MR imaging techniques (described previously) allow comprehensive evaluation of the thoracic aorta in the presence of suspected dissection or intramural hematoma, facilitating confident diagnosis, staging, and follow-up.

SE techniques display the morphology of intimal dissection flaps and may show fenestrations when present. Furthermore, para-aortic hematoma and hemopericardium may be depicted using these techniques. This approach, however, may fail to differentiate blood within the false lumen from intramural thrombus because of spurious high intraluminal signal intensity from slow-flowing blood, thus should be used as a complement to the other MR imaging techniques.[33]

Precontrast T1-weighted gradient-recalled echo (GRE) sequences allow evaluation of the thoracic aortic wall for crescentic high mural signal intensity, consistent with recent intramural thrombus or thrombosis of the false lumen. Complementary postcontrast GRE imaging confirms luminal enhancement, thus differentiating high signal on SE images resulting from slow flow from that relating to intramural thrombus (Fig. 9).[34] Furthermore, the presence of mural enhancement on postcontrast GRE acquisitions may provide evidence as to possible etiology, suggesting the presence of an inflammatory aortitis.[35]

2-D SSFP techniques allow rapid anatomic coverage while exploiting the high inherent T2/T1 ratio of blood, allowing evaluation of the location and extent of an intimal dissection flap, even in the absence of patient respiratory suspension. This is of particular value in this critically ill patient population, many of whom are in considerable physical and emotional distress and unable to cooperate with breath-holding, unless endotracheal intubation is performed.[21]

ECG-gated, respiratory-navigated 3-D SSFP MRA, although time-consuming, allows further characterization of the extent of intimal dissection, with the added advantage of freedom from cardiac pulsation artifact in the region of the aortic root, allowing determination of the proximity of the intimal entry point to the coronary ostia.

Cine SSFP allows evaluation of the effect of dissection on the aortic valve, including the presence of resultant valvular regurgitation evidenced by proximal signal dephasing.[36] Further foci of dephasing may be detected at the locations of dissection entry or re-entry sites.[37] This technique also may be used as an adjunct to SE techniques (described previously) in the differentiation of high signal relating to slow luminal flow from that of luminal thrombosis.

Phase-contrast flow quantification of aortic dissection or intramural hematoma can be used for follow-up of serial patient studies. This velocity-encoded approach allows quantification of the relative blood flow within the true and false lumens (Fig. 10)[38] and confirmation of the presence and degree of flow within the supra-aortic branch vessels (thus calculation of cerebral blood flow). Furthermore, evaluation at the level of the aortic valve enables measurement of the severity of aortic regurgitation, a parameter, which, if determined as increasing on serial examinations, may prompt surgical intervention.

TR-MRA allows demonstration of the dynamics of true and false luminal enhancement in the presence of aortic dissection, information that may only be presumed from multiphase high-resolution 3-D CE-MRA. In so doing, TR-MRA allows confirmation of the patency of both lumens and determination of the location of dissection entry and exit points, providing a surrogate to visceral perfusion when the dissection flap traverses vital arterial origins (eg, hepatic or renal artery ostia).

3-D high-resolution CE-MRA recently has become the gold standard technique for the display of thoracic aortic dissection. Allowing multiplanar reconstruction in any desired plane and the opportunity for data post processing, including maximum intensity projection (MIP) display or volume rendering, CE-MRA enables wide FOV simultaneous depiction of the extent and location of the intimal flap and relationship to and patency of vital aortic branch vessels, pre- and postoperatively.[39] CE-MRA, however, sometimes may provide suboptimal definition of the ascending aorta resulting from pulsation, and gated cine always should be performed in suspected dissection.

Penetrating Atheromatous Ulceration

Penetrating atheromatous ulceration tends to occur in elderly individuals who have extensive atherosclerotic plaque load, in whom plaque ulceration results in luminal extension into the aortic media. Such ulceration may act as a prelude to aortic dissection or intramural hematoma. The imaging features of penetrating ulceration are similar to those of each of these potential complications, with morphologic characterization of the

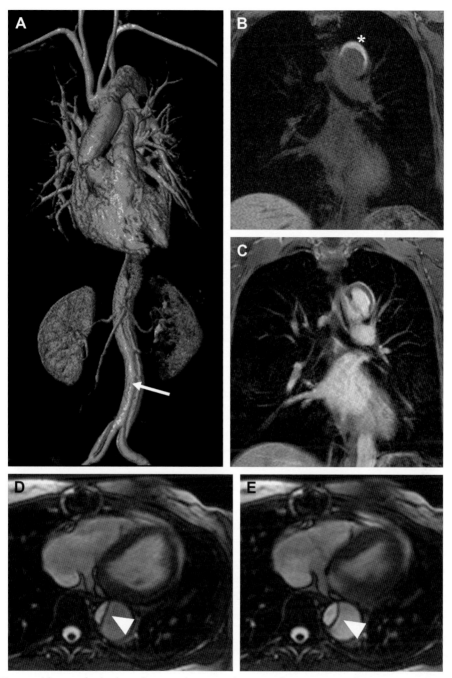

Fig. 9. A 61-year-old man who had previous aortic root replacement for treatment of type A aortic dissection. Volume-rendered full-thickness MIP from CE-MRA (A) shows a residual intimal flap (*arrow*) extending throughout the course of the abdominal aorta and into the right common iliac artery. There is crescentic mural T1 hyperintensity on unenhanced gradient-echo imaging (B), consistent with thrombus within the false lumen (*). This thrombus is hypointense to perfused lumen on postcontrast gradient-echo acquisitions (C). Four-chamber cine SSFP during diastole (D) and systole (E) allows visualization of the degree of flap motion throughout the cardiac cycle (*arrowheads*).

ulceration performed best using T1 SE techniques. Typical appearances include the presence of an ulcerated mural crater, often with adjacent intermediate or high signal intensity on T1 and T2 SE resulting from the presence of a rim of methemoglobin within the involved media.[40] This differs from simple irregular mural atherosclerotic plaque, which is of low signal intensity on both SE

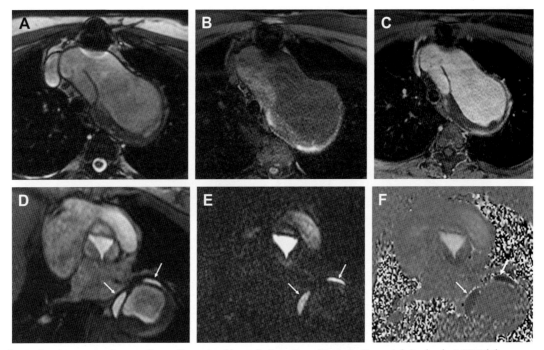

Fig. 10. Previous ascending aortic graft repair of type A dissection. Comparative axial single-shot SSFP (*A*), precontrast T1 fat-saturated gradient-echo (*B*) and postcontrast T1 fat-saturated gradient-echo images (*C*) show a residual dissection flap with T1-hyperintense mural thrombus within the false lumen. Phase-contrast flow quantification at the level of the trileaflet aortic valve (*D–F*) show the presence of two distinct true lumens (*arrows*), which may be quantitatively assessed for their relative contributions to the systemic circulation.

sequences. GRE techniques, particularly when fat saturated and T1 weighted, show similar increased medial signal and rarely provide additional information to that gained using SE sequences.[13]

2D SSFP, although demonstrating the plaque ulceration, may provide little differentiation between this entity and that of simple plaque irregularity and should not be used alone in this capacity. Similarly, 3-D SSFP, TR-MRA, and CE-MRA may allow eloquent depiction of the luminal outpouching at the location of the plaque ulceration, although in the presence of considerable atherosclerotic plaque burden may be of little advantage in the differentiation of true medial ulceration from pseudoulceration, resulting from the approximation of two large focal areas of mural plaque.

Aortic Aneurysms

Aneurysmal dilatation of the thoracic aorta is commonplace, occurring most often as a result of atherosclerosis, and in the presence of hypertension. Less frequently, this entity may be the result of trauma, cystic medial necrosis, connective tissue disorders (including Ehlers-Danlos and Marfan syndromes), inflammatory vasculitis (eg,

Takayasu's arteritis), and infections (such as syphilis). MR imaging is extremely well suited to the evaluation of the thoracic aortic aneurysms.

Black-blood imaging of thoracic aortic aneurysms allows visualization of the involved aortic wall, thus facilitating accurate luminal and wall-to-wall diameter measurement. Furthermore, mural depiction allows evaluation of the extent of coexistent atheroma and confident exclusion of the presence of associated dissection, ulcerated plaque or intramural hematoma, indicating instability.[41]

Pre- and postcontrast fat-saturated T1-weighted GRE acquisitions may be complementary to SE techniques in the exclusion of lesions indicative of aortic mural instability. Furthermore, GRE imaging should be considered in any patients in whom atypical features are present (eg, young or middle-aged patients or those who have saccular rather than fusiform aneurysm, absence of significant atherosclerotic changes, or personal or family history of connective tissue disease), such that dedicated evaluation of mural enhancement, suggesting inflammation, may be performed.[42]

As is the case in the presence of suspected aortic dissection, 2-D and 3-D ECG- and navigator-gated SSFP acquisitions allow detailed anatomic evaluation of thoracic aortic aneurysms, facilitating derivation of diameter measurements. The 3-D approach, although time-consuming, is preferred in the presence of ascending aortic ectasia or aneurysm, allowing evaluation of the Valsalva sinuses and involvement of the coronary ostia, not otherwise achievable with standard 3-D high-resolution CE-MRA. As a result, multiplanar reconstruction of the 3-D dataset may be used to allow true transverse diameter measurements, avoiding the tendency for overestimation of this dimension when derived from transverse axial sections and a reflection of the obliquity of the aortic root.

Cine SSFP imaging may provide key additional information with regard to aortic morphologic characteristics in the presence of a thoracic aneurysm, representing an indicator of aortic mural pulsatility[43] and allowing demonstration of focal high-velocity jets of blood flow, from which aortic ectasia and dilatation may result. Furthermore, the presence of causative valvular stenosis or secondary regurgitation readily may be excluded or evaluated within two to three comfortable breath-holds, providing complementary data to that already obtained with standard morphologic (SE and GRE) techniques.[44]

Phase-contrast techniques allow further quantification of the degree of stenosis or valvular insufficiency detected on cine SSFP imaging. Furthermore, even in the absence of focal stenosis, flow quantification proximal to the aneurysmal segment allows determination of the peak blood velocity entering the aneurysm, thus information regarding potential etiologic factors in the development of this dilatation (**Fig. 11**).[45]

Although inferior to respiratory-navigated 3-D SSFP with regard to imaging of the aortic sinuses and coronary ostia because of the associated absence of ECG gating and potential for respiratory motion, 3-D CE-MRA represents the technique used most commonly for evaluation of thoracic aortic aneurysmal dilatation, allowing comprehensive, detailed imaging within a single breath-hold.[46] CE-MRA now routinely involves exploitation of parallel imaging techniques, such that complete k-space filling during the limited duration allowed by the first pass of the contrast bolus is entirely feasible.[47] Homogeneous opacification of the aortic lumen results, and when imaged at high resolution, provides a comprehensive dataset from which detailed, accurate reconstructions may be derived. It is for this reason that CE-MRA has emerged as the cornerstone of vascular imaging, illustrating the location, extent, morphology, and true dimensions of an aneurysm in any desired plane, irrespective of associated tortuosity.

Aortic Stenosis

Hemodynamically significant stenosis of the thoracic aorta in adults is a rare entity, occurring most often as a result of trauma and on occasion secondary to atherosclerosis or stenosing vasculitis (eg, Takayasu's arteritis). This is seen more often in the pediatric population in the setting of aortic coarctation (discussed later). Irrespective of patient age or underlying etiology, MR imaging is the ideal imaging technique for comprehensive aortic evaluation in the presence of such luminal stenosis, allowing one-stop accurate morphologic and dynamic flow assessment, including simultaneous demonstration of relevant collateral pathways.[48] Each of the imaging techniques discussed previously with respect to aortic aneurysms is equally applicable in the presence of stenosis. Two approaches hold particular value, however, in the evaluation of suspected or known luminal stenosis, namely TR-MRA and phase-contrast flow techniques.

Although the location and caliber of collateral vessels, most often the intercostal and internal mammary vessels, is best depicted with high-resolution CE-MRA, TR-MRA is capable of providing complementary information in the form of dynamic illustration of the direction and temporal attributes of collateral filling.[49] This information may be assumed only from static CE-MRA acquisitions on the basis of collateral location and size.

Phase-contrast velocity-encoded techniques also represent a useful accompaniment to CE-MRA, facilitating multilevel flow quantification proximal and distal to a stenosis, thus derivation of surrogates of pressure gradient, including peak velocity and velocity gradient. Furthermore, this approach allows objective quantification of the degree of collateral circulation, a key factor when intervention is considered.[50]

Valvular Stenosis/Insufficiency

Whether or not a result of inherent cusp pathology or annular distension, aortic valvulopathy drives a significant proportion of decisions regarding surgical intervention. In the presence of ascending aortic ectasia, although luminal diameter and degree of progressive aortic dilatation are key, the development of secondary valvular insufficiency often expedites graft repair, regurgitation heralding the future development of left heart failure.[51]

Cine SSFP imaging represents the cornerstone technique for valvular assessment with MR imaging, allowing concomitant evaluation of cusp morphology, orifice cross-sectional area, and presence of mixed stenosis/regurgitation. High

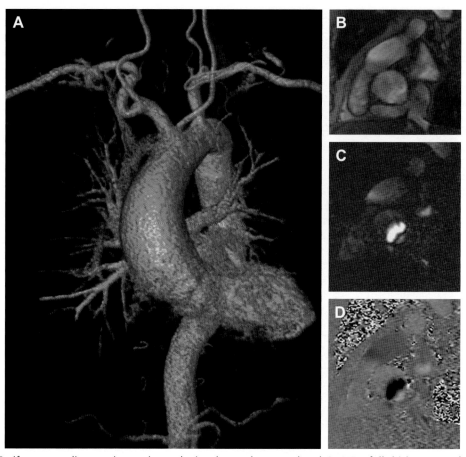

Fig. 11. Fusiform ascending aortic ectasia, as depicted on volume-rendered CE-MRA full-thickness MIP (*A*). Flow quantification at the level of the aortic valve (*B–D*) shows the characteristic fish-mouth appearance of bicuspid aortic valve, a common accompaniment of aortic ectasia and aneurysm.

degrees of valvular stenosis are typified by the presence of an antegrade flame-shaped zone of signal loss on left ventricular outflow SSFP imaging, a result of spin dephasing occurring secondary to disruption of laminar flow (**Fig. 12**).

Phase-contrast flow quantification of valvular stenosis facilitates objective determination of several key flow parameters, most notably peak velocity, a surrogate of stenosis severity. In the presence of such elevated peak velocities, choice of a large VENC is appropriate so that aliasing is avoided.

3-D CE-MRA also is of value in determination of aortic ectasia or aneurysmal dilatation, a not uncommon accompaniment of valvular stenosis.

Aortitis

Inflammatory vasculitis of the thoracic aorta and its supra-aortic branch vessels may occur as a result of many conditions, including Takayasu's arteritis, giant cell arteritis, polyarteritis nodosa,

or syphilitic arteritis. Although certain patterns of vascular involvement may suggest a likely cause (eg, bilateral smooth subclavian artery stenoses in the case of giant cell arteritis), differentiation between these entities may not be radiologically possible, depending instead on histopathologic and serologic investigations for accurate classification. MR imaging does, however, play a key role in the investigation and follow-up of this condition, not least so in the differentiation of active vascular mural inflammation from quiescent residual postinflammatory mural thickening.[52] Furthermore, the versatility of this technique in the detection and characterization of many of the potential complications of aortitis, including aneurysmal dilatation, valvular insufficiency, dissection, intramural hemorrhage, and luminal occlusion, cannot be overlooked.

Postcontrast fat-saturated T1-weighted SE or GRE sequences represent the cornerstone of inflammatory evaluation, allowing rapid large-volume multiplanar coverage of large anatomic

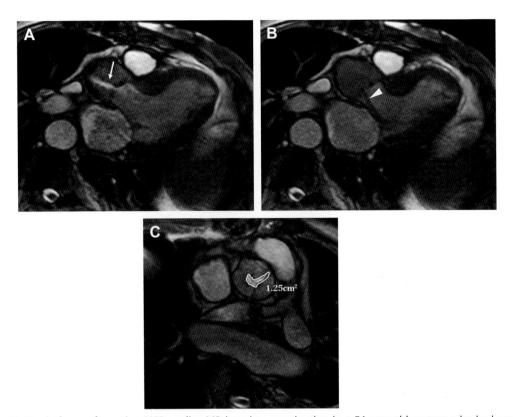

Fig. 12. Single frames from cine SSFP cardiac MR imaging examination in a 54-year-old woman who had severe aortic stenosis. Three-chamber (inflow-outflow view) during systole (*A*) shows flame-shaped area of signal dephasing due to flow acceleration through the stenotic valve level (*arrow*). During diastole (*B*), valvular insufficiency also is identified (*arrowhead*). Transverse image through the aortic valve during peak-systole allows confirmation of the presence of a trileaflet aortic valve and derivation of orifice planimetry (*white margin* in *C*). The calculated value (1.25 cm²) equates with severe aortic stenosis (*C*).

areas for the presence of vascular mural enhancement (**Fig. 13**). Detection of such enhancement allows differentiation between foci of active inflammation and similar regions of inactive postinflammatory thickening. On successful implementation of appropriate medical therapy, a decrease in the degree of enhancement and on occasion resolution of mural thickening may be observed.[53] The specificity of mural enhancement is poor, however, as similar vascular enhancement may occur in the presence of inflammatory atherosclerotic plaque.[54] Discrimination may be hampered by the not infrequent coexistence of these entities.

High-resolution CE-MRA is an essential complement to postcontrast SE or GRE imaging, permitting confirmation of luminal patency over a large FOV. Where clinically indicated, whole-body MRA may be performed using, for example, a double-injection, four-station protocol, as used in the authors' institute (described elsewhere).[55] Acting in its capacity as an overview to vascular patency, subtle mural thickening occurring as a result of aortitis may be appreciated readily on CE-MRA,

a reflection of the high-resolution and near-isotropic voxel acquisition attainable using this technique, and should prompt careful assessment of these regions for the presence of mural enhancement. Such focal mural interrogation optimally is performed on imaging obtained perpendicular to the plane of the vessel in question.

Trauma

Although intimal dissection, intramural hematoma, and subsequent pseudoaneurysm formation may result from blunt thoracic trauma, the most feared complication of such injury is aortic rupture (**Fig. 14**). This life-threatening condition occurs most often immediately distal to the aortic isthmus in the setting of rapid deceleration, where shearing forces are exerted at the junction of the relatively fixed insertion of the ligamentum arteriosum and freely mobile proximal descending thoracic aorta[56] and is invariably associated with para-aortic hematoma. Although MDCT generally is preferred in the acute setting owing to patient

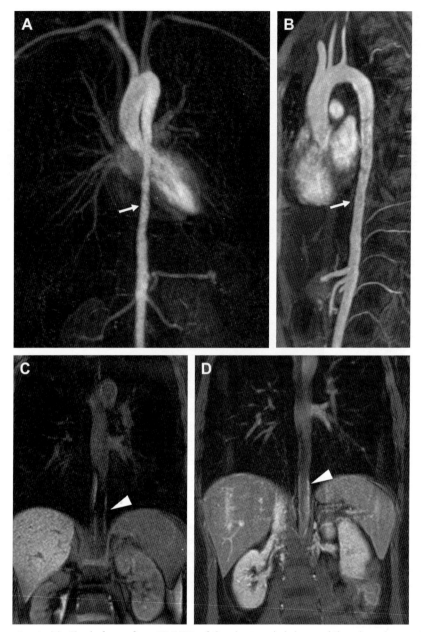

Fig.13. Takayasu's arteritis. Single frame from TR-MRA of the chest and abdomen (*A*) and candy cane CE-MRA MIP reconstruction (*B*) show the presence of luminal irregularity and narrowing at the phrenic level (*arrows*). Precontrast coronal T1 GRE shows corresponding aortic mural thickening (*arrowhead*) (*C*). Administration of Gd contrast agent results in diffuse mural enhancement in the region of abnormal thickening (*arrowhead*) (*D*), consistent with active inflammation (aortitis).

hemodynamic instability, short examination times, and availability, recent advances in MR imaging hardware and software, in particular parallel imaging techniques, have reduced MR imaging scan times considerably, particularly if a targeted approach is adopted.[28] Additionally, this modality is of proved benefit in characterization of the location and extent of injury in patients who are clinically stable.[57]

In addition to standard axial cross-sectional imaging, candy cane sagittal oblique SE imaging is recommended in all cases of suspected aortic rupture for complete evaluation of the aortic isthmus. Although subacute hematoma is characteristically of high signal intensity on T1-weighted imaging, in the hyperacute and acute setting the appearances of para-aortic hematoma may be heterogeneous and complex, comprising hypointense oxy-, and

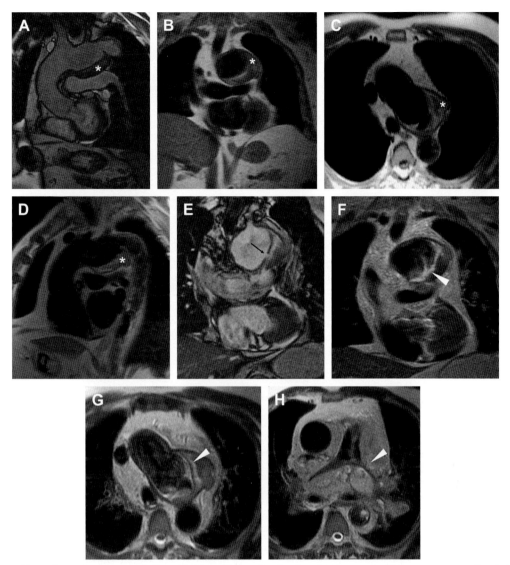

Fig. 14. Thoracic aortic aneurysm before (*A–D*) and immediately after (*E–H*) rupture. This aneurysm previously had been stable in size and configuration over several years. Sagittal oblique single-shot SSFP (*A*), coronal (*B*), axial (*C*), and candy cane HASTE (*D*) acquisitions show the presence of eccentric mural thrombus (*) within this aneurysm. Coronal single-shot SSFP from subsequent MR imaging at the time of acute chest pain (*E*) reveals intimal disruption (*arrow*) with diffusely increased aortic intramural signal and mediastinal signal (*arrowheads*) (*F, G*), consistent with acute rupture. Note the resultant pulmonary arterial compression due to mediastinal hematoma (*arrowhead*) (*H*).

isointense deoxyhemoglobin. Nonetheless, this rarely poses a diagnostic dilemma on SE imaging in the presence of aortic rupture because of frequent visualization of the site of mural disruption and concomitant presence of pleural or pericardial hemorrhagic effusion.

Although CE-MRA may allow demonstration of the location and extent of a traumatic injury and facilitate planning of surgical intervention, this technique often fails to provide information surplus to that gained on SE and GRE imaging. The strength

of this approach lies in its ability to detect further complications of trauma, including intimal dissection and vascular pathology occurring remote to the site of aortic rupture.

Congenital Anomalies

As the most significant of congenital anomalies of the thoracic aorta, including aortic coarctation and double aortic arch with tracheal or esophageal compression, tend to manifest in childhood, noninvasive cross-sectional MR imaging in the absence of ionizing radiation exposure is wholly desirable. As a result, MR imaging has become an essential component and alternative to catheter angiography in the evaluation of such anomalies, many of which may be evaluated only partially on TTE or TEE. A comprehensive examination of suspected congenital aortic disease should include complementary SE and MRA techniques, allowing determination of aortic and supra-aortic vascular configuration, luminal and mural integrity, and the relationship of these structures to adjacent mediastinal soft tissues.[58]

Aortic coarctation

Considerable variation may exist in the appearance of aortic coarctation, including its location (preductal, ductal, and postductal), extent (focal and diffuse), and effect on aortic lumen (a spectrum from mild to complete aortic interruption). Given this inconsistency, the various imaging approaches allowed during MR imaging provide an ideal opportunity for full characterization of such a stenosed segment, irrespective of aortic morphology.[59] High-resolution 3-D CE-MRA is the mainstay of this evaluation, providing an array of postprocessing options capable of displaying the coarctation and associated collateral pathways in a variety of projections and formats, allowing derivation of accurate measurements and planning of surgical repair (**Figs. 15 and 16**).[60] SE black-blood imaging allows evaluation of the mural characteristics at the location of the coarctation and should include a candy cane sagittal oblique view for optimal visualization of the affected segment. Although these techniques provide key morphologic information, determination of the hemodynamic significance of a coarctation and, thus, requirement for surgical intervention may prove difficult on this imaging alone. The authors have found sagittal oblique TR-MRA of considerable value in this regard, particularly in the presence of suspected short segment aortic interruption, opacification of the descending thoracic aorta occurring via a patent ductus arteriosus before arrival of contrast within the ascending aorta. Phase-contrast flow quantification also has proved useful in the preoperative period to assess MR imaging–estimated pressure gradients across the coarctation and in the postoperative period in exclusion of recoarctation (**Fig. 17**).[61] This technique also has proved useful in the quantitative evaluation of associated collateral flow.[50] Cine SSFP evaluation of the aortic valve also should be considered in this population, given the high incidence (approximately 50%) of bicuspid aortic valve in association with coarctation.

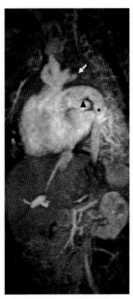

Fig. 15. Sagittal oblique CE-MRA MIP reconstruction in an infant who had interruption of the aortic arch (immediately distal to the origin of the left subclavian artery) (*arrow*). The descending thoracic aorta (*) is supplied by a large patent ductus arteriosus (*arrowhead*).

Aortic pseudocoarctation

Aortic pseudocoarctation, a developmental anomaly of the thoracic aorta, manifests as an elongation of the transverse arch, characteristically associated with a kinked appearance at the location of the ligamentum arteriosum. attachment. Although of no hemodynamic consequence, the major significance of this entity is that its differentiation from true coarctation has in the past on occasion proved difficult, particularly when aortic tortuosity is associated with turbulent flow. This rarely is the case in present times owing to the considerable morphologic and dynamic information provided by the techniques for aortic coarctation (described previously). Phase-contrast flow mapping is diagnostic, revealing the absence of a significant velocity or estimated pressure gradient across the affected segment.[62]

The Postoperative Aorta

Consideration of the spectrum of operative procedures in current practice for the management of various thoracic aorta disorders is beyond the scope of this text. Patch aortoplasty, subclavian-flap arterioplasty, and, more recently, balloon angioplasty for aortic coarctation pose little difficulty with regard to postoperative imaging and the previous discussion applies equally to these postoperative patients as to those in the preoperative

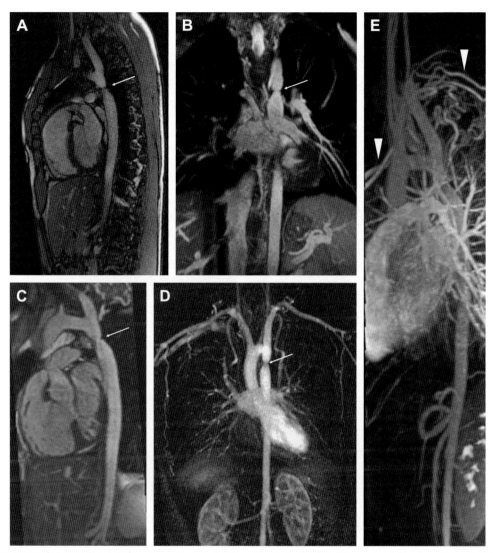

Fig. 16. Hemodynamically significant aortic coarctation. Single-shot SSFP (*A*), coronal free-breathing 3-D SSFP-MRA (*B*), candy cane reconstruction from the same free-breathing 3-D SSFP-MRA examination (*C*), and single-frame from dynamic TR-MRA examination (*D*) show the location, extent, and significance of the coarcted segment (*arrows*). Sagittal full-thickness CE-MRA MIP (*E*) reveals the presence of extensive scapular collateral vessels and dilated internal mammary arteries (*arrowheads*), indicating hemodynamically significant stenosis.

setting. Several interventions are worthy of particular reference, however, because of the frequency with which they are encountered or the challenges inherent to their subsequent imaging.

Endovascular stent/stent grafts

A trend has occurred in recent years toward endovascular, rather than open, repair of a variety of vascular disorders, a reflection of the less invasive nature and lower morbidity and mortality associated with this approach. In many cases, such stent or stent-graft deployment acts to exclude an aneurysm sac from the high-pressure thoracic aortic circulation, addressing the significant risk for

further luminal dilatation associated with this entity. Intimal dissection, the presence of a pseudoaneurysm, and recurrent coarctation represent but a few other indications for this technique (**Fig. 18**). Metallic susceptibility artifact occurring secondary to the presence of an endovascular stent has long been recognized as a potential limiting factor in the evaluation of postoperative luminal patency. Depending on stent composition, a spectrum of imaging manifestations may result, ranging from minimal to complete loss of luminal signal.[63] This may be the case particularly when the diameter of the vessel in question is diminutive, as in the pelvis or extremities. With regard to the

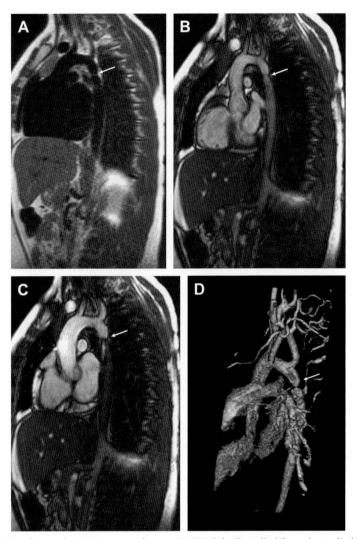

Fig. 17 Aortic coarctation (*arrows*) as seen on candy cane HASTE (*A*), diastolic (*B*), and systolic (*C*) images from cine SSFP acquisition and reconstructed CE-MRA MIP (*D*). Note the signal loss relating to turbulence within the aorta distal to the level of the coarctation during the systolic phase, not present during diastole when the resistance to flow is lower. CE-MRA also demonstrates many dilated intercostal collateral vessels. This diseased segment was treated successfully with balloon angioplasty and stenting (conventional angiographic images) (*E–I*).

thoracic aorta, this signal loss rarely is of such a degree to interfere with diagnostic interpretation;[64,65] thus MR imaging represents an ideal means of morphologic and dynamic postoperative evaluation. High-resolution CE-MRA should represent a central component to such imaging, facilitating 3-D reconstruction in a variety of imaging planes, as often is required for comprehensive evaluation of these curved grafts. The value of phase-contrast MR imaging in the assessment of changes in collateral blood flow also has been shown, allowing confirmation of hemodynamic improvement after stenting of recurrent aortic coarctation.[66] Transverse black-blood SE and pre- and postcontrast GRE imaging also may

have a role to play in the assessment of stent-graft internal architecture, particularly when the presence of mural atheroma is suspected.

Aortic root repairs

Open surgical repair of the ascending aortic root often is indicated in the presence of type A intimal dissection, such that proximal extension of the flap to involve coronary ostia and the valve annulus may be avoided. As a result, it is not uncommon for such repair to incorporate aortic valve replacement, often prosthetic. Comprehensive postsurgical evaluation of such a repair should involve valvular and graft interrogation, thus a combination of cine SSFP and 3-D MRA techniques. Particular

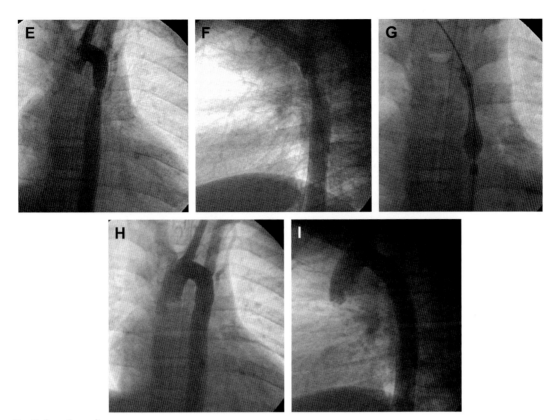

Fig. 17 (*continued*)

attention should be paid to valvular competency, the presence of graft mural atheroma, and the integrity of the proximal and distal graft anastomoses. Reproducible depiction of a residual distal intimal flap, present in excess of 75% of cases,[67] also is of primary concern in order that the presence of flow within the false lumen may be differentiated from thrombosis of this lumen. Although SSFP imaging represents the current standard approach to cine imaging, the susceptibility of

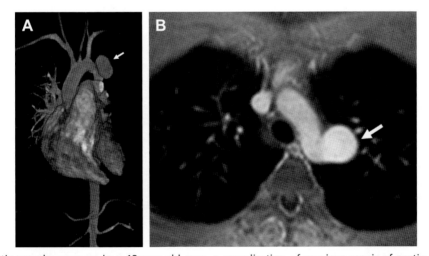

Fig. 18. Aortic pseudoaneurysm in a 13-year-old man, a complication of previous repair of aortic coarctation. Volume-rendered full-thickness MIP from CE-MRA examination (*A*) displays the morphology and location of the pseduoaneurysm. Direct communication with the true aortic lumen is confirmed on subsequent postcontrast T1-weighted axial gradient-echo acquisitions (*B*).

this technique to off-resonance and metallic susceptibility artifacts may render it inferior to standard cine GRE techniques in the presence of a metallic valve prosthesis.[68]

SUMMARY/KEY POINTS

- Currently available MR imaging and MRA techniques allow for comprehensive thoracic aortic evaluation in the preoperative and postoperative settings, with complete morphologic and functional investigation within a reasonable time period.
- Although fundamental components may remain unchanged, the requirement for fine tuning to suit the customized needs of individual patients is not uncommon; thus, familiarity with each of the approaches (described previously) is important.

REFERENCES

1. Blockmans D. The use of (18F)fluoro-deoxyglucose positron emission tomography in the assessment of large vessel vasculitis. Clin Exp Rheumatol 2003; 21(6 Suppl 32):S15–22.
2. Carr JC, Finn JP. MR imaging of the thoracic aorta. Magn Reson Imaging Clin N Am 2003;11(1):135–48.
3. Carr JC, Simonetti O, Bundy J, et al. Cine MR angiography of the heart with segmented true fast imaging with steady-state precession. Radiology 2001; 219(3):828–34.
4. Bradley WG Jr, Waluch V. Blood flow: magnetic resonance imaging. Radiology 1985;154(2):443–50.
5. Matsunaga N, Hayashi K, Okada M, et al. Magnetic resonance imaging features of aortic diseases. Top Magn Reson Imaging 2003;14(3):253–66.
6. von Scholthess GK, Fisher M, Crooks LE, et al. Gated MR imaging of the heart: intracardiac signals in patients and healthy subjects. Radiology 1985; 156(1):125–32.
7. Edelman RR, Chien D, Kim D. Fast selective black blood MR imaging. Radiology 1991;181(3):655–60.
8. Simonetti OP, Finn JP, White RD, et al. "Black blood" T2-weighted inversion-recovery MR imaging of the heart. Radiology 1996;199(1):49–57.
9. Stehling MK, Holzknecht NG, Laub G, et al. Single-shot T1- and T2-weighted magnetic resonance imaging of the heart with black blood: preliminary experience. MAGMA 1996;4(3–4):231–40.
10. Winterer JT, Lehnhardt S, Schneider B, et al. MRI of heart morphology. Comparison of nongradient echo sequences with single and multislice acquisition. Invest Radiol 1999;34(8):516–22.
11. Wallis F, Roditi GH, Redpath TW, et al. Inflammatory abdominal aortic aneurysms: diagnosis with gadolinium enhanced T1-weighted imaging. Clin Radiol 2000; 55(2):136–9.
12. Kelekis NL, Semelka RC, Molina PL, et al. Immediate postgadolinium spoiled gradient-echo MRI for evaluating the abdominal aorta in the setting of abdominal MR examination. J Magn Reson Imaging 1997;7(4):652–6.
13. Yucel EK, Steinberg FL, Egglin TK, et al. Penetrating aortic ulcers: diagnosis with MR imaging. Radiology 1990;177(3):779–81.
14. Gebker R, Gomaa O, Schnackenburg B, et al. Comparison of different MRI techniques for the assessment of thoracic aortic pathology: 3D contrast enhanced MR angiography, turbo spin echo and balanced steady state free precession. Int J Cardiovasc Imaging 2007;23(6):747–56.
15. Wansapura J, Fleck R, Crotty E, et al. Frequency scouting for cardiac imaging with SSFP at 3 Tesla. Pediatr Radiol 2006;36:1082–5.
16. Bi X, Deshpande V, Simonetti O, et al. Three-dimensional breathhold SSFP coronary MRA: a comparison between 1.5T and 3.0T. J Magn Reson Imaging 2005;22(2):206–12.
17. Weber OM, Pujadas S, Martin AJ, et al. Free-breathing, three-dimensional coronary artery magnetic resonance angiography: comparison of sequences. J Magn Reson Imaging 2004;20(3): 395–402.
18. Dumoulin CL, Souza SP, Walker MF, et al. Three-dimensional phase contrast MR angiography. Magn Reson Med 1989;9:139–49.
19. Markl M, Harloff A, Bley RA, et al. Time-resolved 3D MR velocity mapping at 3T: improved navigator-gated assessment of vascular anatomy and blood flow. J Magn Reson Imaging 2007;25(4):824–31.
20. Tomiguchi S, Morishita S, Nakashima R, et al. Usefulness of turbo-FLASH dynamic MR imaging of dissecting aneurysms of the thoracic aorta. Cardiovasc Intervent Radiol 1994;17(1):17–21.
21. Pereles FS, McCarthy RM, Baskaran V, et al. Thoracic aortic dissection and aneurysm: evaluation with non-enhanced true FISP MR angiography in less than 4 minutes. Radiology 2002;223(1):270–4.
22. Kunz RP, Oberholzer K, Kuroczynski W, et al. Assessment of chronic aortic dissection: contribution of different ECG-gated breath-hold MRI techniques. AJR Am J Roentgenol 2004;182(5):1319–26.
23. Givehchian M, Kramer U, Miller S, et al. Aortic root remodeling: functional MRI as an accurate tool for complete follow-up. Thorac Cardiovasc Surg 2005; 53(5):267–73.
24. Michaely HJ, Nael K, Schoenberg SO, et al. Renal perfusion: comparison of saturation-recovery Turbo-flash measurements at 1.5T with saturation-recovery Turboflash and time-resolved echo-shared angiographic technique (TREAT) at 3.0T. J Magn Reson Imaging 2006;24(6):1413–9.

25. Finn JP, Baskaran V, Carr JC, et al. Thorax: low-dose contrast-enhanced three-dimensional MR angiography with subsecond temporal resolution—initial results. Radiology 2002;224(3):896–904.
26. Pruessmann KP, Weiger M, Scheidegger MB, et al. SENSE: sensitivity encoding for fast MRI. Magn Reson Med 1999;42(5):952–62.
27. Schoenberg SO, Wunsch C, Knopp MV, et al. Abdominal aortic aneurysm. Detection of multilevel vascular pathology by time-resolved multiphase 3D gadolinium MR angiography: initial report. Invest Radiol 1999;34(10):648–59.
28. Sodickson DK, McKenzie CA, Li W, et al. Contrast-enhanced 3D MR angiography with simultaneous acquisition of spatial harmonics: a pilot study. Radiology 2000;217(1):284–9.
29. Chung T, Muthupillai R. Application of SENSE in clinical pediatric body MR imaging. Top Magn Reson Imaging 2004;15(3):187–96.
30. De Sanctis RW, Doroghazi RM, Austen WG, et al. Aortic dissection. N Engl J Med 1987;317(17):1060–7.
31. DeBakey ME, Henly WS, Cooley DA, et al. Surgical management of dissecting aneurysm involving the ascending aorta. J Cardiovasc Surg (Torino) 1964;5:200–11.
32. Miller DC, Stinson EB, Oyer PE, et al. Operative treatment of aortic dissections. Experience with 125 patients over a sixteen-year period. J Thorac Cardiovasc Surg 1979;78(3):365–82.
33. Kersting-Sommerhoff BA, Higgins CB, White RD, et al. Aortic dissection: sensitivity and specificity of MR imaging. Radiology 1988;166(3):651–5.
34. Wolff KA, Herold CJ, Tempany CM, et al. Aortic dissection: atypical patterns seen at MR imaging. Radiology 1991;181(2):489–95.
35. Narvaez J, Narvaez JA, Nolla JM, et al. Giant cell arteritis and polymyalgia rheumatic: usefulness of vascular magnetic resonance imaging studies in the diagnosis of aortitis. Rheumatology (Oxford) 2005;44(4):479–83.
36. Pflugfelder PW, Landzberg JS, Cassidy MM, et al. Comparison of cine MR imaging with Doppler echocardiography for the evaluation of aortic regurgitation. AJR Am J Roentgenol 1989;152(4):729–35.
37. Nitatori T, Yokoyama K, Hachiya J, et al. Fast dynamic MRI of aortic dissection: flow assessment by subsecond imaging. Radiat Med 1999;17(1):9–14.
38. Strotzer M, Aebert H, Lenhart M, et al. Morphology and hemodynamics in dissection of the descending aorta. Assessment with MR imaging. Acta Radiol 2000;41(6):594–600.
39. Cesare ED, Giordano AC, Cerone G, et al. Comparative evaluation of TEE, conventional MRI and contrast-enhanced 3D breath-hold MRA in the post-operative follow-up of dissecting aneurysms. Int J Card Imaging 2000;16(3):135–47.
40. Harris JA, Bis KG, Glover JL, et al. Penetrating atherosclerotic ulcers of the aorta. J Vasc Surg 1994;19(1):90–8.
41. Link KM, Lesko NM. The role of MR imaging in the evaluation of acquired diseases of the thoracic aorta. AJR Am J Roentgenol 1992;158(5):1115–25.
42. Desai MY, Stone JH, Foo TK, et al. Delayed contrast-enhanced MRI of the aortic wall in Takayasu's arteritis: initial experience. AJR Am J Roentgenol 2005;184(5):1427–31.
43. Vos AW, Wisselink W, Marcus JT, et al. Aortic aneurysm pulsatile wall motion imaged by cine MRI: a tool to evaluate efficacy of endovascular aneurysm repair? Eur J Vasc Endovasc Surg 2002;23(2):158–61.
44. Krombach FA, Kuhl H, Bucker A, et al. Cine MR imaging of heart valve dysfunction with segmented true fast imaging with steady state free precession. J Magn Reson Imaging 2004;19(1):59–67.
45. Markl M, Draney MT, Hope MD, et al. Time-resolved 3-dimensional velocity mapping in the thoracic aorta: visualization of 3-directional blood flow patterns in healthy volunteers and patients. J Comput Assist Tomogr 2004;28(4):459–68.
46. Nael K, Laub G, Finn JP. Three-dimensional contrast-enhanced MR angiography of the thoraco-abdominal vessels. Magn Reson Imaging Clin N Am 2005;13(2):359–80.
47. Nael K, Fenchel M, Krishnam M, et al. High-spatial resolution whole-body MR angiography with high-acceleration parallel acquisition and 32-channel 3.0-T unit: initial experience. Radiology 2007;242(3):865–72.
48. Salanitri GC. Intercostal artery aneurysms complicating thoracic aortic coarctation: diagnosis with magnetic resonance angiography. Australas Radiol 2007;51(1):78–82.
49. Rebergen SA, de Roos A. Congenital heart disease. Evaluation of anatomy and function by MRI. Herz 2000;25(4):365–83.
50. Holmqvist C, Stahlberg F, Hanseus K, et al. Collateral flow in coarctation of the aorta with magnetic resonance velocity mapping: correlation to morphological imaging of collateral vessels. J Magn Reson Imaging 2002;15(1):39–46.
51. Cotrufo M, Agozzino L, De Feo M, et al. Aortic valve dysfunction and dilated ascending aorta. A complex and controversial association. Ital Heart J 2003;4(9):589–95.
52. Bley TA, Uhl M, Venhoff N, et al. 3-T MRI reveals cranial and thoracic inflammatory changes in giant cell arteritis. Clin Rheumatol 2007;26(3):448–50.
53. Tanigawa E, Eguchi K, Kitamura Y, et al. Magnetic resonance imaging detection of aortic and pulmonary artery wall thickening in the acute stage of

Takayasu arteritis. Improvement of clinical and radiologic findings after steroid therapy. Arthritis Rheum 1992;35(4):476–80.

54. Weiss CR, Arai AE, Bui MN, et al. Arterial wall MRI characteristics are associated with elevated serum markers of inflammation in humans. J Magn Reson Imaging 2001;14(6):698–704.

55. Nael K, Fenchel MC, Kramer U, et al. Whole-body contrast-enhanced magnetic resonance angiography: new advances at 3.0 T. Top Magn Reson Imaging 2007;18(2):127–34.

56. Russo V, Renzulli M, Buttazzi K, et al. Acquired diseases of the thoracic aorta: role of MRI and MRA. Eur Radiol 2006;16(4):852–65.

57. Fattori R, Celletti F, Bertaccini P, et al. Delayed surgery of traumatic aortic rupture. Role of magnetic resonance imaging. Circulation 1996; 94(11):2865–70.

58. Russo V, Renzulli M, La Palombara C, et al. Congenital diseases of the thoracic aorta. Role of MRI and MRA. Eur Radiol 2006;16(3):676–84.

59. Didier D, Saint-Martin C, Lapierre C, et al. Coarctation of the aorta: pre and postoperative evaluation with MRI and MR angiography; correlation with echocardiography and surgery. Int J Cardiovasc Imaging 2006;22(3–4):457–75.

60. Godart F, Labrot G, Devos P, et al. Coarctation of the aorta: comparison of aortic dimensions between conventional MR imaging, 3D MR angiography, and conventional angiography. Eur Radiol 2002; 12(8):2034–9.

61. Euchhorn JG, Fink C, Delorme S, et al. Magnetic resonance blood flow measurements in the follow-up of

pediatric patients with aortic coarctation—a re-evaluation. Int J Cardiol 2006;113(3):291–8.

62. Hope MD, Levin JM, Markl M, et al. Images in cardiovascular medicine. Four-dimensional magnetic resonance velocity mapping in a healthy volunteer with pseduocoarctation of the thoracic aorta. Circulation 2004;109(25):3221–2.

63. Wang Y, Truong RN, Yen C, et al. Quantitative evaluation of susceptibility and shielding effects of nitinol, platinum, cobalt-alloy and stainless steel stents. Magn Reson Med 2003;49(5):972–6.

64. Farhat F, Attia C, Boussel L, et al. Endovascular repair of the descending thoracic aorta: mid-term results and evaluation of magnetic resonance angiography. J Cardiovasc Surg (Torino) 2007;48(1):1–6.

65. Merkle EM, Klein S, Wisianowsky C, et al. Magnetic resonance imaging versus multislice computed tomography of thoracic aortic endografts. J Endovasc Ther 2002;9(Suppl 2):I12–3.

66. Pujadas S, Reddy GP, Weber O, et al. Phase contrast MR imaging to measure changes in collateral blood flow after stenting of recurrent aortic coarctation: initial experience. J Magn Reson Imaging 2006; 24(1):72–6.

67. Riley P, Rooney S, Bonser R, et al. Imaging the postoperative thoracic aorta: normal anatomy and pitfalls. Br J Radiol 2001;74(888):1150–8.

68. Deutsch HJ, Bachmann R, Sechtem U, et al. Regurgitant flow in cardiac valve prostheses: diagnostic value of gradient echo nuclear magnetic resonance imaging in reference to transesophageal two-dimensional color Doppler echocardiography. J Am Coll Cardiol 1992;19(7):1500–7.

Time-Resolved MR Angiography of the Thorax

Derek G. Lohan, MD*, Mayil Krishnam, MD, Anderanik Tomasian, MD, Roya Saleh, MD, J. Paul Finn, MD

KEYWORDS

- MR • Angiography • Dynamic
- Imaging

Recent developments in contrast-enhanced magnetic resonance angiography (CE-MRA) have fostered the ambitious goals of submillimeter voxel dimensions comparable to CT, extended fields-of-view (FOV), and practical breath-hold acquisition times. These goals have been realized by the development of increasingly powerful gradient hardware, multiarray receiver coils, and parallel imaging techniques.[1,2] The increased signal-to-noise ratio (SNR) available at 3 tesla[3–5] has further improved sequence performance and these developments have collectively contributed to the widespread acceptance of CE-MRA as a safe and reliable tool for a variety of clinical applications. CE-MRA is now capable of high-resolution isotropic voxel acquisition, facilitating subsequent image reconstruction in any desired plane without compromise of in-plane spatial resolution, offering advantages over conventional "projectional" digital subtraction angiography (DSA).

Despite potentially exquisite 3-D vascular depiction, conventional CE-MRA provides little dynamic information relating to direction or rate of vascular enhancement, features that are readily apparent on DSA. The requirement for improved temporal resolution fueled the development of time-resolved MRA (TR-MRA) techniques. This article considers the evolution of TR-MRA to date, providing clinical examples of scenarios in which this technique may play a complementary or alternative role to CE-MRA.

Regardless of the technique used, TR-MRA involves rapid sequential imaging of an anatomic volume during the dynamic intravascular passage of a contrast bolus (**Fig. 1**).[6,7] When the acquisition time window is narrow, this approach mitigates the requirement for accurate positioning of central k-space points relative to peak contrast opacification, a persistent source of potential error during CE-MRA.[8–10] Imaging begins before arrival of contrast agent and continues for as many volume measurements as required to suit the clinical application. As a result, arterial and venous phases of luminal opacification are clearly discriminated. This approach may aid identification and evaluation of transient vascular phenomena or complex vascular flow kinetics[11,12] too rapid for detection on standard CE-MRA owing to long acquisition times of 20 to 40 seconds.

As required by the uncertainty principle, improvements in temporal resolution invoke a penalty with regard to spatial resolution, a reflection of the inverse relationship between these parameters. Improved spatial resolution, as a rule, requires increased k-space data sampling to maintain adequate SNR; thus, more prolonged acquisition times result. Alternatively, should the clinical indication allow for reduction in through-plane resolution, in-plane resolution, or coverage, more modest requirements for k-space filling can be used for faster acquisition. Even without view-sharing or parallel data acquisition techniques

Department of Radiology, David Geffen School of Medicine at the University of California, Los Angeles, 10945 Le Conte Avenue, Suite 3371, Peter V. Ueberroth Building, Los Angeles, CA 90095-7206, USA
* Corresponding author.
E-mail address: derek.lohan@gmail.com (D.G. Lohan).

Magn Reson Imaging Clin N Am 16 (2008) 235–248
doi:10.1016/j.mric.2008.02.015

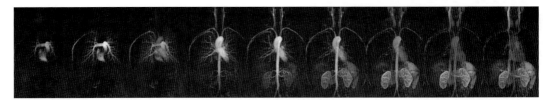

Fig. 1. Normal TR-MRA examination, illustrating dynamic sequential opacification of the pulmonary arterial, pulmonary venous, systemic arterial, and systemic venous circulations.

(discussed later), dynamic 3-D MRA may be performed with true frame rates of 1 second or less.[13]

2-D (UNSUBTRACTED) TEST BOLUS TIME-RESOLVED MAGNETIC RESONANCE ANGIOGRAPHY

Initial applications of TR-MRA occurred in the form of a 2-D technique. Although 3-D TR-MRA applications have since been developed and are increasingly available, 2-D TR-MRA remains widely used for the purpose of CE-MRA contrast bolus timing (Fig. 2).[8,14] Test bolus TR-MRA involves the use of a T1-weighted gradient-recalled echo (GRE) sequence with sufficiently short repetition time so as to allow repeated imaging at 1- to 2-second intervals. The imaging section is chosen to encompass at least a portion of the vessel of clinical concern; arrival of the contrast bolus is evidenced by a transient, readily appreciable increase in intraluminal signal intensity. Such a test bolus allows derivation of dynamic enhancement curves upon which timing calculations for CE-MRA may be made.[15] A saline flush, administered at the same rate as the gadolinium test bolus, typically follows to prevent pooling of the often minute contrast bolus (1–2 mL) within the injected extremity venous system.

2-D TIME-RESOLVED MAGNETIC RESONANCE ANGIOGRAPHY

Mask image subtraction, analogous to conventional DSA, may be used during TR-MRA. This approach involves the acquisition of an image dataset obtained before arrival of contrast, which is subtracted from subsequent contrast-enhanced frames. Subtraction initially was performed offline and used complex algorithms, although successfully allowing for "projectional" 2-D TR-MRA while removing potential interference from soft tissue signal.[16] Subsequent technical refinements allowed for temporal imaging at rates of 0.5 to 1 second per frame.[17] This approach initially was met with considerable enthusiasm concerning potential applications, including preclusion of the need for invasive conventional DSA.[18] Restrictions in spatial resolution and SNR, an inability to discern between superimposed vascular structures, and

potential for exclusion of pathology lying peripheral to the slab volume, however, limited its widespread clinical adoption. Investigators attempted to overcome these limitations by using more restricted slab volumes to prevent vascular overlap, correlation analysis for improvements in SNR, and administration of multiple contrast boluses while imaging in various anatomic planes, all with limited success.

3-D TIME-RESOLVED MAGNETIC RESONANCE ANGIOGRAPHY

A 3-D approach to TR-MRA offers several theoretic advantages over its 2-D counterpart, including improved SNR relating to averaging of partition data, greater tissue volume coverage, and potential for retrospective multiplanar reconstruction, which allows separation of overlapping vessels. Each of these improvements, however, necessitates a longer duration of imaging; thus, not all are clinically achievable without compromises elsewhere.

Although several approaches to 3-D TR-MRA are described, each represents a modification of 3-D high-resolution CE-MRA and involves a T1-weighted rapid GRE sequence.[19] 3-D TR-MRA, however, involves the use of ultrafast repetition and echo times of 2 milliseconds and 1 millisecond or less, respectively, to allow for rapid data refreshment and thus improved temporal resolution when compared with conventional CE-MRA. In so doing, this approach demands concessions with regard to the number of phase- and slice-encoding steps of k-space sampling allowed, thus compromising in spatial resolution. One approach is to compromise on through-plane resolution, allowing subsecond temporal imaging while maintaining the advantages of 3-D TR-MRA (Fig. 3).[13] Using a partial-Fourier scheme of 80% in the in-plane phase-encoding direction and only 62.5% of the full k-space vector in the slice-select direction, Finn and colleagues achieved volume acquisition times of approximately 800 milliseconds. Although the limited through-plane resolution of this approach precluded viewing of maximum intensity projection (MIP) reconstructions off-axis, careful preselection of imaging plane to suit the clinical situation often was sufficient to obviate

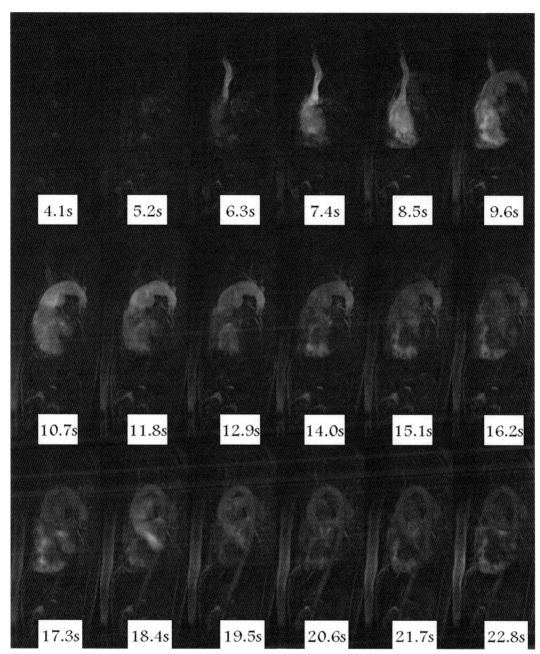

Fig. 2. Timing bolus TR-MRA. Sequential sagittal frames, separated by time interval of 1.1 seconds and performed for the purpose of CE-MRA timing calculation. The peak of aortic opacification occurs at 19.5 seconds after commencement of the contrast injection.

subsequent reconstruction. Furthermore, as these investigators indicated, with compact bolus injection and sufficiently rapid imaging, differences in temporal vascular enhancement may allow separation of overlying vessels in the absence of off-axis reconstructions. In unusual situations where a single imaging plane is insufficient, a second contrast bolus injection with alteration of imaging plane remains a reasonable option.

A separate approach to 3-D TR-MRA, TR imaging of contrast kinetics (TRICKS), was introduced by Korosec and coworkers.[20] TRICKS involves the use of temporal interpolation, whereby the low spatial-frequency data within the center of k-space is sampled more frequently than is the higher spatial-frequency data, located further peripherally. This method then shares high spatial-frequency data between adjacent frames, such

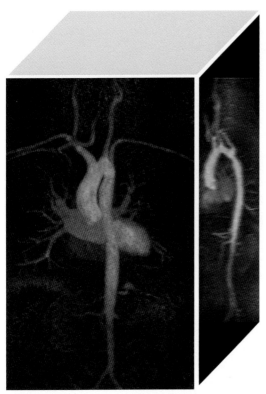

Fig. 3. One approach to TR-MRA. Note the high in-plane spatial resolution, allowing confident diagnostic interpretation. Through-plane resolution is relatively compromised, however, limiting useful off-axis data reconstruction.

that a full k-space complement is available for each individual frame. In contrast to the technique described by Finn and colleagues, this approach provides images of sufficiently high through-plane spatial resolution to allow off-axis MIP reconstruction, although at the expense of involving significantly larger datasets, thus considerably more complex image processing algorithms.[21]

Although several variations of the 3-D TR-MRA techniques (described previously) have been investigated since the inception of TR imaging, those in current use include TRICKS, projection reconstruction TRICKS, CE timing-robust angiography (CENTRA), TR echo-shared angiographic technique (TREAT), and TR angiography with interleaved stochastic trajectories (TWIST).

RECENT DEVELOPMENTS

Several key advances in MR imaging hardware and software have contributed in recent times to significant improvements in the implementation of CE-MRA. The introduction of parallel imaging techniques, whereby signal integration from multiple individual elements within a phased-array receiver coil is used to expedite data sampling,[1,2,22] has resulted in vast improvements in the speed of k-space filling and subsequent data reconstruction.[23] As a result, increased volume coverage or further improvements in spatial resolution can be achieved without prolongation of acquisition time. Alternatively, the combination of parallel imaging with TR-MRA may facilitate increased temporal resolution, typically by a factor of 30%.[24,25] Currently available parallel acquisition techniques used for this purpose include sensitivity encoding (SENSE) and generalized autocalibrating partially parallel acquisition (GRAPPA).

The successful application of parallel imaging techniques is heavily reliant, however, on the presence of high-performance gradient coils with slew rates now as high as 200 millitesla per meter per millisecond.[26] Exploitation of the benefits of such rapid gradients, particularly when implemented with high field-strength scanners, allows improvements in spatial resolution, FOV, or temporal resolution or combinations thereof. Imaging at high field strengths, such as 3 tesla, also holds considerable advantage with regard to SNR, providing a theoretic doubling in signal, thus offering the potential for contrast dose-reduction during TR-MRA.

CLINICAL APPLICATIONS

The attributes of TR-MRA (discussed previously) have resulted in its application to a wide range of clinical scenarios. Given the heightened sensitivity to T1-shortening agents experienced at 3 tesla, TR-MRA may be used as a routine supplement to high-resolution CE-MRA without overall increase in administered gadolinium dose. As a result, complementary TR-MRA and CE-MRA allow definitive, comprehensive dynamic, and morphologic vascular evaluation to a degree immensely superior to that provided by either technique alone. A variety of implementations of TR-MRA, images that exemplify the value of this approach, pertinent literature, and consideration of the potential future applications of this technique are discussed.

Pulmonary Time-Resolved Magnetic Resonance Angiography

It has long been recognized that assessment of pulmonary integrity must involve morphologic and functional evaluation, most commonly in the forms of conventional chest radiography and pulmonary function tests, respectively. The same approach holds true with regard to pulmonary vascular interrogation, high-resolution CE-MRA allowing eloquent confirmation of vascular patency although providing little, if any, essential dynamic information. The application of TR-MRA to pulmonary imaging is particularly appropriate for several reasons. First, the configuration of the chest is such that a coronal 2-D or 3-D acquisition facilitates single-volume imaging of the central and majority of the peripheral extents of both lungs, allowing comparison between right and left pulmonary perfusion. Furthermore, such an imaging plane by default includes the heart and mediastinum in the FOV. As a result, this permits evaluation of the entire course of the contrast bolus, including systemic venous return to the right atrium and ventricle, the pulmonary arterial phase, pulmonary parenchymal enhancement, pulmonary venous return to the left atrium, and systemic arterial perfusion from the left ventricle to ascending aorta. Finally, TR-MRA is of benefit in pulmonary imaging owing to the nature of the flow characteristics involved. Pulmonary perfusion time, from the arterial phase of vascular enhancement to atrial venous return, normally is in the region of 3 to 4 seconds[27] (or longer in the presence of pulmonary arterial hypertension) (**Fig. 4**). Hence the 1- to 2-second temporal resolution routinely obtained during TR-MRA is ideal for this purpose, providing multiple frames

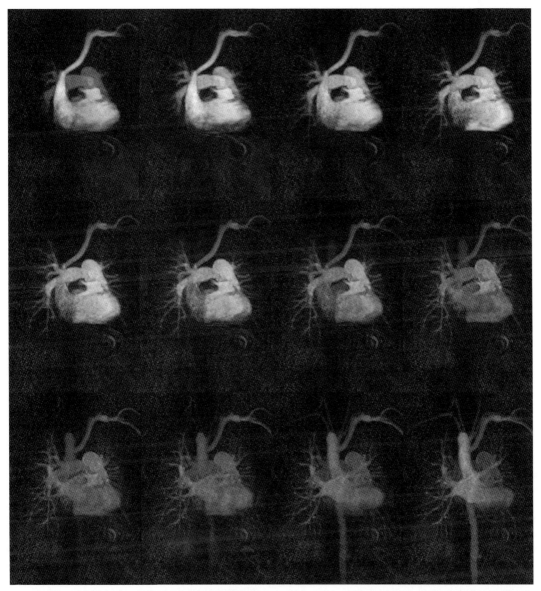

Fig. 4. A 54-year-old male patient who had pulmonary hypertension. Although the sequence of opacification (pulmonary arterial, pulmonary venous, and systemic arterial) is preserved, a marked prolonged pulmonary arterial-to-pulmonary venous perfusion time of 10 seconds is present, consistent with pulmonary hypertension.

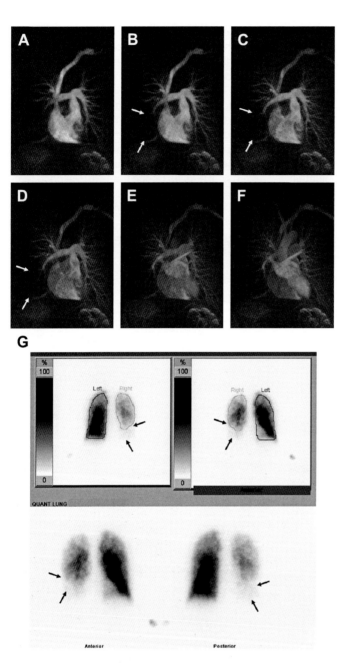

Fig. 5. TR-MRA (*A–F*) and scintigraphic pulmonary perfusion study (*G*) from a 49-year-old woman who had chest pain and subsequent confirmation of pulmonary embolus. There is globally reduced right lung perfusion, particularly that of the right lower lobe (*white arrows*). This perfusion defect was confirmed on [99m]technetium–macroaggregated albumin scintigraphy (*black arrows*).

that allow confident segmentation of the pulmonary arterial, parenchymal, and venous phases of vascular enhancement.

Goyen and colleagues[28] were among the first to evaluate the value of dynamic pulmonary imaging and its potential in patients in whom lengthy respiratory suspension commanded by high-resolution CE-MRA could not be tolerated. TR-MRA allowed depiction of the pulmonary arterial tree to the subsegmental branch level in all subjects, with concordance between dynamic TR-MRA findings and those of corroborative studies in patients

who have suspected pulmonary embolus. More recently, Nael and coworkers,[29] confirmed the usefulness of this technique in at 1.5 tesla, while also demonstrating comparable diagnostic quality imaging when assessing pulmonary perfusion at 3 tesla.

Initial reports regarding the clinical applicability of TR-MRA in the evaluation of patients who have pulmonary hypertension are encouraging, allowing differentiation between idiopathic and chronic thromboembolic pulmonary arterial hypertension, thus having an impact on the management algorithm.[30,31] TR-MRA also has been assessed with regard to investigation of suspected acute pulmonary embolic disease (**Fig. 5**). In their study of 27 patients who had contraindications to iodinated contrast medium, Ersoy and coworkers[32] determined TR-MRA as allowing diagnostic pulmonary segmental arterial visualization in 94% to 95% of subjects and confident inclusion or exclusion of pulmonary embolism in 96% of patients (**Fig. 6**). These investigators used a 3-D TR-MRA sequence with a temporal resolution of 3.3 seconds and 1.3 × 1.8 × 3.0–mm voxel resolution on a 1.5-tesla MR imaging system.

Catheter-guided radiofrequency ablation of the pulmonary venous ostia is an efficient treatment option in the management of atrial fibrillation.[33] Secondary pulmonary venous stenosis is a well-recognized complication of this technique, however,[34] and may necessitate endovascular stent deployment to maintain luminal patency. The reliability of TR-MRA in allowing confident separation of the arterial and venous phases of pulmonary opacification has been exploited in this regard, confirming its ability to provide accurate ostial measurements, depict differential pulmonary perfusion, and allow visualization of the offending stenosis (**Figs. 7 and 8**).[35,36]

Arteriovenous malformations (AVMs), in particular those associated with a high degree of hemodynamic shunting, pose a particular challenge for high-resolution CE-MRA, a reflection of the vastly longer acquisition time required for CE-MRA relative to the bolus transit time through such an anomaly. As a result, isolated arterial or venous opacification cannot be achieved in the majority of cases, the presence of contrast within afferent and efferent conduits rendering morphologic evaluation of such an AVM difficult, if not impossible, in the case of complex lesions. Dynamic assessment of pulmonary AVMs, however, is a valuable complement to CE-MRA, and on occasion may afford morphologic evaluation superior to that of high-resolution imaging owing to reduction or elimination of venous contamination.[37]

Congenital Heart Disease

Appraisal of congenital cardiac conditions, invasively or noninvasively, may represent one of the most challenging facets of diagnostic imaging owing to the vast realm of potential anomalies, several of which may coexist within a single patient. Perhaps more so than any other area of medical imaging, it is vital that the location, patency, direction, and magnitude of flow within the atria and ventricles, great vessels, collateral channels, and anomalous conduits are accurately known, such that a complete appreciation of the hemodynamic significance of the congenital abnormality is gained. ECG-gated segmented steady-state free precession (SSFP) gradient-echo sequences represent the mainstay of intracardiac morphologic evaluation, allowing determination of the presence and secondary effects of septal and endocardial cushion defects, valvular abnormalities, or atrioventricular discordance.[38] This approach also is capable of indicating the hemodynamic consequences of such anomalies, including visualization of flow across a tissue defect or focal signal dephasing, indicating the presence of stenosis or insufficiency.[39] Cine SSFP may suffice for simple congenital conditions in which an abnormal communication is present between two otherwise unremarkable cavities or structures. A comprehensive evaluation of complex congenital heart disease, however, using this approach would necessitate an inconceivable number of acquisitions and imaging planes, rendering it impractical, particularly in the presence of extracardiac vascular anomalies. High-resolution 3-D CE-MRA addresses the limitations of cross-sectional imaging to a certain degree,

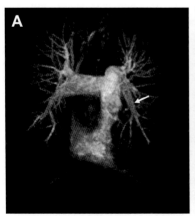
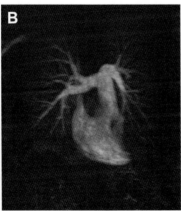

Fig. 6. Comparable CE-MRA and TR-MRA frames during the pulmonary arterial phase of opacification in a patient who had suspected pulmonary embolus. Note the presence of a possible intraluminal filling defect in the left lower lobe pulmonary artery on CE-MRA (*arrow*) (*A*). TR-MRA (*B*) confirmed the absence of such a filling defect that actually represented a pseudoembolus related to improper coordination of the contrast bolus peak and filling of the center of k-space.

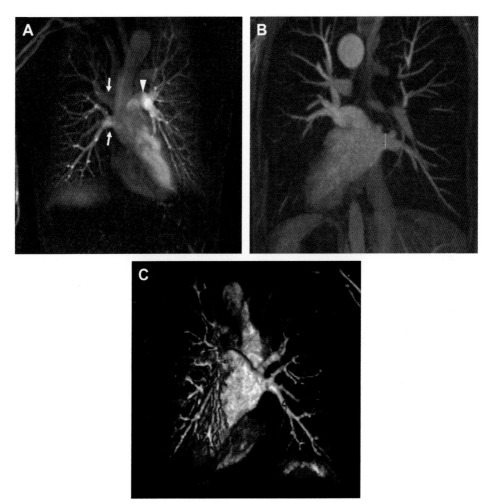

Fig. 7. Pulmonary venous phase frame from TR-MRA examination (*A*) shows the presence of two pulmonary venous ostia on the right (*arrows*) and a single ostium on the left (*arrowhead*). Depiction of pulmonary veins is comparable to that of CE-MRA (posterior view) (*B*). (*C*) Posterior volume-rendered TR-MRA frame, illustrating pulmonary venous morphology.

allowing confirmation of the presence and patency of vascular conduits. CE-MRA is incapable, however, of demonstrating transient events, such as intracardiac shunts or directional flow within a patent ductus arteriosus (PDA) (**Fig. 9**).

TR-MRA offers the unique opportunity to combine 3-D large FOV morphologic evaluation with dynamic functional assessment that includes detection of short-lived hemodynamic phenomena. Optimization of temporal resolution to achieve repeated data acquisition in times approaching 1 second is key, a reflection of the rapid rates of blood flow within the heart and great vessels. In their evaluation of 81 patients who had congenital heart disease that included aortic coarctation, tetralogy of Fallot, and transposition of the great arteries and truncus arteriosus, Fenchel and colleagues[12] gained important functional information

from TR-MRA, information that was not available on CE-MRA, in 63% of cases. This included transient intracardiac and extracardiac shunts in 22% and 2.5%, respectively. Balci and coworkers[40] found similarly encouraging results when implementing TR-MRA in the assessment of anomalous pulmonary venous return.

The authors' experience is that TR-MRA may be of particular value in the evaluation of congenital heart disease in the postoperative period. Determination of shunt patency and integrity, indication of the sequence of chamber and conduit opacification, assessment of visceral enhancement, and confirmation that a physiologically preferable hemodynamic circulation has been restored are a few of the factors that may be assessed readily and rapidly using this technique during the injection of a minimal dose of contrast agent.[41]

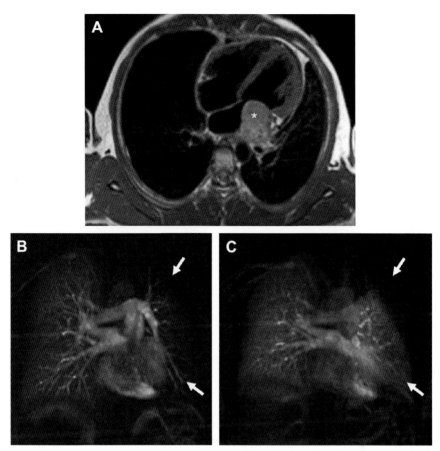

Fig. 8. Primary cardiac osteosarcoma in a 19-year-old man. (*A*) Four-chamber T1-turbo spin-echo image shows a left atrial mass invading the left pulmonary veins (*). TR-MRA images before (*B*) and after (*C*) surgical intervention show interval improvement in left pulmonary (in particular the left upper lobe) parenchymal perfusion (*arrows*).

Thoracic Aorta and Supra-Aortic Branch Vessels

Isotropic 3-D high-resolution CE-MRA, in the absence of specific contraindications to MR imaging, has become the gold standard imaging technique for the evaluation of the thoracic aorta. The data provided is readily amenable to postprocessing, yielding reconstructions of exquisite detail and allowing a high level of diagnostic interpretation as to the presence and morphology of aortic pathology. The authors recommend the

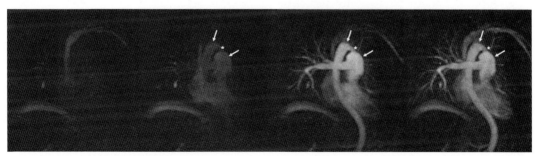

Fig. 9. Sequential coronal TR-MRA frames from a patient who had PDA. There is simultaneous opacification of the pulmonary arteries and descending thoracic aorta (*arrows*), bypassing the pulmonary venous phase of opacification. The large PDA is readily appreciable (*).

routine use of TR-MRA to provide complementary data relevant to thoracocervicocranial pathology, allowing increasingly comprehensive patient evaluation (**Fig. 10**). Lenhart and colleagues[42] were among the first to recognize the potential value of this approach when imaging the carotid circulation, determining a sensitivity and specificity of 98% and 86%, respectively, when compared with selective catheter angiography in the grading of significant carotid stenoses. Subsequent introduction of parallel imaging techniques significantly improved the temporal resolution from 10 seconds per dataset, as described in the study of Lenhart and colleagues, to 1.5 seconds, described by Meckel and colleagues.[43] As a result, multiple arterial and venous phases of vascular enhancement were obtained, allowing a greater degree of vascular interrogation and improvements in diagnostic confidence. Jaspers and cowokers[44] successfully applied this technique to spinal cord arterial and venous phase separation, confirming its ability to confidently differentiate the artery of Adamkiewicz and great anterior radiculomedullary vein. Other potentially useful applications include the evaluation of suspected subclavian steal syndrome,[45] head and neck vascular malformations,[46] spinal arteriovenous shunts, and fistulas.[47,48]

TR-MRA also shows considerable promise in the postoperative setting in the evaluation of treated intracranial AVMs and extracranial to intracranial bypass shunts.[49,50] More recently, further improvements in image quality and temporal resolution have proved possible at higher field strengths, a reflection of the heightened sensitivity to T1-shortening agents and superior SNR experienced at 3 tesla.[51–53]

Central Venous Imaging

Despite the absence of relevant studies within the current medical literature, the authors' experience with thoracic dynamic TR venography has been encouraging. Imaging during upper-extremity venous contrast administration allows confirmation of the presence of central venous patency, stenosis, or occlusion and demonstration of the course and significance of dominant collateral venous pathways (**Fig. 11**). A comprehensive evaluation may necessitate bilateral upper-extremity injection, although this may occur as two separate injections. Although failure of venous luminal opacification is highly suggestive of occlusion, complementary thoracic postcontrast T1 GRE sections are recommended to confirm the presence of occlusive intraluminal thrombus or extrinsic compressing mass lesion.

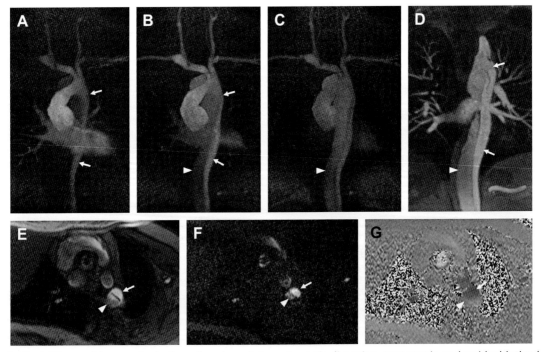

Fig. 10. A 72-year-old man who had previous type A thoracic aortic dissection, root repair, and residual intimal dissection flap. TR-MRA (*A–C*), CE-MRA (*D*), and phase-sensitive flow quantification (*E–G*) analyses show disparity between rates of true luminal (*arrows*) and false luminal (*arrowheads*) opacification.

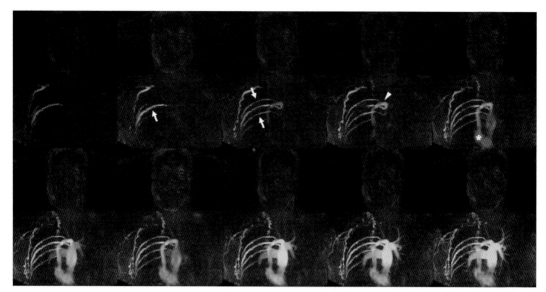

Fig. 11. A 57-year-old man who had central venous occlusion. Contrast injection via the right upper extremity drains to the right intercostal veins (*arrows*), a result of right axillary and subclavian vein occlusion, and then to the azygos system (*arrowhead*), with subsequent venous return to the right atrium (*).

Pediatric Time-Resolved Magnetic Resonance Angiography

MRA continues to prove difficult in the pediatric population for a variety of reasons. Among these is the requirement for intravenous sedation, degradation in image quality often resulting from an ability to achieve respiratory suspension. Diminutive patient size, restrictions in the allowable contrast dose, and high-flow circulatory hemodynamics renders imaging of infants and children challenging, even in the most controlled of conditions. As considered by Muthupillai and colleagues,[54] one important exception exists: spatial resolution requirements are more modest in the pediatric population compared with adult imaging. This allowance stems from the contrast between pediatric and adult pathologies, namely that imaging of the former is concerned primarily with conduit patency and integrity, whereas atherosclerotic irregularities and luminal stenoses are of primary importance in older age groups. Using the parallel imaging technique, SENSE, with an acceleration factor of two, in-plane and through-plane resolutions of 1.4 mm × 1.7 mm and 3.1 mm, respectively, these investigators performed TR-MRA with a temporal resolution of 6.8 seconds in 22 pediatric patients. Clinical indications for MR imaging evaluation in this study included vascular rings, systemic arterial aneurysms, issues with central venous access, pulmonary venous anomalies, and postoperative aortic coarctation assessments. These investigators reported diagnostic quality examinations in all cases, despite the absence of respiratory suspension, capable of allowing confident arterial-to-venous separation. The experience described by Chung was similarly encouraging, also in a pediatric population and for a variety of clinical indications.[55]

Incidental Lesions

The potential significance of soft tissue enhancement, as observed during lower-extremity dynamic MRA has been described elsewhere.[56] Given the fundamental basis of this imaging technique, any tissue demonstrating rapid parenchymal perfusion might be readily appreciable during the time period allowed by thoracic TR-MRA. This holds true particularly regarding the thyroid gland, where homogeneous arterial-phase parenchymal enhancement commonly is seen during TR-MRA. The authors' experience suggests that TR-MRA may be of value in the incidental detection of previously unsuspected thyroid abnormalities, including focal hyperenhancing nodules, diffuse parenchymal heterogeneity accompanying multinodular goiter, and hypoenhancement in the presence of hypothyroidism. This potential for incidental lesion detection is not confined to the thyroid gland, TR-MRA possessing the capability of demonstrating hypervascular lesions throughout the imaging FOV, including meningiomas (**Fig. 12**) and visceral branch aneurysms.

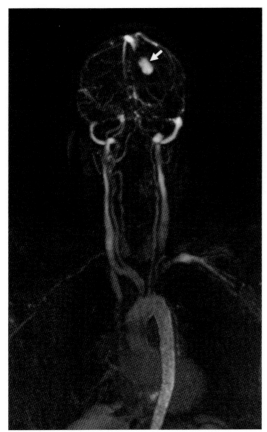

Fig. 12. A 72-year-old female patient undergoing TR-MRA for carotid-vertebral analysis. Note intense enhancement of an incidental meningioma (*arrow*).

SUMMARY/KEY POINTS

- Comprehensive thoracic vascular evaluation necessitates morphologic and functional assessment, clearly within the capabilities of CE-MRA and TR-MRA.
- Dynamic evaluation may complement high-resolution angiography, providing additional information relating to transient flow phenomena while incurring few penalties in the form of slightly increased contrast dose requirements and study durations, both of which may be offset by imaging at higher field strengths. Although still in its infancy, this technique is becoming widely accepted as of considerable potential value in pediatric and adult imaging.
- The authors advocate the routine use of TR-MRA in all cases of thoracic vascular evaluation and consider the potential benefits of this approach to significantly outweigh its risks in all but the most exceptional of cases.
- The future for TR-MRA remains promising, with increasing field and gradient strengths, parallel imaging techniques, and temporal echo sharing offering the potential for further improvements in matrix and temporal imaging.

REFERENCES

1. Pruessman KP. Parallel imaging at high field strength: synergies and joint potential. Top Magn Reson Imaging 2004;15:237–44.
2. Sodickson DK, McKenzie CA, Li W, et al. Contrast-enhanced 3D MR angiography with simultaneous acquisition of spatial harmonics: a pilot study. Radiology 2000;217:284–9.
3. Leiner T, de Vries M, Hoogeveen R, et al. Contrast-enhanced peripheral MR angiography at 3.0 Tesla: initial experience with a whole-body scanner in healthy volunteers. J Magn Reson Imaging 2003; 17(5):609–14.
4. Allkemper T, Heindel W, Kooijman H, et al. Effect of field strengths on magnetic resonance angiography: comparison of an ultrasmall superparamagnetic iron oxide blood-pool contrast agent and gadopentetate dimeglumine in rabbits at 1.5 and 3.0 Tesla. Invest Radiol 2006;41(2):97–104.
5. Nael K, Ruehm SG, Michaely HJ, et al. High spatial resolution CE-MRA of the carotid circulation with parallel imaging: comparison of image quality between 2 different acceleration factors at 3.0 Tesla. Invest Radiol 2006;41(4):391–9.
6. Krings T, Hans F. New developments in MRA: time-resolved MRA. Neuroradiology 2004;46(Suppl 2): s214–22.
7. Sohn CH, Sevick RJ, Frayne R. Contrast-enhanced MR angiography of the intracranial circulation. Magn Reson Imaging Clin N Am 2003;11(4):599–614.
8. Cai Z, Stolpen A, Sharafuddin MJ, et al. Bolus characteristics based on magnetic resonance angiography. Biomed Eng Online 2006;5:53.
9. Hood MN, Ho VB, Foo TK, et al. High-resolution gadolinium-enhanced 3D MRA of the infrapopliteal arteries. Lessons for improving bolus-chase peripheral MRA. Magn Reson Imaging 2002;20(7):543–9.
10. Heverhagen JT, Funck RC, Schwarz U, et al. Kinetic evaluation of an i.v. bolus of MR contrast media. Magn Reson Imaging 2001;19(7):1025–30.
11. Nael K, Michaely HJ, Lee M, et al. Dynamic pulmonary perfusion and flow quantification with MR imaging, 3.0T vs. 1.5T: initial results. J Magn Reson Imaging 2006;24(2):333–9.
12. Fenchel M, Saleh R, Dinh H, et al. Juvenile and adult congenital heart disease: time-resolved 3D contrast-enhanced MR angiography. Radiology 2007;244(2): 399–410.
13. Finn JP, Baskaran V, Carr JC, et al. Thorax: low-dose contrast-enhanced three-dimensional MR angiography with subsecond temporal resolution—initial results. Radiology 2002;224(3):896–904.

14. Earls JP, Rofsky NM, DeCorato DR, et al. Breath-hold single-dose gadolinium-enhanced three-dimensional MR aortography: usefulness of a timing examination and MR power injector. Radiology 1996;201(3):705–10.

15. Kreitner KF, Kunz RP, Weschler C, et al. Systematic analysis of the geometry of a defined contrast-medium bolus—implications for contrast enhanced 3D MR-angiography of the thoracic vessels. Rofo 2005;177(5):646–54.

16. Wang Y, Johnston DL, Breen JF, et al. Dynamic MR digital subtraction angiography using contrast enhancement, fast data acquisition, and complex subtraction. Magn Reson Med 1996;36(4):551–6.

17. Hennig J, Scheffler K, Laubenberger J, et al. Time-resolved projection angiography after bolus injection of contrast agent. Magn Reson Med 1997;37(3):341–5.

18. Klisch J, Strecker R, Hennig J, et al. Time-resolved projection MRA: clinical application in intracranial vascular malformations. Neuroradiology 2000;42(2):104–7.

19. Frayne R, Grist TM, Korosec FR, et al. MR angiography with three-dimensional MR digital subtraction angiography. Top Magn Reson Imaging 1996;8(6):366–88.

20. Korosec FR, Frayne R, Grist TM, et al. Time-resolved contrast-enhanced 3D MR angiography. Magn Reson Med 1996;36(3):345–51.

21. Mistretta CA, Grist TM, Korosec FR, et al. 3D time-resolved contrast-enhanced MR DSA: advantages and tradeoffs. Magn Reson Med 1998;40(4):571–81.

22. Wilson GJ, Hoogeveen RM, Willinek WA, et al. Parallel imaging in MR angiography. Top Magn Reson Imaging 2004;15(3):169–85.

23. Kressler B, Spincemaille P, Prince MR, et al. Reduction of reconstruction time for time-resolved spiral 3D contrast-enhanced magnetic resonance angiography using parallel computing. Magn Reson Med 2006;56(3):704–8.

24. Fink C, Ley S, Kroeker R, et al. Time-resolved contrast-enhanced three-dimensional magnetic resonance angiography of the chest: combination of parallel imaging with view sharing (TREAT). Invest Radiol 2005;40(1):40–8.

25. Brauck K, Maderwald S, Vogt FM, et al. Time-resolved contrast-enhanced magnetic resonance angiography of the hand with parallel imaging and view sharing: initial experience. Eur Radiol 2007;17(1):183–92.

26. Nael K, Fenchel M, Krishnam M, et al. High-spatial-resolution whole-body MR angiography with high-acceleration parallel acquisition and 32-channel 3.0-T unit: initial experience. Radiology 2007;242(3):865–72.

27. Fishman AP. Dynamics of the pulmonary circulation. In: Hamilton WF, editor. Handbook of physiology, section 2: circulation. Washington, DC: American Physiological Society; 1963. p. 1708.

28. Goyen M, Laub G, Ladd ME, et al. Dynamic 3D MR angiography of the pulmonary arteries in under four seconds. J Magn Reson Imaging 2001;13(3):372–7.

29. Nael K, Saleh R, Nyborg GK, et al. Pulmonary MR perfusion at 3.0 Tesla using a blood pool contrast agent: Initial results in a swine model. J Magn Reson Imaging 2007;25(1):66–72.

30. Ley S, Fink C, Zaporozhan J, et al. Value of high spatial and high temporal resolution magnetic resonance angiography for differentiation between idiopathic and thromboembolic pulmonary hypertension: initial results. Eur Radiol 2005;15(11):2256–63.

31. Nikolaou K, Schoenberg SO, Attenberger U, et al. Pulmonary arterial hypertension: diagnosis with fast perfusion MR imaging and high spatial-resolution MR angiography—preliminary experience. Radiology 2005;236(2):694–703.

32. Ersoy H, Goldhaber SZ, Cai T, et al. Time-resolved MR angiography: a primary screening examination of patients with suspected pulmonary embolism and contraindications to administration of iodinated contrast material. AJR Am J Roentgenol 2007;188(5):1246–54.

33. Haissaguerre M, Shah DC, Jais P, et al. Mapping-guided ablation of pulmonary veins to cure atrial fibrillation. Am J Cardiol 2000;86(9A):9K–19K.

34. Robbins IM, Colvin EV, Doyle TP, et al. Pulmonary vein stenosis after catheter ablation of atrial fibrillation. Circulation 1998;98(17):1769–75.

35. Kluge A, Dill T, Ekinci O, et al. Decreased pulmonary perfusion in pulmonary vein stenosis after radiofrequency ablation: assessment with dynamic magnetic resonance perfusion imaging. Chest 2004;126(2):428–37.

36. Korperich H, Gieseke J, Esdorn H, et al. Ultrafast time-resolved contrast-enhanced 3D pulmonary venous cardiovascular magnetic resonance angiography using SENSE combined with CENTRA-keyhole. J Cardiovasc Magn Reson 2007;9(1):77–87.

37. Goyen M, Ruehm SG, Jagenburg A, et al. Pulmonary arteriovenous malformation: characterization with time-resolved ultrafast 3D MR angiography. J Magn Reson Imaging 2001;13(3):458–60.

38. Pereles FS, Kapoor V, Carr JC, et al. Usefulness of segmented trueFISP cardiac pulse sequence in evaluation of congenital and acquired adult cardiac abnormalities. AJR Am J Roentgenol 2001;177(5):1155–60.

39. Colletti PM. Evaluation of intracardiac shunts with cardiac magnetic resonance. Curr Cardiol Rep 2005;7(1):52–8.

40. Balci NC, Yalcin Y, Tunaci A, et al. Assessment of the anomalous pulmonary circulation by dynamic

contrast-enhanced MR angiography in under four seconds. Magn Reson Imaging 2003;21(1):1–7.

41. Goo HW, Yang DH, Park IS, et al. Time-resolved three-dimensional magnetic resonance angiography in patients who have undergone a Fontan operation or bidirectional cavopulmonary connection: initial experience. J Magn Reson Imaging 2007;25(4):727–36.

42. Lenhart M, Framme N, Volk M, et al. Time-resolved contrast-enhanced magnetic resonance angiography of the carotid arteries: diagnostic accuracy and inter-observer variability compared with selective catheter angiography. Invest Radiol 2002; 37(10):535–41.

43. Meckel S, Mekle R, Taschner C, et al. Time-resolved 3D contrast-enhanced MRA with GRAPPA on a 1.5-T system for imaging of craniocervical vascular disease: initial experience. Neuroradiology 2006; 48(5):291–9.

44. Jaspers K, Nigenhuis RJ, Backes WH. Differentiation of spinal cord arteries and veins by time-resolved MR angiography. J Magn Reson Imaging 2007; 26(1):31–40.

45. Virmani R, Carroll TJ, Hung J, et al. Diagnosis of subclavian steal syndrome using dynamic time-resolved magnetic resonance angiography: a technical note. Magn Reson Imaging 2008;26(2):287–92.

46. Ziyeh S, Schumacher M, Strecker R, et al. Head and neck vascular malformations: time-resolved MR projection angiography. Neuroradiology 2003;45(10): 681–6.

47. Ali S, Cashen RA, Carroll TJ, et al. Time-resolved spinal MR angiography: initial clinical experience in the evaluation of spinal arteriovenous shunts. AJNR Am J Neuroradiol 2007;28(9):1806–10.

48. Meckel S, Maier M, Ruiz DS, et al. MR angiography of dural arteriovenous fistulas: diagnosis and follow-up after treatment using a time-resolved 3D contrast-enhanced technique. AJNR Am J Neuroradiol 2007;28(5):877–84.

49. Shim YW, Chung TS, Kang WS, et al. Non-invasive follow-up evaluation of post-embolized AVM with time-resolved MRA: a case report. Korean J Radiol 2002;3(4):271–5.

50. Tsuchiya K, Honya K, Fujikawa A, et al. Postoperative assessment of extracranial-intracranial bypass by time-resolved 3D contrast-enhanced MR angiography using parallel imaging. AJNR Am J Neuroradiol 2005;26(9):2243–7.

51. Nael K, Michaely HJ, Villablanca P, et al. Time-resolved contrast-enhanced magnetic resonance angiography of the head and neck at 3.0 Tesla: initial results. Invest Radiol 2006;41(2):116–24.

52. Cashen TA, Carr JC, Shin W, et al. Intracranial time-resolved contrast-enhanced MR angiography at 3T. AJNR Am J Neuroradiol 2006;27(4):822–9.

53. Frydrychowicz A, Bley TA, Winterer JT, et al. Accelerated time-resolved 3D contrast-enhanced MR angiography at 3T: clinical experience in 31 patients. MAGMA 2006;19(4):187–95.

54. Muthupillai R, Vick GW 3rd, Flamm SD, et al. Time-resolved contrast-enhanced magnetic resonance angiography in pediatric patients using sensitivity encoding. J Magn Reson Imaging 2003;17(5): 559–64.

55. Chung T. Magnetic resonance angiography of the body in pediatric patients: experience with a contrast-enhanced time-resolved technique. Pediatr Radiol 2005;35(1):3–10.

56. Zhang HL, Kent KC, Bush HL, et al. Soft tissue enhancement on time-resolved peripheral magnetic resonance angiography. J Magn Reson Imaging 2004;19(5):590–7.

MR Imaging of Thoracic Veins

Navid Rahmani, MD, Charles S. White, MD*

KEYWORDS

- MR imaging • Magnetic • Thoracic veins
- Congenital • Vessels

MR imaging is an excellent imaging modality for identifying and characterizing the thoracic veins. These vessels include, but are not limited to, the inferior and superior vena cava (SVC), the brachiocephalic veins, and the pulmonary veins. Typical MR imaging sequences include black and bright blood sequences, which have traditionally been spin-echo and gradient-echo sequences, respectively.[1] These sequences have been largely replaced with double inversion recovery (IR) and steady-state free precession (SSFP) sequences because of faster image acquisition in the former and better internal contrast in the latter.

The authors review the classic and newer MR imaging techniques for the evaluation of the thoracic veins and provide a description of the normal appearance of the veins on these sequences. They also describe various thoracic vein congenital and acquired diseases.

MR IMAGING TECHNIQUES

MR imaging sequences used to evaluate the thoracic vessels and the heart can be generically divided into black and bright blood sequences.

Multislice T1-weighted spin-echo sequences have traditionally been used as the primary dark blood sequence for evaluating the thoracic vessels. The sequence is based on the signal void produced by the flowing and constantly moving blood.[2] These sequences can be performed with cardiac gating to reduce motion artifact, especially for vessels located near the heart. The larger vessels in the upper chest, which are more removed from the heart, can be evaluated without cardiac gating. Cardiac-gated T1 spin-echo sequences should

have the repetition time set to approximately 85% to 90% of the patient's R-to-R interval. Consequently, they are highly dependent on the heart rate.[3] The echo time is sufficiently short to produce the desired T1 weighting but long enough to prevent loss of signal void.[1]

Black blood sequences are excellent for anatomic delineation between the blood vessels and the adjacent structures; however, flow-related enhancement of unsaturated blood and respiratory motion artifact are potential limitations of this sequence. Enhancement of unsaturated blood results in increased blood signal, decreasing contrast between the vessels and the adjacent structures. Saturation bands outside the field of view have been used to reduce flow-related enhancement. Respiratory compensation algorithm or navigator echo pulses based on diaphragmatic motion can minimize respiratory motion artifact.[4]

Recently, multislice T1-weighted spin-echo sequences have been replaced largely by double IR sequences,[5] which are T2-weighted dark blood sequences with longer repetition times covering two heartbeats. Advantages include faster image acquisition within one breath-hold, thus reducing respiratory motion artifact.

Bright blood sequences, in which inflowing blood is displayed as white, are a critical supplement to the black blood sequences for evaluation of the thoracic veins. They have generally been gradient-echo sequences. Fast image acquisitions and the ability to acquire physiologic information are some of the advantages of the bright blood sequences. Additionally, images obtained through the different phases of the cardiac cycle on the

Department of Radiology, University of Maryland Medical Center, 22 S. Greene Street, Baltimore, MD 21201, USA
* Corresponding author.
E-mail address: cwhite@umm.edu (C.S. White).

Magn Reson Imaging Clin N Am 16 (2008) 249–262
doi:10.1016/j.mric.2008.02.017

mri.theclinics.com

gated studies can be viewed in a cine format to illustrate cardiac motion. Turbulent flow can also be recognized on these sequences, and is an important diagnostic clue in the setting of vessel stenosis or regurgitation through a cardiac valve. Turbulent flow is seen as loss of signal in the midst of bright inflowing blood.[5]

Gradient-echo techniques are also valuable for determining quantitative information regarding blood flow and velocity by using phase-encoded or phase-contrast sequences. Velocity and direction are encoded in every pixel of the images on these sequences, allowing measurement of velocity, magnitude, and direction of blood flow.[1]

Gradient-echo imaging, also known as MR angiographic imaging or time-of-flight (TOF) imaging, is based on the concept of flow-related enhancement of proton spins entering an imaging slice. The images can be displayed using maximum intensity projection (MIP) reconstruction. A ray-tracing technique is used to construct a three-dimensional (3D) data set, analogous to conventional angiography, allowing visualization from multiple planes. Arterial inflow is usually nulled by using presaturation bands, which allows evaluation of the relevant thoracic veins on MIP images.[4] Multiple thin imaging slices are obtained in two-dimensional TOF, in contrast to 3D TOF, in which a volume of images is obtained simultaneously. Three-dimensional TOF demonstrates greater spatial resolution. Its major limitation is the loss of signal with a thick volume of images and slow-flowing blood.

Contrast-enhanced gradient-echo images can also be obtained using intravascular gadolinium administration. Gadolinium increases image signal-to-noise ratio by means of T1 shortening; therefore, artifacts resulting from slow flow are minimized.[6,7] Three-dimensional MR angiography following gadolinium injection has been shown to be a valuable tool for studying thoracic vessels. In a study evaluating pulmonary veins on MR imaging, Pilleul and Merchant[8] demonstrated that 3D MR angiography showed a significant advantage over spin-echo MR imaging in identifying normal pulmonary veins. All four pulmonary veins were identified on spin-echo imaging in only 55% of the 40 patients they studied. In contrast, they identified all four pulmonary veins in 92.5% of patients on 3D MR angiography. Recently, reports of a rare condition, nephrogenic systemic fibrosis, have led to concern about using gadolinium-based contrast agents in patients who have renal compromise.

SSFP sequences represent a recent advance and produce bright blood sequences. These sequences demonstrate even greater contrast between the blood pool and adjacent structures and they have largely replaced older gradient-echo images because of desirable features such as speed, contrast, and signal-to-noise ratio. Limitations of this type of sequence are related to its extreme sensitivity to field inhomogeneity, which can be seen in the setting of metallic artifacts. Image quality can be significantly degraded secondary to these artifacts, particularly when using 3-T magnets. SSFP is also less sensitive to turbulent flow in the context of stenotic vessels or abnormal valves, possibly resulting in less accurate studies. As a result, it may be prudent to perform a traditional gradient-echo sequence for detecting subtle flow abnormalities or in the presence of overwhelming artifacts due to field inhomogeneity.[9]

NORMAL THORACIC VEINS

A brief review of the normal embryogenesis of the systemic and pulmonary venous system in the thorax can aid in the understanding of the complex congenital diseases described later.

The embryonic paired anterior and posterior cardinal veins give rise to the systemic thoracic veins. The right anterior cardinal vein forms the SVC by anastomosing with the left anterior cardinal vein through a bridging vessel persisting as the left brachiocephalic vein. The distal aspect of the left anterior cardinal vein, also known as the left common cardinal vein, persists as the coronary sinus, whereas the proximal portion of the left anterior cardinal vein normally involutes. The right posterior cardinal vein gives rise to the root of the azygos vein. The left posterior cardinal vein degenerates.

The supracardinal system gives rise to the inferior part of the azygos vein and the hemiazygos vein, and the upper portion of the inferior vena cava (IVC). The more caudal IVC above the renal veins is derived from the subcardinal venous system.[1] The right vitelline vein, which embryologically drains the yolk sac, the gastrointestinal system, and the portal circulation, also forms part of the IVC. Thus, the embryogenesis of the IVC is constructed through multiple differing venous systems.

A bulge at the sinoatrial region of the heart during the fourth week of embryogenesis gives rise to the pulmonary venous system, which eventually loses its connection to the cardinal veins and is integrated with the left atrium. The most common pulmonary venous anatomy consists of two superior and two inferior pulmonary veins on each side of the left atrium. The left upper lobe, including the lingula, drains into the left superior pulmonary vein. The middle and right upper lobes drain into the right superior pulmonary vein. The lower lobes are connected to the inferior pulmonary veins on their respective sides.[10] The configuration of normal pulmonary venous anatomy has substantial variation. Mansour and colleagues[11] demonstrated that only 56% of the 105 patients they studied with MR imaging had the typical pattern of four pulmonary veins; 29% of the patients had five pulmonary veins, and 17% had a common left pulmonary venous trunk. A smaller study of 58 patients found that the most common atypical variation of the pulmonary veins, which was found in 16% of the patients, involved three right and two left pulmonary veins. The third right vein drained the right middle lobe in this group.[12]

The larger caliber veins are well seen on the basic dark blood sequences. McMurdo and colleagues[13] studied 25 patients and demonstrated that the vena cava and the brachiocephalic, jugular, and azygos veins are visible on all the axial images that included the relevant vessel. The smaller veins, including the hemiazygos and the internal mammary veins, had variable visualizations among the MR studies. Cardiac-gated studies allowed better identification of these smaller vessels.

Usually, the ostia of the pulmonary veins are well visualized on dark blood sequences. Masui and colleagues[14] demonstrated that in 88% of the 56 patients they studied, all four pulmonary venous connections were visualized with dark blood spin-echo sequences. Additionally, at least three of the four pulmonary vein ostia were identified in all their patients. Imaging accuracy is undoubtedly improved with the newer dark blood double IR sequences.

Because of the limited spatial resolution of MR imaging, identification of the segmental and subsegmental branches of the pulmonary veins may be difficult. In addition, on dark blood sequences, the low signal within the branching vessels blends in with the surrounding low-signal, air-containing lung parenchyma, making identification of the distal branching pulmonary veins even more difficult. Bright blood sequences, however, have the advantage of the internal image contrast, which refers to vessel intraluminal high signal intensity against the low signal intensity of the adjacent structures such as myocardium and air within the lung parenchyma.[1] SSFP sequences have further augmented the temporal and spatial resolution of bright blood sequences relative to gradient echo, allowing easier identification of the smaller thoracic veins (**Fig. 1**).

It is important to be aware of some pitfalls when evaluating normal thoracic veins. The azygos arch can sometimes have an invisible lateral wall because both margins are adjacent to air-filled lung on dark blood sequences. For similar reasons, an azygos fissure can be imperceptible on spin-echo images. The anterior wall of the inferior left pulmonary vein can sometimes insert into the left atrium more medial than usual and abut the posterior wall of the left atrium, giving the impression of a left atrial nodule or mass.[1]

CONGENITAL ANOMALIES

White and colleagues[15] have proposed a classification scheme separating the thoracic vein congenital abnormalities into systemic and pulmonary divisions. The classification scheme is shown in **Box 1**.

DIAGNOSTIC ALGORITHM OF CONGENITAL THORACIC VENOUS ANOMALIES

Patients who have suspicion of thoracic venous anomalies are usually first evaluated with multidetector CT or ultrasound. The advantages of

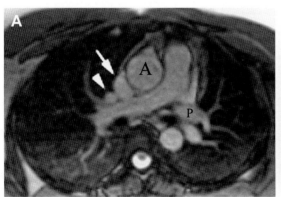
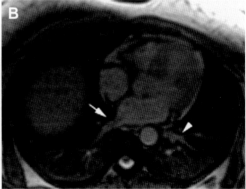

Fig. 1. Normal anatomy of the pulmonary veins. (*A*) Axial bright blood MR image at the level of the right pulmonary artery demonstrates the right superior pulmonary vein (*arrowhead*) lateral to the SVC (*arrow*) and anterior to the right pulmonary artery. The left superior pulmonary vein (P) is posterior to the main pulmonary artery, and (A) is the aorta. (*B*) Axial bright blood image through the left atrium demonstrates the right inferior pulmonary vein (*arrow*) entry into the left atrium. Portions of the left inferior pulmonary vein are also noted (*arrowhead*).

Box 1
Classification scheme for thoracic vein congenital anomalies

I. Systemic venous anomalies

  A. Anomalies of the superior vena cava

    1. Left SVC

      a. Connection to coronary sinus

      b. Connection to coronary sinus, unroofed coronary sinus

      c. Persistent left SVC terminating in left atrium

    2. Right SVC

      a. Absent right SVC with persistent left SVC

      b. Right SVC connecting to left atrium

      c. Aneurysmal right SVC

      d. Anomalous low insertion

  B. Anomalies of IVC

    1. Intrahepatic interruption of IVC with azygous continuation

    2. Intrahepatic interruption of IVC with hemizygous continuation to left SVC

    3. Anomalous connection of IVC to left atrium

    4. Anomalous connection of IVC to coronary sinus

    5. Anomalous high insertion of IVC to right atrium

  C. Miscellaneous thoracic venous disorders

    1. Absent left brachiocephalic vein with venous return through left superior intercostal vein

    2. Anomalous hepatic venous connection to right atrium

    3. Anomalous hepatic venous connection to left atrium

II. Pulmonary venous anomalies

  A. Total anomalous pulmonary venous connection or return

    1. Supracardiac

      a. Left innominate vein

      b. Right SVC

      c. Azygos vein

    2. Cardiac

      a. Coronary sinus

      b. Right atrium

    3. Infracardiac

      a. Portal vein or tributary

      b. Ductus venosus

      c. IVC

      d. Left gastric vein

    4. Mixed

  B. Partial anomalous pulmonary venous return

    1. Right veins

      a. SVC

      b. Right atrium

      c. Both

    2. Right veins to IVC (scimitar)

    3. Right veins to azygos vein

    4. Left veins

  C. Pulmonary lesions associated with anomalous pulmonary venous connection

    1. Bronchopulmonary sequestration

      a. Extralobar

      b. Interlobar (rare)

    2. Pulmonary arteriovenous malformation

    3. Congenital cystic adenomatoid malformation

---

multidetector CT scanning include noninvasiveness, excellent spatial resolution, and easy accessibility. It also allows for concomitant evaluation of the lungs. Ionizing radiation, especially in the pediatric patient population, is the main disadvantage. The advantages of echocardiography include noninvasiveness and fast and direct visualization of venous anomalies in most instances. Occasionally, however, evaluation of venous anomalies can be limited because of lack of penetration of the ultrasound beam through the lungs, bones, and other factors related to patient body habitus.[1]

Angiography provides excellent evaluation of complex thoracic venous anomalies. Its disadvantages include invasiveness and the use of ionizing radiation. The use of intravascular contrast material can also limit the use of angiography and multidetector CT in certain situations.

The combination of echocardiography and CT scan usually provides adequate information regarding thoracic venous anomalies. However, in certain situations, MR imaging is performed to delineate further the extent of the venous abnormalities and concomitant congenital cardiac anomalies, which may not be adequately documented on the other studies. MR imaging is often favored in the pediatric population because of its lack of ionizing radiation. However, the prolonged imaging time may preclude this modality as an option in some pediatric patients or may require the use of sedation.

Although the algorithm for evaluating suspected thoracic venous anomalies should be individualized, evaluation of these patients can be separated roughly into systemic and pulmonary divisions.

At times, systemic thoracic vein congenital anomalies can manifest in conjunction with other cardiovascular abnormalities. Most patients, however, are asymptomatic. In contrast, patients who have pulmonary venous anomalies often present early in life because of pulmonary venous flow obstruction or physiologic shunting resulting in cyanosis. These patients may also have associated intracardiac defects.[15]

Asymptomatic systemic venous anomalies may come to attention as a result of an abnormal contour on a chest radiograph. These patients are usually evaluated further with CT. In many instances, systemic anomalies are noted incidentally on CT performed for other reasons. Echocardiography can also be the initial study for detecting anomalous systemic veins. MR imaging, however, can be performed to delineate the course of the anomalous vein and to characterize concomitant cardiac and noncardiac abnormalities.

Symptomatic patients who have pulmonary venous anomalies usually receive their initial diagnosis on echocardiography because they present during infancy or earlier in life than those who have systemic venous anomalies. Again, MR imaging can delineate the extent of the anomalous veins and other associated congenital diseases. In addition, functional analysis and hemodynamic information can be obtained through MR imaging.[1]

CONGENITAL SYSTEMIC THORACIC VENOUS ANOMALIES
Anomalies of the Superior Vena Cava

A common anomaly involving the SVC is a left-sided SVC, which occurs in 0.3% of normal individuals and in 4.4% of patients who have congenital heart disease.[16–18] It is the persistence of the left anterior cardinal vein that results in the left-sided SVC. The vessel is seen lateral to the aortic arch and anterior to the left hilum, usually draining into the right atrium by way of an enlarged coronary sinus (**Fig. 2**). In rare instances, the anomalous SVC drains into the left atrium with the physiologic sequela of a right-to-left shunt (Raghib complex). These latter patients have a substantially higher incidence of concomitant congenital heart disease (**Fig. 3**).[1]

This anomaly is sometimes detected following insertion of a central venous catheter or pacemaker, where the tip is visualized in an unusual location on radiographs corresponding to the left SVC. Persistent left-sided SVC should also be considered following the diagnosis of a dilated coronary sinus noted on transthoracic echocardiogram.[19,20]

Patients who have left-sided SVC have an absent right SVC in 10% to 18% of cases. Patients who have bilateral SVCs usually have a small-caliber right SVC. The left brachiocephalic vein is absent in 65% of patients who have left SVC.[18,19] Gonzalez-Juanatey and colleagues[20] studied 10 patients who had persistent left SVC, 5 of whom had absent left brachiocephalic veins. In their study, 3 patients had an absent right

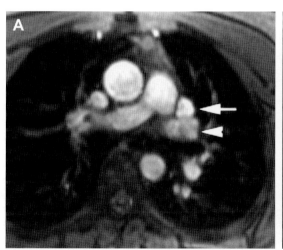
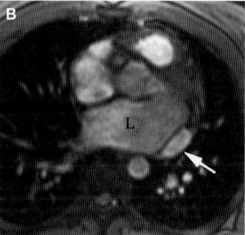

Fig. 2. Persistent left SVC. (*A*) Axial bright blood image through the level of the main pulmonary artery demonstrates two vessels, the left SVC (*arrow*) and left superior pulmonary vein (*arrowhead*), anterior to the left main stem and left upper lobe bronchi and lateral to the main pulmonary artery and aorta. (*B*) More caudal axial bright blood image through the left atrium (L) demonstrates an enlarged coronary sinus (*arrow*) that subsequently drains the left SVC into the right atrium.

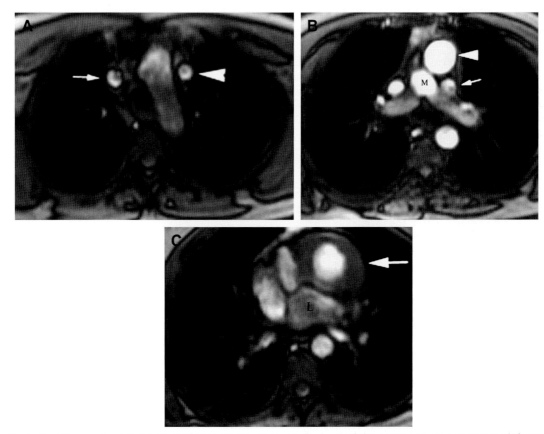

Fig. 3. Raghib complex. (*A*) Axial bright blood image through the level of the aortic arch demonstrates a left SVC (*arrowhead*). A right SVC is also present (*arrow*). (*B*) Caudal axial image demonstrates the left SVC (*arrow*) immediately anterior to the left pulmonary artery. The left SVC enters the left atrial appendage immediately caudal to this axial image, consistent with the Raghib complex. The ascending aorta (*arrowhead*) is anterior and to the left of the main pulmonary artery (*M*), compatible with transposition of great vessels. (*C*) Axial image through the left atrium (*L*) demonstrates the connection between the morphologic right ventricle, defined by the infundibulum (*arrow*), and the ascending aorta, compatible with the diagnosis of corrected transposition of the great vessels.

SVC, and predictably, these patients also demonstrated enlarged coronary sinuses.

Atrial septal defect and azygos continuation of IVC are other congenital abnormalities that can coexist with left-sided SVC.[17]

Isolated anomalies of a right SVC are rare. Right SVC may drain into the left atrium, have a low insertion into the right atrium, or be congenitally dilated.[21–24] Right SVC can also be congenitally dilated and can be detected as an incidental mediastinal mass. SVC thrombosis or an association with cystic hygromas has been reported in patients who have congenitally dilated SVC.[25]

MR imaging is excellent in delineating the full extent of the anomalous left SVC, including its origin and termination. The origin is usually at the confluence of the left internal jugular and the left subclavian veins, whereas its termination is within one of the atria. MR imaging also allows the detection of associated anomalies, which may involve the right SVC, the left brachiocephalic vein, or the heart.[1]

Anomalies of the Inferior Vena Cava

It is surprising that anomalies of the IVC are uncommon because embryogenesis of this vessel requires coherent development of four separate vascular systems, as described earlier.

The most common anomaly to involve the IVC is azygos continuation of the IVC. This anomaly is defined by interruption of the intrahepatic IVC. As a result, blood is directed posteriorly toward an enlarged azygos vein along the right paraspinal location draining into the SVC.[18] On MR imaging, the intrahepatic IVC is absent, whereas an enlarged azygos or hemiazygos vessel is present, coursing superiorly along the spine. The enlarged azygos vein lies in its normal anatomic position, posterior to the heart, and subsequently arches anteriorly over the right main stem bronchus to drain into the SVC (**Fig. 4**). The intrahepatic veins drain into the right atrium directly by way of the suprahepatic IVC.[26]

Interrupted IVC can occasionally be associated with hemiazygos continuation, where the blood is directed into an enlarged hemiazygos vein along the left paraspinal location, draining into the azygos vein by crossing from left to right at T8-T9. The azygos vein then drains into the SVC. The hemiazygos vein can also drain into a persistent enlarged left SVC.[25]

Azygos continuation of IVC results from the persistence of the right supracardinal vein and the lack of the development of the suprarenal component of the subcardinal vein. Concomitant associated anomalies are common and may include heterotaxia syndromes, particularly polysplenia and persistent left SVC.[27]

Other rare anomalies involving the IVC include connection to the coronary sinus or left atrium, or high insertion into the right atrium. Communication of the IVC with the left atrium results in a variable degree of cyanosis because of the high degree of physiologic shunting.[28]

Miscellaneous Systemic Thoracic Venous Anomalies

Other rare systemic thoracic venous anomalies that can be studied with MR imaging include the retroaortic innominate vein, characterized by the left brachiocephalic vein coursing posterior to the ascending aorta. This anomaly can be associated with abnormalities of the aortic arch.[29] The absent left brachiocephalic vein is another rare thoracic venous anomaly. These patients divert their left upper extremity venous return through the left superior intercostal vein to the azygos system. Abnormal hepatic venous connections to the right or left atrium have also been reported.[30]

CONGENITAL PULMONARY VENOUS ANOMALIES
Total Anomalous Pulmonary Venous Return

Total anomalous pulmonary venous connection or return (TAPVR) usually manifests in infancy, typically as cyanosis during the first year of life. It is characterized by complete pulmonary venous return to the systemic venous system. It is invariably associated with a right-to-left shunt, usually an interatrial shunt. Asplenia is also a common association, although the anomaly is more often isolated. TAPVR accounts for about 2% of all congenital heart disease.[31] Failure of the embryologic common pulmonary vein to join the primitive sinus venosus in conjunction with persistent communication between the pulmonary venous plexus and the cardinal, cardiac, or portal venous system gives rise to TAPVR.[32,33]

TAPVR can be divided into three broad categories, which include supracardiac, cardiac, and infracardiac types. In the supracardiac variant, which is the most common, the anomalous pulmonary vein communicates with the left brachiocephalic vein in 80% of cases. In the remainder of cases, the pulmonary venous drainage is directly into the right SVC (**Fig. 5**) or the azygos vein.[1]

The anomalous vessel in the cardiac type drains into the coronary sinus in about 80% of cases and into the right atrium in about 20%. Often, the cardiac variant of TAPVR has several distinct draining veins.[1]

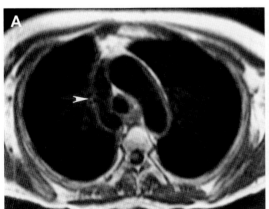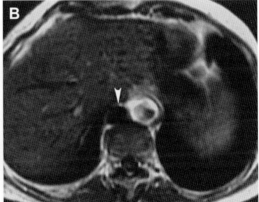

Fig. 4. Azygos continuation of the IVC. (*A*) Axial black blood image demonstrates a dilated azygos arch (*arrowhead*). (*B*) Axial T1-weighted MR image shows the dilated azygos vein (*arrowhead*) to the right of the descending aorta. Note the absence of the intrahepatic IVC. (*From* White CS. MR imaging of the thoracic veins. Magn Reson Imaging Clin N Am 2000;8:17–32; with permission.)

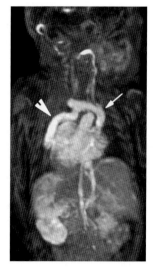

Fig. 5. TAPVR (supracardiac type). Postgadolinium coronal MIP image demonstrates the anomalous pulmonary vein (*arrowhead*) draining into the brachiocephalic vein and, subsequently, the left SVC (*arrow*) in a patient who has situs inversus. Patient also has a single ventricle and a single atrium (not shown). Note abdominal situs with left-sided liver.

In the subdiaphragmatic of infracardiac, the anomalous vessel communicates most commonly with the portal vein and occasionally with the ductus venosus, IVC, or left gastric vein. Pulmonary venous congestion is noted as an early manifestation in this latter subtype, caused by obstruction of the venous flow through the diaphragm.[34] A mixed type of TAPVR may also occur, consisting of some combination of the previous three variants.

At times, TAPVR can be diagnosed accurately with echocardiography. CT, particularly with electrocardiography gating, may demonstrate the

course of the aberrant vessel; however, complete evaluation may occasionally be difficult. Visualization of the pulmonary veins into the left atrium can also be suboptimal. MR imaging can be an excellent adjunct in these circumstances. In addition to demonstrating the anatomy, direction of flow within these anomalous veins and the site of interatrial shunts or other cardiac abnormalities can be ascertained on phase-contrast sequences.

Partial Anomalous Pulmonary Venous Return

In contrast to TAPVR, partial anomalous pulmonary venous return (PAPVR) or connection commonly leads to clinical symptoms at a later age and is often an incidental finding. It can be an isolated finding or associated with other intracardiac defects.[35] A frequency of 0.5% to 0.7% of PAPVR has been reported in patients who have congenital heart disease.[36,37] Physiologically, this anomaly can be viewed as a left-to-right shunt, and patients usually present with clinical symptoms similar to atrial septal defect.

The most common type of PAPVR is a right upper pulmonary vein connecting to the right atrium or the SVC. This type of anomaly has a high association with the sinus venosus type of atrial septal defect (**Fig. 6**). A less common type occurs when the anomalous right pulmonary vein drains into the IVC. On chest radiography, this anomalous vessel has a characteristic tubular or curvilinear scimitar appearance at the right lung base as it courses toward the right hemidiaphragm before draining into the IVC. Based on the appearance of the vessel, the term "scimitar syndrome" is used to describe the anomaly, which is also associated with a hypogenetic or small right lung. Associated cardiac defects, usually atrial

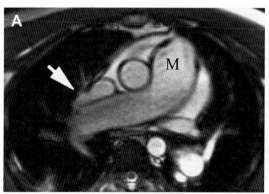

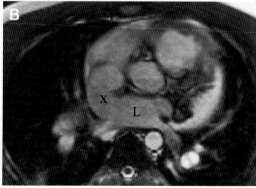

Fig. 6. Right upper lobe PAPVR with sinus venosus atrial septal defect. (*A*) Axial bright blood image through the main pulmonary artery (M) demonstrates the anomalous pulmonary vein (*arrow*) connecting to the SVC. Note enlarged main and bilateral pulmonary arteries due to left-to-right shunt and increased flow. (*B*) Axial bright blood image caudal to the previous image through the left atrium (L) demonstrates sinus venosus atrial septal defect (X) between the superior aspects of the atria.

septal defects, have been reported in about 25% of patients who have the scimitar syndrome.[38,39]

One third of PAPVRs involve the left pulmonary veins.[33] PAPVR involving the left upper lobe, which is more common in the adult population, can be seen as an anomalous vessel lateral to the aortic arch, known as a vertical vein (**Fig. 7A**). This structure can be confused with persistent left-sided SVC on axial images.[19] However, the direction of blood flow in PAPVR is cranial because the vessel drains into the left brachiocephalic vein. In persistent left-sided SVC, the direction of blood flow is caudal because the left SVC usually connects to the coronary sinus (**Fig. 7B**). In addition, as one proceeds caudally, the anomalous vein in PAPVR branches within the lung parenchyma, whereas a left SVC enlarges within the mediastinum as it courses toward the coronary sinus.

The advantages of MR imaging for the evaluation of PAPVR are similar to those described for TAPVR. Bright blood and, to a lesser degree, black blood sequences can be used to demonstrate the anomalous vessel with great accuracy. White and colleagues demonstrated in a study of 14 patients that 79% and 93% of anomalous pulmonary veins were identified on spin-echo and gradient-echo images, respectively.[39]

Findings that distinguish left upper lobe PAPVR from a persistent left SVC include absence of the left superior pulmonary vein anterior to the left main stem bronchus in PAPVR. Instead, in left-sided SVC, two vessels are present anterior

to the left main stem bronchus. The two vessels are the normal left superior pulmonary vein and the persistent left SVC.[25] Another differentiating clue is a normal, or probably dilated, left innominate vein and SVC seen in the left upper lobe PAPVR due to increased flow. Dilated coronary sinus in combination with a small or absent left innominate vein can be seen in persistent left SVC.[19] In PAPVR, the left upper lobe vein communicates with the anomalous vertical vein in the aortopulmonary window. The direction of blood flow on phase-contrast MR can also be used to differentiate the two entities.[1]

PULMONARY LESIONS ASSOCIATED WITH ABNORMAL PULMONARY VEINS

Pulmonary lesions known to be associated with abnormal pulmonary venous return include bronchopulmonary sequestration, particularly the extralobar type, and cystic adenomatoid malformation.[40] An enlarged pulmonary vein is seen in pulmonary arteriovenous malformation, which can be adequately demonstrated with MR imaging.[41,42]

A pulmonary varix is characterized by a focal dilatation of a pulmonary vein. An acquired form is often associated with mitral valve disease. The most commonly affected vessels are the right lower or left upper lobe pulmonary veins. When congenital, it is believed to be caused by incomplete fusion of the primitive pulmonary plexus

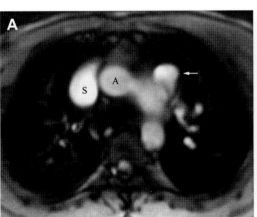
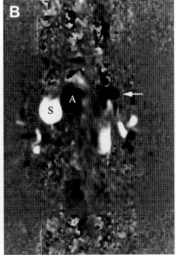

Fig. 7. Left upper lobe PAPVR. (*A*) Axial gradient-echo image demonstrates the anomalous left upper lobe pulmonary vein (*arrow*) lateral to the aortopulmonary window. The SVC (S) is dilated because of increased flow. A, aorta. (*B*) Axial phase-contrast MR image demonstrates low signal within the anomalous left pulmonary vein (*arrow*), indicating cephalic flow, distinguishing this anomaly from left SVC. Note similar flow direction within the ascending aorta (A). S, SVC. (*From* White CS. MR imaging of the thoracic veins. Magn Reson Imaging Clin N Am 2000;8:17–32; with permission.)

and the pulmonary vein. MR imaging may demonstrate a dilated vascular structure in continuity with the pulmonary vein. The low blood flow nature of the anomaly is also evident on black and bright blood sequences.[43,44]

ACQUIRED ABNORMALITIES OF THE THORACIC VENOUS SYSTEM

As with any other organ system, the thoracic venous vasculature can be affected by neoplasm, infection, thrombosis, trauma, and hemodynamic effects.[1] The vessels may become occluded or stenosed. Iatrogenic causes of stenoses or occlusion include atrial fibrillation radiofrequency ablation, which affects the pulmonary veins, as will be described. These vascular abnormalities and their causes can usually be demonstrated adequately on MR imaging.

Systemic Veins

SVC obstruction is one of the most common entities within the acquired thoracic systemic venous diseases and is a common indication for MR imaging. Neoplasm, most commonly lung cancer, followed by lymphoma or metastatic breast cancer, has been historically thought of as the most common cause. In an evaluation of 86 patients who had SVC obstruction diagnosed in the 1960s and 1970s, Parish and colleagues[45] demonstrated that malignant lesions accounted for 78% of the obstructions, with less than 10% of cases resulting from venous thrombosis. Recently, with the increased widespread use of central venous catheters, the frequency of

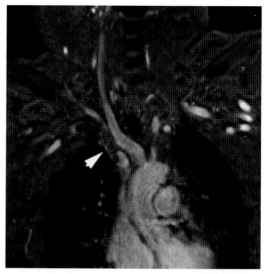

Fig. 8. SVC thrombus. Coronal MRV two-dimensional TOF demonstrates a filling defect (*arrow*) extending from the right brachiocephalic vein to the SVC, consistent with thrombus in a patient who has compromised renal function presenting with facial swelling. Contrast-enhanced MR imaging was not performed because of concern about nephrogenic systemic fibrosis.

nonneoplastic or thrombotic SVC obstruction has dramatically increased (**Fig. 8**). Other nonmalignant causes of SVC obstruction include fibrosing mediastinitis (**Fig. 9**).[1]

SVC obstruction can usually be visualized and studied adequately with contrast-enhanced CT. The degree of vessel luminal narrowing and the cause are well demonstrated with CT. Collateral

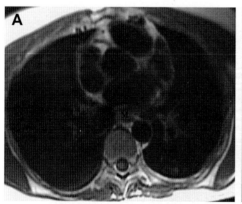 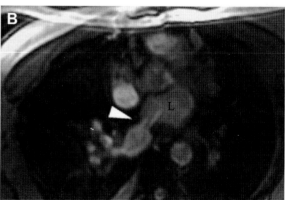

Fig. 9. Fibrosing mediastinitis with pulmonary vein occlusion and stenosis. (*A*) Axial T1-weighted black blood image through the left atrium shows a dilated right inferior pulmonary vein entering the left atrium. The left inferior pulmonary vein and the upper lobe pulmonary veins were occluded. The lower part of the fibrotic mass (M) is visible behind the left atrium. (*B*) Axial gradient-echo MR image through the left atrium (L) shows the dilated right inferior pulmonary vein with mild ostial narrowing (*arrowhead*). Left inferior pulmonary vein is absent. (*From* White CS. MR imaging of the thoracic veins. Magn Reson Imaging Clin N Am 2000;8:17–32; with permission.)

vessels can also be seen as stronger evidence for hemodynamically significant stenosis. CT can also demonstrate the presence of mediastinal and hilar calcifications, which may be seen with fibrosing mediastinitis. The most important limitation to CT scanning for suspected SVC obstruction is the need for administration of intravenous contrast. Therefore, MR imaging has its role in evaluating SVC obstruction in the presence of renal compromise or allergies to iodinated contrast.[1] Weinreb and colleagues[46] studied 14 patients who had SVC obstruction with MR imaging demonstrating the exact location of the obstruction in these patients. Specific causes were noted in 2 patients, which were teratoma and postradiation fibrosis. Dilated collateral vessels were demonstrated in 4 patients. This information was collected without the use of gradient-echo techniques or bright blood sequences. One would expect even better results with advanced bright blood sequences, which delineate flow more optimally. The use of these bright blood sequences would allow one to differentiate slow flow from thrombosis and to show the extent of stenosis and collateral vessels.[47]

The recently described risk for nephrogenic systemic fibrosis associated with gadolinium has limited the use of MR imaging contrast in patients who have elevated creatinine; however, valuable information can be obtained even from unenhanced MR imaging sequences, including TOF MR angiography (see **Fig. 8**).

Primary neoplasms of the thoracic systemic veins are rare. The most common primary neoplasm is leiomyosarcoma. Secondary tumors, commonly renal cell carcinomas, can extend into the systemic veins by extension into the IVC and the right atrium. The amount of venous involvement can be readily determined with the use of MR imaging.[48] Other tumors that can have a similar growth pattern include hepatocellular carcinoma, adrenal carcinoma, Wilms tumor, and pancreatic carcinoma.[49] The extent of heart involvement, including myocardial penetration, can be evaluated with MR imaging, with substantial implications for treatment and prognosis.

Other thoracic systemic venous abnormalities that can be imaged with MR imaging include rare aneurysmal dilatation of the vessels and penetrating or blunt trauma.

Pulmonary Veins

Either MR imaging or CT can be used to assess the left atrium and the pulmonary veins in patients who have atrial fibrillation, who are being considered for radiofrequency ablation. Radiofrequency ablation of the left atrium and the pulmonary vein ostia has recently evolved into a commonly used therapy for atrial fibrillation that is refractory to antiarrhythmic medications.[50] The technique is based on the finding that more than 90% of atrial fibrillation initiation foci originate within the pulmonary veins. Consequently, MR imaging has recently assumed an important role in this therapy. MR imaging is used to provide accurate baseline preprocedural anatomic information about the left atrium and the pulmonary veins, and their variations (**Fig. 10**). Such baseline information, including the number and diameter of the pulmonary ostia, can provide a road map for the electrophysiologists to determine the type and size of catheters to use during the procedure. Other valuable information includes the left atrial dimension and the presence of left atrial thrombi. Contrast-enhanced pulmonary venous MR angiography with a T1-weighted 3D gradient-echo sequence can be used for pulmonary venous mapping.[51]

Postprocedural MR imaging can also provide valuable information. Pulmonary vein stenosis or thrombosis due to the application of radiofrequency energy is a well-known complication of radiofrequency ablation. Patients can present with shortness of breath, hemoptysis, or dyspnea. Controlled delivery of this energy to the ostial

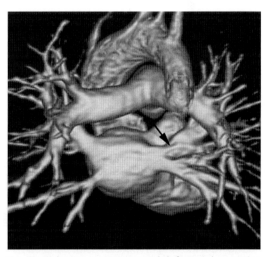

Fig. 10. Pulmonary venous and left atrial mapping with MR imaging. Volume-rendered gadolinium-enhanced MR image of the left atrium and pulmonary veins for preprocedural anatomic evaluation for atrial fibrillation radiofrequency ablation demonstrates two right and three left pulmonary veins. The smaller left pulmonary vein is marked with the arrow. (*Courtesy of* D. Bluemke, MD, PhD, Johns Hopkins Medical Institutions, Baltimore, MD.)

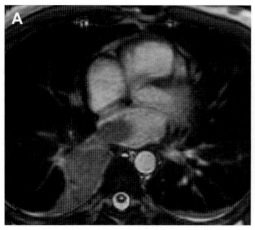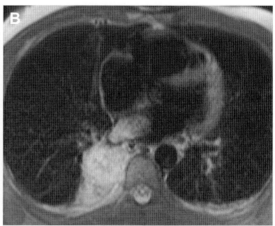

Fig. 11. Lung cancer with pulmonary venous infiltration. Axial bright (*A*) and black (*B*) blood sequences demonstrate a right posterior lung cancer with invasion into the right inferior pulmonary vein and extension into the left atrium.

segment of the pulmonary veins has shown decreased risk for pulmonary venous stenosis. The degree of stenosis relative to baseline can be demonstrated accurately with MR imaging. Anselme and colleagues[52] used MR imaging to show that up to 38% of pulmonary veins treated with radiofrequency ablation had mild ostial diameter reduction. Subsequent improvements in catheter technique appear to have decreased this number.

In addition to the above MR indications related to radiofrequency ablation, detection and evaluation of left atrial and pulmonary vein scar following radiofrequency ablation have been investigated. This application is based on the well-established concept that fibrotic tissue or scar demonstrates delayed hyperenhancement. Peters and colleagues[50] noted that delayed images of the left atrium and pulmonary vein ostia following injection of gadolinium demonstrated hyperenhancement in each of their patients. This information may guide subsequent radiofrequency ablation in patients who have recurrent arrhythmia. Scar morphology on MR imaging may also be useful for predicting atrial fibrillation recurrence.[51]

Other acquired conditions that involve the pulmonary veins include obstruction by neoplasm arising from the lung or mediastinum. Lung cancer can reach the left atrium by infiltrating the pulmonary veins (**Fig. 11**).

Similar to the systemic veins, fibrosing mediastinitis may involve the pulmonary veins and the left atrium. It may cause narrowing or occlusion of the vessels, resulting in pulmonary arterial hypertension (see **Fig. 9**). MR imaging is an effective modality to study the pulmonary veins and the left atrium in this condition to assess the degree of obstruction and to confirm the cause.[1]

SUMMARY

MR imaging is an excellent modality for the assessment of congenital and acquired abnormalities of the thoracic venous system, and is often used in conjunction with echocardiography, angiography, and CT to evaluate thoracic veins and delineate the extent of disease by providing excellent anatomic and physiologic information.

The classification system for thoracic venous anomalies proposed herein provides a construct for an organized approach to the diagnosis of thoracic venous anomalies on MR imaging.

REFERENCES

1. White CS. MR imaging of the thoracic veins. Magn Reson Imaging Clin N Am 2000;8:17–32.
2. Julsrud PR. Magnetic resonance imaging of the pulmonary arteries and veins. Semin Ultrasound CT MR 1990;11:184–205.
3. Poustchi-Amin M, Gutierez FR, Brown JJ, et al. How to plan and perform a cardiac MR imaging examination. Radiol Clin North Am 2004;42:497–514.
4. Felmlee JP, Ehman RL. Spatial presaturation: a method for suppressing flow artifacts and improving depiction of vascular anatomy in MR imaging. Radiology 1987;164:559–64.
5. Boiselle PM, White CS. New techniques in cardiothoracic imaging. New York: Informa Healthcare USA, Inc.; 2007. p. 81–2.

6. Gilfeather M, Roberts ED. Pulmonary MRA and venous MRV. Seminars of Interventional Radiology 1998;15:205–14.

7. Prince MR. Gadolinium-enhanced MR aortography. Radiology 1994;191:155–64.

8. Pilleul F, Merchant N. MRI of the pulmonary veins: comparison between 3D MR angiography and T1-weighted spin echo. J Comput Assist Tomogr 2000;24(5):683–7.

9. Lee VS. Cardiovascular MRI: physical principles to practical protocols. Philadelphia: Lippincott Williams and Wilkins; 2006. p. 293–5.

10. Burdorick NE, Mcdonald V, Flisak ME, et al. The pulmonary veins. Semin Roentgenol 1989;24:127–40.

11. Mansour M, Holmvang G, Sosnovik D, et al. Assessment of pulmonary vein anatomic variability by magnetic resonance imaging: implications for catheter ablation techniques for atrial fibrillation. J Cardiovasc Electrophysiol 2004;15(4):387–93.

12. Scharf C, Sneider M, Case I, et al. Anatomy of the pulmonary veins in patients with atrial fibrillation and effects of segmental ostial ablation analyzed by computed tomography. J Cardiovasc Electrophysiol 2003;14:150–5.

13. McMurdo KK, deGeer G, Webb WR, et al. Normal and occluded mediastinal veins: MR imaging. Radiology 1986;159:33–8.

14. Masui T, Seelos KC, Kersting-Sommerhoff BA, et al. Abnormalities of the pulmonary veins: evaluation with MR imaging and comparison with cardiac angiography and echocardiography. Radiology 1991;181:645–9.

15. White CS, Baffa JM, Haney PJ, et al. MR imaging of congenital anomalies of thoracic veins. Radiographics 1997;17:595–608.

16. Campbell M, Deuchar DC. The left-sided superior vena cava. Br Heart J 1994;16:423–39.

17. Cha EM, Khoury GH. Persistent left superior vena cava. Radiologic and clinical significance. Radiology 1972;103:375–81.

18. Webb WR, Gamsu G, Speckmen JM, et al. Computed tomographic demonstration of mediastinal venous anomalies. AJR Am J Roentgenol 1982;139:157–61.

19. Dillon EH, Camputaro C. Partial anomalous pulmonary venous drainage of the left upper lobe vs. duplication of the superior vena cava: distinction based on CT findings. AJR Am J Roentgenol 1993;160:375–8.

20. Gonzalez-Juanatey C, Testa A, Vidan J, et al. Persistent left superior vena cava draining into the coronary sinus: report of 10 cases and literature review. Clin Cardiol 2004;27(9):515–8.

21. Cormier MG, Yedlicka JW, Gray RJ, et al. Congenital anomalies of the superior vena cava: a CT study. Semin Roentgenol 1989;24:77–83.

22. Freedom RM, Schaffer MS, Rowe RD. Anomalous low insertion of right superior vena cava. Br Heart J 1982;48:601–3.

23. Modry DL, Hidvegi RS, La Fleche LR. Congenital saccular aneurysm of the superior vena cava. Ann Thorac Surg 1980;29:258–62.

24. Park HY, Summerer MH, Preuss K, et al. Anomalous drainage of the right superior vena cava into the left atrium. J Am Coll Cardiol 1983;2:358–62.

25. Demos TC, Posniak HV, Pierce KL, et al. Venous anomalies of the thorax. AJR Am J Roentgenol 2004;182(5):1139–50.

26. Kellman GM, Alpern MB, Sandler MA, et al. Computed tomography of vena caval anomalies with embryologic correlation. Radiographics 1988;8:533–56.

27. Winer-Muram HT. Adult presentation of heterotaxic syndromes and related complexes. J Thorac Imaging 1995;10:43–57.

28. Gardner DL, Cole L. Long survival with inferior cava into the left atrium. Br Heart J 1955;17:93–7.

29. Minami M, Noda M, Kawauchi N, et al. Post-aortic innominate vein: radiological assessment and pathogenesis. Clin Radiol 1993;48:52–6.

30. Fisher MR, Hricak H, Higgins CB. Magnetic resonance imaging of developmental venous anomalies. AJR Am J Roentgenol 1985;145:705–9.

31. Kastler B, Livolsi A, Germain P, et al. Contribution of MR in supracardiac total anomalous pulmonary venous drainage. Pediatr Radiol 1992;22:262–3.

32. Oropeza G, Hernandez FA, Callard GM, et al. Anomalous pulmonary venous drainage of the left upper lobe. Ann Thorac Surg 1970;9:180–5.

33. Pennes DR, Ellis JH. Anomalous pulmonary venous drainage in relation to left superior vena cava and coronary sinus. Radiology 1986;159:23–4.

34. Livolsi A, Kastler B, Marcellin L, et al. MR diagnosis of subdiaphragmatic anomalous pulmonary venous drainage in a newborn. J Comput Assist Tomogr 1991;15:1051–3.

35. Vesely TM, Julsrud PR, Brown JJ, et al. MR imaging of partial anomalous pulmonary venous connections. J Comput Assist Tomogr 1991;15:752–6.

36. Healey JE. An antomic survey of anomalous pulmonary veins: their clinical significance. J Thorac Cardiovasc Surg 1952;23:433–44.

37. Kalke BR, Carlson RG, Ferlic RM, et al. Partial anomalous pulmonary venous connections. Am J Cardiol 1967;20:91–101.

38. Baxter R, McFadden PM, Gradman M, et al. Scimitar syndrome: cine magnetic resonance imaging demonstration of anomalous pulmonary venous drainage. Ann Thorac Surg 1990;50:121–3.

39. Kivelitz DE, Scheer I, Taupitz M. Scimitar syndrome: diagnosis with MR angiography. AJR Am J Roentgenol 1999;172:1700.

40. Felker RE, Tonkin ILD. Imaging of pulmonary sequestration. AJR Am J Roentgenol 1990;154:241–9.

41. White CS, Templeton PA, Pais OS, et al. Anomalies of pulmonary veins: usefulness of spin-echo and

gradient-echo imaging. AJR Am J Roentgenol 1998; 170:1365–8.

42. Donovan CB, Edelman RR, Vrachliotis TG, et al. Bronchopulmonary sequestration with MR angiographic evaluation: a case report. Angiology 1994; 14:239–44.

43. Bhaktaram VJ, Asirvatham S, Sebastian C, et al. Large pulmonary vein varix diagnosed by echocardiography: an unusual site for thrombus in atrial fibrillation. J Am Soc Echocardiogr 1998;11:213–5.

44. Wildenhain PM, Boureleas EC. Pulmonary varix: magnetic resonance findings. Cathet Cardiovasc Diagn 1991;24:268–70.

45. Parish JM, Marschke RF, Dines DE, et al. Etiologic considerations in superior vena cava syndrome. Mayo Clin Proc 1981;56:407–13.

46. Weinreb JC, Mootz A, Cohen JM. MRI evaluation of mediastinal and thoracic inlet venous obstruction. AJR Am J Roentgenol 1986;146:679–84.

47. Hansen ME, Spritzer CE, Sostman HD. Assessing the patency of mediastinal and thoracic inlet veins:

value of MR imaging. AJR Am J Roentgenol 1990; 155:1177–82.

48. Roubidoux MA, Dunnick NR, Sostman HD, et al. Renal carcinoma: detection of venous extension with gradient echo MR imaging. Radiology 1992;182:269–72.

49. Sonin AH, Mazer MJ, Powers TA. Obstruction of the inferior vena cava: a multiple modality demonstration of causes, manifestations, and collateral pathways. Radiographics 1992;12:309–22.

50. Peters DC, Wylie JV, Hauser TH, et al. Detection of pulmonary vein and left atrial scar after catheter ablation with three-dimensional navigator-gated delayed enhancement MR imaging: initial experience. Radiology 2007;243:690–5.

51. Ishihara Y, Nazafat R, Wylie JV, et al. MRI evaluation of RF ablation scarring for atrial fibrillation treatment. Medical Imaging 2007;6509:65090Q1–65090Q12.

52. Anselme F, Gahide G, Savouré A, et al. MR evaluation of pulmonary vein diameter reduction after radiofrequency catheter ablation of atrial fibrillation. Eur Radiol 2006;16(11):2505–11.

MR Imaging/Magnetic Resonance Angiography of the Pulmonary Arteries and Pulmonary Thromboembolic Disease

Sebastian Ley, MD[a],*, Hans-Ulrich Kauczor, MD[b,c]

KEYWORDS

- Resonance angiography • Pulmonary arteries
- Pulmonary perfusion • Acute pulmonary embolism
- Chronic thromboembolic hypertension

Direct visualization of the pulmonary arteries can be performed using invasive techniques, digital subtraction angiography (DSA), and noninvasive modalities, such as CT and MR imaging. With development of modern multidetector CT (MDCT) scanners, MDCT has become the noninvasive gold standard for imaging of the pulmonary arteries.[1,2] CT, however, has the inherent risk for radiation and need for nephrotoxic contrast agents and the amount of functional information that can be obtained is limited.

During the past few years MR imaging has undergone significant technical improvements, such as faster acquisitions, larger coverage, and faster reconstruction, which have substantially improved patient acceptance of this modality. Furthermore, the availability of MR imaging systems has improved over the past years. These factors positively influenced developments of MR imaging applications of the chest. The implementation of magnetic resonance angiography (MRA), lung perfusion imaging, and the assessment of right heart function seem promising techniques for a comprehensive evaluation in patients who have congenital or acquired pulmonary arterial pathologies.[3]

This review highlights the current state of various MRA techniques for the diagnosis of pulmonary vascular disorders with a special focus on the most common acquired diseases of the pulmonary arteries: acute and chronic thromboembolic disease.

TECHNIQUE

Different imaging strategies are available for imaging the pulmonary arteries: contrast-enhanced (CE) and non–contrast-enhanced (non-CE) acquisitions. The technique used most often is a high spatial resolution CE-MRA.

CONTRAST-ENHANCED MAGNETIC RESONANCE ANGIOGRAPHY WITH HIGH SPATIAL RESOLUTION

CE-MRA consists of heavily T1-weighted gradient-echo MR imaging sequences after an intravenous

a Department of Pediatric Radiology, University Hospital Heidelberg, Im Neuenheimer Feld 153, 69120 Heidelberg, Germany
b Department of Diagnostic Radiology, University Hospital Heidelberg, Im Neuenheimer Feld 110, 69120 Heidelberg, Germany
c German Cancer Research Center, Im Neuenheimer Feld 400, 69120 Heidelberg, Germany
* Corresponding author.
E-mail address: ley@gmx.de (S. Ley).

Magn Reson Imaging Clin N Am 16 (2008) 263–273
doi:10.1016/j.mric.2008.02.012

injection of a paramagnetic MR imaging contrast agent.[4] In general, 3-D techniques with a minimum relaxation time (TR) of less than 5 ms and an echo time (TE) of less than 2 ms are used for CE-MRA of the pulmonary arteries.[5] A short TR allows for short breath-hold acquisitions. A short TE minimizes background signal and susceptibility artifacts. Nowadays, acquisition time has been shortened further using parallel imaging.[6] In parallel imaging, the entire image is reconstructed from an under-sampled k-space in the phase-encoding direction; thus, acquisition time decreases. With a typical acceleration factor of 2, every second line in k-space is skipped, leading to reduction of scan time of approximately 50%.[7] This reduced acquisition time also can be traded for higher spatial resolution. This tradeoff, which the user has to accept for the reduction of scan time or the higher spatial resolution, is a decreased signal-to-noise ratio (SNR). SNR is inversely proportional to the square root of the acceleration factor times, a geometry factor determined mainly by the coil design.[8] In the case of an acceleration factor of 2, the resulting signal is at best 71% of the original signal.[8] Although an acceleration factor of 3 seems acceptable for the renal arteries,[9] an acceleration factor of 2 usually is recommended for the pulmonary arteries. This leads to high spatial resolution with a voxel size of 1.2 mm × 1.0 mm × 1.6 mm, requiring an acquisition period and a breath-hold of 20 to 30 seconds. Backfolding artifacts in the center of the image can appear if acceleration factors of 2 are used in a coronal acquisition. To overcome this problem, patients are scanned with their arms above their heads, which might cause discomfort in some patients.[6] More

recently, the use of novel, non-Cartesian, k-space filling techniques, such as radial and spiral image data acquisition, also has been proposed for use in the chest.[10,11] As the breath-hold is crucial for image quality, the scan generally is acquired in the coronal orientation because the number of slices required for full coverage is lower than in other orientations (**Figs. 1 and 2**). Additionally, a single injection of contrast is sufficient. To improve spatial resolution or reduce the duration of the breath-hold, the sequential acquisition of two sagittal slabs covering the right and left lung separately has been used successfully in patients who have chronic thromboembolic pulmonary hypertension (CTEPH) (**Fig. 3**).[12]

With combination of the latest technical developments, such as a 32-channel chest coil, 3-T MR imaging, high relaxivity contrast agents, and acceleration factors of 6, the acquisition of isotropic ($1 \times 1 \times 1$ mm^3) voxels covering the entire pulmonary circulation in 20 seconds is feasible.[13]

CONTRAST ADMINISTRATION

For T1 shortening of blood, a gadolinium compound (Gd) is injected in a peripheral vein as a bolus, preferable by an automated power injector. Mostly standard-strength Gds in a standard dose (0.1 mL/kg bodyweight) are used for optimal opacification of the pulmonary arteries. To guarantee an optimal bolus profile, the administration of the contrast agent with flow rates between 2 and 5 mL per second is mandatory. The bolus geometry is determined mainly by injection parameters; cardiac function is of minor importance.[14] An injection scheme with a flow rate of 2 mL per

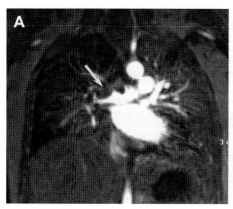
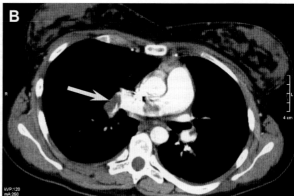

Fig. 1. (A) MRA in a 26-year-old female patient who had central acute PE (*arrow*). The dataset was acquired in a coronal orientation with a spatial resolution of 2.3 × 2.3 × 6 mm. As the patient was dyspneic, a high temporal resolution technique was performed first (20 datasets were acquired in 20 seconds). The embolic material is located in the main right pulmonary artery. (B) Corresponding axial CTA image (same day) showing the same findings (*arrow*).

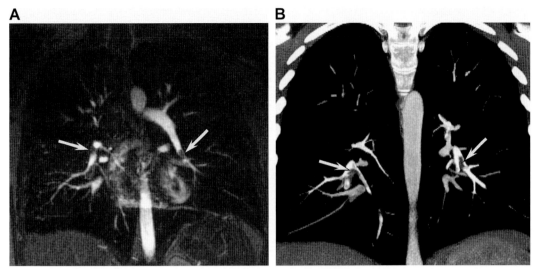

Fig. 2. A 25-year-old female patient who had segmental emboli (*arrows*) in both lower lobes. (*A*) MRA with high spatial resolution (1.3 × 1.3 × 1.6 mm, time of acquisition 20 seconds) allowed for detailed evaluation of the pulmonary arteries. The same finding (*arrows*) is demonstrated at CT (*B*) (same day, hours earlier). Because of less severe pulmonary arterial obstruction, the patient could hold her breath during the acquisition.

second results in a mean transit time of the contrast agent through the pulmonary circulation of 14 seconds; mean pulmonary transit time may be reduced to 9 seconds using an injection speed of 4 mL per second. The administration of a saline flush using a minimum 20 mL injected at the same flow rate immediately after contrast administration is strongly recommended to achieve a compact bolus profile. The saline chaser ensures that the entire contrast bolus contributes to vessel opacification. Adequate timing of the contrast agent together with an adapted flow rate is essential to achieve high contrast between pulmonary artery branches and surrounding structures. The Gd concentration should be optimized to the time of central k-space acquisition, as this determines the vascular signal intensity. Because a significant number of patients referred for MRA of the pulmonary arteries presents with right heart compromise or pulmonary hypertension, the scan delay should be adjusted individually using a care bolus procedure or a test bolus examination. In general, arterial enhancement should be predominant because overlay of pulmonary veins might impair the selective assessment of arteries.

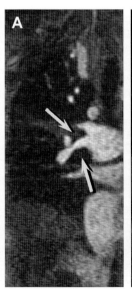 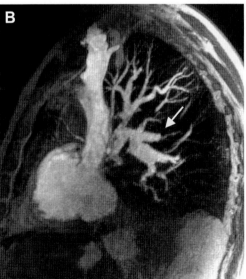

Fig. 3. Chronic thromboembolic disease. High spatial resolution MRA dataset was acquired in sagittal orientation (shown here for the right lung). In a 17-second breathhold, a spatial resolution of 1 × 1 × 1.2 mm was achieved. (*A*) Coronal reformatted image showing the wall adherent thrombotic material in the right pars intermedia. (*B*) The sagittal MIP demonstrates the typical finding of abrupt vessel diameter changes (ie, for segment 6) (*arrow*).

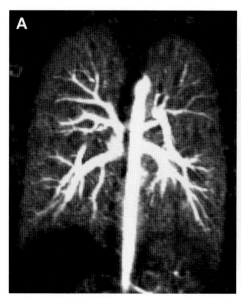
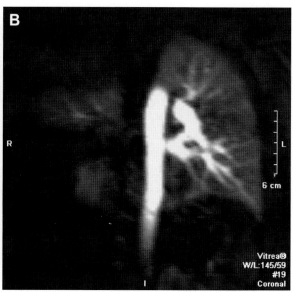

Fig. 4. (A) 3-D pulmonary perfusion (20-mm MIP) in a healthy volunteer. (B) Perfusion MR imaging in the same patient as Fig. 1A (who had acute PE), showing large perfusion defects in the right lower lobe and minor perfusion reduction in the right upper lobe (2.3 × 2.3 × 6 mm). The left lung showed normal a perfusion, and no thrombotic material was seen at CT in the left lung.

CONTRAST-ENHANCED HIGH SPATIAL RESOLUTION MAGNETIC RESONANCE ANGIOGRAPHY WITH HIGH TEMPORAL RESOLUTION

An alternative approach is to optimize the MR imaging sequence for high temporal resolution and to apply it as a multiphasic acquisition.[15,16] In time-resolved MRA, the scan time for the individual 3-D dataset is reduced to less than 5 seconds. The rationale is threefold:

1. Patients who have severe respiratory disease and very limited breath-hold capabilities can be examined;
2. The arteriovenous discrimination is improved. This allows for characterization of vascular territories, especially in anomalies and shunts, and;
3. Time-resolved multiphasic CE-MRA is independent of the bolus timing, because the contrast injection and the MR imaging sequence are started simultaneously. Advanced time-resolved imaging techniques integrate a view-sharing approach to achieve a temporal resolution of 3.3 seconds for a 3-D dataset with a relatively high spatial resolution of, for example, 1.3 × 1.8 × 3 mm^3.[17]

Recent experimental approaches combine view-sharing with spiral k-space filling, allowing for even higher spatial resolution images with shorter acquisition times.[18] If the temporal resolution is substantially reduced further (ie, 1 second per 3-D dataset), the perfusion of the lung parenchyma can be assessed parallel to the central pulmonary arteries.[19] This allows for easy depiction of perfusion deficits as a result of vascular obstruction (Fig. 4).

NON–CONTRAST-ENHANCED OVERLAPPING STEADY-STATE FREE PRECESSION SEQUENCES

Critically ill patients do not tolerate even a short breath-hold time of 5 to 10 seconds for CE-MRA. The same is true for CT angiography (CTA), and its imaging results might be suboptimal. For these patients, free-breathing real-time imaging techniques based on steady-state free precession (SSFP), also called balanced fast-field echo or fast imaging using steady-state acquisition (FISP), are available.[20,21] The entire chest can be covered in all three orientations in less than 180 seconds with 50% slice overlap resulting from an acquisition time per image of approximately 0.4 to 0.5 seconds (Fig. 5). This approach allows for a lobar and segmental evaluation of the pulmonary arteries. Real-time MR imaging showed a high specificity (98%) and sensitivity (89%) in a study of patients who had acute pulmonary embolism (PE) with 16-slice MDCT serving as the reference modality (see Fig. 5).[22]

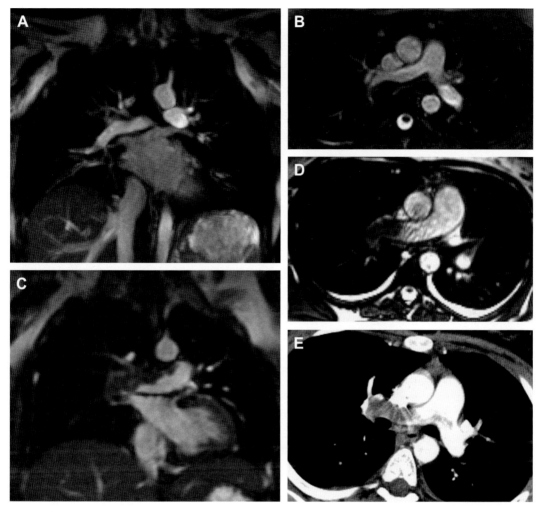

Fig. 5. Capabilities of real-time, overlapping true FISP MR imaging without breath-hold. (*A*) Coronal MIP in a healthy volunteer and (*B*) axial image at the level of the pulmonary arterial bifurcation showing normal findings. (*C, D*) Coronal and transversal slice demonstrating the large central emboli. The spatial resolution of the coronal slice was 1.9 × 1.9 × 4 mm. Note that the sequence is acquired with 50% overlap in z-direction, that a "real" slice thickness of 2 mm results. (*E*) CTA showing the thromboembolic material.

NON–CONTRAST-ENHANCED RESPIRATORY-GATED STEADY-STATE FREE PRECESSION

One technique that may offer an alternative to breath-hold imaging is navigator-gated MR imaging, in which imaging is performed during free breathing. The navigator was first described in 1989 by Ehman and Felmlee[23] and has been used primarily to image blood vessels that are subject to respiratory and cardiac motion, in particular the coronary arteries.[24] This method, however, rarely has been used for pulmonary imaging.[25] With the advent of faster gradient systems and continued development of SSFP, it has become possible to perform rapid 3-D imaging.

The faster gradient systems allow for reduced repetition times, making SSFP practical. Further, the refocusing nature of SSFP, as opposed to the standard spoiled gradient-echo technique, allows for a higher flip angle and many more views per segment before significant signal decay is seen.[26] In a study in healthy volunteers, a breath-hold SSFP sequence was compared with a navigator-gated SSFP (**Fig. 6**). Both sequences resulted in a comparable image quality with the same SNR level; however, no analysis was performed regarding vessel conspicuity on a segmental level. Image acquisition was approximately 29 seconds for the breath-hold and 180 seconds for the navigator technique.[27] Therefore, in critically ill patients, this technique may be worth trying as an alternative.

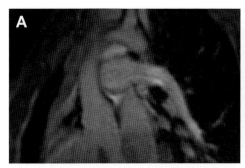
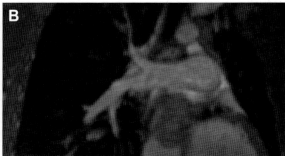

Fig. 6. Cardiac and respiratory-gated 3-D SSFP technique (1.1 × 1.1 × 1 mm) in a volunteer. Multiplanar reformatted image of the left (A) and right (B) pulmonary arteries showing normal findings. Because of ECG and respiratory gating, the acquisition time is approximately 5 to 7 minutes for the region demonstrated.

MAJOR ACQUIRED PATHOLOGIES OF THE PULMONARY ARTERIES: ACUTE AND CHRONIC THROMBOEMBOLISM
Acute Pulmonary Embolism

Most frequently, the pulmonary arteries are examined because of a clinical suspicion of PE, one of the most common medical problems in the Western world.[28] Because of the robustness and speed of examination, pulmonary CTA is the recommended standard protocol of care in patients suspected of having PE[29] and it might be complemented by CT venography. Because of the inherent advantage of MR imaging with stepwise protocols and the possibility of functional evaluation of the burden on the right ventricle, MR imaging also is used for diagnosis of PE (see Figs. 1 and 2). Comprehensive overviews in recent literature of MR imaging for diagnosis of acute PE recently have been published.[3,19] Therefore, only the latest studies using of state-of-the-art scanner technology are discussed in detail.

In 2005, 89 patients who had suspected PE were examined using coronal-, axial-, and sagittal-orientated CE-MRA. The images were interpreted independently by two teams of radiologists. A heterogeneous combination of clinical probability, D-dimer testing, spiral CT, compression venous ultrasound, and pulmonary DSA served as the gold standard.[30] The study cohort had high prevalence of PE (71%). Depending on the team of readers, the sensitivity and specificity of CE-MRA ranged between 31% and 71% and 85% and 92%, respectively. In a study investigating CE-MRA in 48 patients who had suspected PE, Pleszewski, and colleagues[31] reported a sensitivity and specificity of 82% and 100%, respectively, and overall a slightly lower sensitivity than CTA. A high spatial resolution (0.7 × 1.2 × 1.5 mm) CE-MRA acquired in a 15-second breath-hold time was performed in 62 patients who had suspected PE and revealed a sensitivity of 81% and specificity of 100% when compared with CTA acquired with a 16-slice MDCT.[22] In a different study, eight dyspneic patients who had known or suspected PE were examined using a time-resolved CE-MRA with a scan time of less than 4 seconds per 3-D dataset. Pulmonary CE-MRA allowed for the assessment of the pulmonary arterial tree to the subsegmental level and identified PE in all cases in which PE subsequently was confirmed. All patients could hold their breath for at least 8 seconds, during which a dataset with an angiogram of the pulmonary arteries could be obtained.[16] In another study, conventional pulmonary DSA served as the gold standard in 48 patients who had suspected acute PE. A time-resolved CE-MRA with parallel imaging resulted in a high sensitivity (92%) and specificity (94%) for the detection of PE.[32]

In 41 patients who had suspected PE, perfusion MR imaging showed a high intermodality agreement with single photon emission CT for perfusion defects (kappa value per examination was 0.98).[33] The visualization of the typical wedge-shaped parenchymal perfusion defects (see Fig. 4) allows for a fast and reliable detection of vascular obstruction (even at the subsegmental level); however, direct visualization of the thrombotic material often is not possible. Perfusion MR imaging had the highest sensitivity in detection of PE in comparison with three different MR imaging techniques.[22] In clinical practice, however, pulmonary perfusion MR imaging and high-resolution CE-MRA usually are acquired in a combined protocol, which is more accurate than individual examinations.[22,34,35] A combined protocol of pulmonary perfusion MR imaging and high-resolution CE-MRA provides a sensitivity and specificity for the detection of acute PE of over 90% and agrees closely with CTA.[22]

As it has been shown that some patients who have acute PE show incomplete thrombus resolution or even development of chronic PE despite appropriate anticoagulation therapy, treatment response monitoring of these patients should be performed.[36] The combination of a high diagnostic sensitivity with a radiation-free technique makes perfusion MR imaging a highly appropriate tool for monitoring thrombus resolution during anticoagulation therapy.[37,38] In a follow-up study, 33 patients who had acute PE were examined with pulmonary perfusion MR imaging initially and 1 week after initiation of therapy. A subgroup of eight patients also underwent a second follow-up examination. Between examinations, pulmonary perfusion changed noticeably (ie, the time-to-peak enhancement decreased and the peak enhancement of the affected areas increased).[38]

Chronic Thromboembolic Pulmonary Hypertension

Overall, the exact pathologic pathways of the development of CTEPH are not yet fully understood.[39] In the THESEE study, a perfusion lung scan was performed in 157 patients 8 days and 3 months after acute PE. After 3 months, a residual obstruction was found in 66% of patients and 10% had no resolution at all.[40] Based on these data, Pengo and colleagues[41] found a cumulative incidence of symptomatic CTEPH of 3.8% after 2 years in patients who had an acute episode of PE. Instead of thrombolysis, the thromboembolic material follows an aberrant path of organization and recanalization leading to the characteristic abnormalities, such as intraluminal webs and bands, pouch-like endings of arteries, irregularities of the arterial wall, and stenotic lesions (see **Fig. 3**; **Fig 7**).[42–44] This aberrant path of obstruction and reopening occurs in repeated cycles over many years. Other data suggest that in situ thrombosis may play a major role in the development of CTEPH.[45,46] Additionally, small-vessel hypertensive arteriopathy, similar to that seen in other forms of pulmonary hypertension, develops in small unobstructed vessels.[43,44] Patients become symptomatic if approximately 60% of the total diameter of the pulmonary arterial bed is obstructed. This obstruction led to an increase in pulmonary arterial pressure and vascular resistance with subsequent cor pulmonale, ending in right heart failure with a corresponding 5-year survival rate of only 30%.[42–44] The primary treatment of CTEPH is surgical pulmonary endarterectomy (PEA), which leads to a permanent improvement of the pulmonary hemodynamics.[47–49] The technical feasibility and success of surgery mainly depend on the localization of the thromboembolic material: surgical accessibility is possible if the organized thrombi are not located distal to the lobar arteries or the origin of the segmental vessels, such that a safe dissection plane for endarterectomy is feasible.[50]

On occasion, however, patients who have CTEPH have disease that is not accessible to surgery (distal obstructive changes), or patients themselves are unsuitable for surgery because of significant comorbidity. In these situations, pulmonary arterial hypertension-specific drug treatment can reduce the symptoms.[51] In rare cases, balloon angioplasty may be considered. Lung (or heart-lung) transplantation also can be considered in selected cases where PEA is not indicated, or when significant pulmonary hypertension persists after PEA.[46]

MR imaging is well suited for diagnosis and follow-up of CTEPH patients.[52] There are few studies, however, available that explore the usefulness of CE-MRA in the diagnostic evaluation of CTEPH. One study of 34 CE-MRAs successfully depicted findings of CTEPH,[53] including wall-adherent thromboembolic material in the central parts of the pulmonary arteries to the segmental level, intraluminal webs and bands, abnormal proximal-to-distal tapering, and abrupt vessel cutoffs (see **Fig. 3**). A thorough analysis of source images and the creation of multiplanar reformations are most important for the exact assessment of the morphologic findings. Maximum intensity projections (MIPs), alternatively, provide an overview and an impression of the arterial vascular tree comparable to those provided by the DSA images. In that study, pulmonary MRA depicted all patent vessel segments to the level of segmental arteries (533/533 vessel segments) when compared with selective DSA. For subsegmental arteries, DSA detected significantly more patent vessel segments than MRA (733 versus 681). MRA was superior to DSA in delineating the exact central beginning of the thromboembolic material. In all cases, the most proximal site as assessed by MRA corresponded to the beginning of the dissection procedure during PEA. As all patients suffered from CTEPH and were candidates for surgery, however, there was no statement possible regarding the ability of CE-MRA in the differentiation of other causes of pulmonary hypertension. Postoperatively, CE-MRA enabled the delineation of reopened segmental arteries and a decrease in the diameter of the central pulmonary arteries. A complete normalization of pulmonary arterial vasculature was not documented in any case.

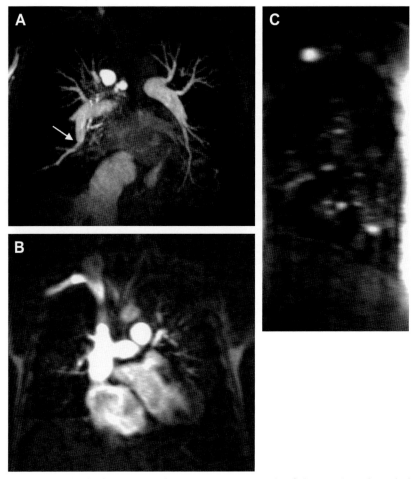

Fig. 7. A 58-year-old man who had pulmonary hypertension as a result of chronic thromboembolic disease. (*A*) MRA showing the typical webs (*arrow*) and vessel cutoffs. (*B*) Perfusion study of this patient demonstrating the typical wedge shaped perfusion defects (ie, right lower lobe). (*C*) Sagittal reformation of the 3-D perfusion dataset (right lung). Here the perfusion defects are better to be delineated; even a segmental assignment is possible.

In a study of 29 patients who had CTEPH or primary pulmonary hypertension (PPH), CE-MRA (1.0 × 0.7 × 1.6 mm³) was compared with DSA or CTA.[35] CE-MRA had sensitivities ranging between 83% and 86% for detection of complete vessel obstructions and free-floating thrombi and sensitivities ranging between 50% and 71% for the depiction of older or organized thrombi, webs, and bands. The specificities ranged between 73% and 95% for nonobstructing findings and from 91% to 96% for occluding findings, respectively. CE-MRA enabled correct differentiation of PPH and CTEPH in 24 of 29 patients (83%). As with acute PE, pulmonary perfusion MR imaging should be performed for identification of the typical wedge-shaped perfusion defects. This was also done in the study (discussed previously) by Nikolaou and colleagues.[35] Perfusion defects were classified as patchy or diffuse (indicative of PPH) or segmental or circumscribed (indicative of CTEPH) (see **Fig. 7**). Compared with perfusion scintigraphy as the standard of reference, MR imaging had an overall sensitivity of 77% in detecting perfusion defects on a per-patient basis. Compared with the final diagnosis, perfusion MR imaging enabled a correct diagnosis of PPH or CTEPH in 20 (69%) of 29 patients. The combined interpretation of perfusion MR imaging and MRA led to a correct diagnosis of PPH or CTEPH in 26 (90%) of 29 patients when compared with the final reference diagnosis (combination of perfusion scintigraphy with DSA or CTA). In another series, perfusion MR imaging was used to differentiate patients who had idiopathic pulmonary arterial hypertension (IPAH), CTEPH, and healthy volunteers.[34] Based on a per-segment analysis, patients who had PPH showed a patchy or diffuse reduction of perfusion in 71 (79%) of 90 segments, a normal finding in 18 (20%) of 90 segments, and one focal defect (1%). Patients who had CTEPH showed focal perfusion defects in 47 (52%), absent segmental perfusion in 23 (26%), and a normal perfusion in 20 (22%) of 90 segments. On a per-patient basis, there was no difficulty in differentiating the two pathologic entities and in depicting the healthy volunteers. Semiquantitative analysis showed that healthy volunteers demonstrated a significantly shorter transit time of the contrast agent through the pulmonary circulation than patients who had IPAH and CTEPH (14 $\pm$ 1 second versus 22 $\pm$ 4 seconds and 25 $\pm$ 11 seconds, respectively). No difference was found between both patient populations.

SUMMARY

- MRA of the pulmonary arteries still is a rapidly evolving technique with already proved high clinical usefulness.
- Multiple step protocols, such as perfusion MR imaging followed by high spatial resolution MRA, seem to provide a satisfactory clinical approach for the assessment of different vascular diseases affecting the pulmonary arteries. These magnetic resonance protocols, particularly in combination with additional cardiovascular sequences, make MR imaging a powerful noninvasive imaging technique for the investigation of pulmonary arterial diseases.

REFERENCES

1. Bruzzi JF, Remy-Jardin M, Delhaye D, et al. When, why, and how to examine the heart during thoracic CT: part 2, clinical applications. AJR Am J Roentgenol 2006;186:333–41.
2. Schoepf UJ, Costello P. CT angiography for diagnosis of pulmonary embolism: state of the art. Radiology 2004;230:329–37.
3. Pedersen MR, Fisher MT, van Beek EJ. MR imaging of the pulmonary vasculature—an update. Eur Radiol 2006;16:1374–86.
4. Prince MR. Gadolinium-enhanced MR aortography. Radiology 1994;191:155–64.
5. Zhang H, Maki JH, Prince MR. 3D contrast-enhanced MR angiography. J Magn Reson Imaging 2007;25:13–25.
6. Oosterhof T, Mulder BJ. Magnetic resonance angiography for anatomical evaluation of the great arteries. Int J Cardiovasc Imaging 2005;21:323–4.
7. Sodickson DK, Griswold MA, Jakob PM, et al. Signal-to-noise ratio and signal-to-noise efficiency in SMASH imaging. Magn Reson Med 1999;41:1009–22.
8. Pruessmann KP, Weiger M, Scheidegger MB, et al. SENSE: sensitivity encoding for fast. Magn Reson Med 1999;42:952–62.
9. Michaely HJ, Herrmann KA, Kramer H, et al. High-resolution renal MRA: comparison of image quality and vessel depiction with different parallel imaging acceleration factors. J Magn Reson Imaging 2006;24:95–100.
10. Kressler B, Spincemaille P, Prince MR, et al. Reduction of reconstruction time for time-resolved spiral 3D contrast-enhanced magnetic resonance angiography using parallel computing. Magn Reson Med 2006;56:704–8.
11. Yeh EN, Stuber M, McKenzie CA, et al. Inherently self-calibrating non-Cartesian parallel imaging. Magn Reson Med 2005;54:1–8.
12. Oberholzer K, Romaneehsen B, Kunz P, et al. [Contrast-enhanced 3D MR angiography of the pulmonary arteries with integrated parallel acquisition technique (iPAT) in patients with chronic-thromboembolic pulmonary hypertension CTEPH—sagittal or coronal acquisition]. Rofo 2004;176:605–9.
13. Nael K, Fenchel M, Krishnam M, et al. 3.0 Tesla high spatial resolution contrast-enhanced magnetic resonance angiography (CE-MRA) of the pulmonary circulation: initial experience with a 32-channel phased array coil using a high relaxivity contrast agent. Invest Radiol 2007;42:392–8.
14. Kreitner KF, Kunz RP, Weschler C, et al. [Systematic analysis of the geometry of a defined contrast medium bolus—implications for contrast enhanced 3D MR-angiography of thoracic vessels]. Rofo 2005;177:646–54.
15. Fink C, Ley S, Kroeker R, et al. Time-resolved contrast-enhanced three-dimensional magnetic resonance angiography of the chest: combination of parallel imaging with view sharing (TREAT). Invest Radiol 2005;40:40–8.
16. Goyen M, Laub G, Ladd ME, et al. Dynamic 3D MR angiography of the pulmonary arteries in under four seconds. J Magn Reson Imaging 2001;13:372–7.
17. Ersoy H, Goldhaber SZ, Cai T, et al. Time-resolved MR angiography: a primary screening examination of patients with suspected pulmonary embolism and contraindications to administration of iodinated contrast material. AJR Am J Roentgenol 2007;188:1246–54.
18. Du J, Bydder M. High-resolution time-resolved contrast-enhanced MR abdominal and pulmonary angiography using a spiral-TRICKS sequence. Magn Reson Med 2007;58:631–5.
19. Fink C, Ley S, Schoenberg SO, et al. Magnetic resonance imaging of acute pulmonary embolism. Eur Radiol 2007;17:2546–53.

20. Kluge A, Muller C, Hansel J, et al. Real-time MR with TrueFISP for the detection of acute pulmonary embolism: initial clinical experience. Eur Radiol 2004;14:709–18.

21. Pereles FS, McCarthy RM, Baskaran V, et al. Thoracic aortic dissection and aneurysm: evaluation with nonenhanced true FISP MR angiography in less than 4 minutes. Radiology 2002;223:270–4.

22. Kluge A, Luboldt W, Bachmann G. Acute pulmonary embolism to the subsegmental level: diagnostic accuracy of three MRI techniques compared with 16-MDCT. AJR Am J Roentgenol 2006;187:W7–14.

23. Ehman RL, Felmlee JP. Adaptive technique for high-definition MR imaging of moving structures. Radiology 1989;173:255–63.

24. Spuentrup E, Bornert P, Botnar RM, et al. Navigator-gated free-breathing three-dimensional balanced fast field echo (TrueFISP) coronary magnetic resonance angiography. Invest Radiol 2002;37:637–42.

25. Wang Y, Rossman PJ, Grimm RC, et al. 3D MR angiography of pulmonary arteries using real-time navigator gating and magnetization preparation. Magn Reson Med 1996;36:579–87.

26. Deshpande VS, Shea SM, Laub G, et al. 3D magnetization-prepared true-FISP: a new technique for imaging coronary arteries. Magn Reson Med 2001; 46:494–502.

27. Hui BK, Noga ML, Gan KD, et al. Navigator-gated three-dimensional MR angiography of the pulmonary arteries using steady-state free precession. J Magn Reson Imaging 2005;21:831–5.

28. Stein PD, Beemath A, Matta F, et al. Clinical characteristics of patients with acute pulmonary embolism: data from PIOPED II. Am J Med 2007;120:871–9.

29. Stein PD, Hull RD. Multidetector computed tomography for the diagnosis of acute pulmonary embolism. Curr Opin Pulm Med 2007;13:384–8.

30. Blum A, Bellou A, Guillemin F, et al. Performance of magnetic resonance angiography in suspected acute pulmonary embolism. Thromb Haemost 2005;93:503–11.

31. Pleszewski B, Chartrand-Lefebvre C, Qanadli SD, et al. Gadolinium-enhanced pulmonary magnetic resonance angiography in the diagnosis of acute pulmonary embolism: a prospective study on 48 patients. Clin Imaging 2006;30:166–72.

32. Ohno Y, Higashino T, Takenaka D, et al. MR angiography with sensitivity encoding (SENSE) for suspected pulmonary embolism: comparison with MDCT and ventilation-perfusion scintigraphy. AJR Am J Roentgenol 2004;183:91–8.

33. Kluge A, Gerriets T, Stolz E, et al. Pulmonary perfusion in acute pulmonary embolism: agreement of MRI and SPECT for lobar, segmental and subsegmental perfusion defects. Acta Radiol 2006;47:933–40.

34. Ley S, Mereles D, Puderbach M, et al. Value of MR phase-contrast flow measurements for functional assessment of pulmonary arterial hypertension. Eur Radiol 2007;17:1892–7.

35. Nikolaou K, Schoenberg SO, Attenberger U, et al. Pulmonary arterial hypertension: diagnosis with fast perfusion MR imaging and high-spatial-resolution MR angiography—preliminary experience. Radiology 2005;236:694–703.

36. Remy-Jardin M, Louvegny S, Remy J, et al. Acute central thromboembolic disease: posttherapeutic follow-up with spiral CT angiography. Radiology 1997;203:173–80.

37. Fink C, Risse F, Semmler W, et al. [MRI of pulmonary perfusion]. Radiologe 2006;46:290–9.

38. Kluge A, Gerriets T, Lange U, et al. MRI for short-term follow-up of acute pulmonary embolism. Assessment of thrombus appearance and pulmonary perfusion: a feasibility study. Eur Radiol 2005;15:1969–77.

39. Peacock A, Simonneau G, Rubin L. Controversies, uncertainties and future research on the treatment of chronic thromboembolic pulmonary hypertension. Proc Am Thorac Soc 2006;3:608–14.

40. Wartski M, Collignon MA. Incomplete recovery of lung perfusion after 3 months in patients with acute pulmonary embolism treated with antithrombotic agents. THESEE Study Group. Tinzaparin ou Heparin Standard: evaluation dans l'Embolie Pulmonaire Study. J Nucl Med 2000;41:1043–8.

41. Pengo V, Lensing AW, Prins MH, et al. Incidence of chronic thromboembolic pulmonary hypertension after pulmonary embolism. N Engl J Med 2004; 350:2257–64.

42. Auger WR, Kerr KM, Kim NH, et al. Chronic thromboembolic pulmonary hypertension. Cardiol Clin 2004; 22:453–66, vii.

43. Dartevelle P, Fadel E, Mussot S, et al. Chronic thromboembolic pulmonary hypertension. Eur Respir J 2004;23:637–48.

44. Frazier AA, Galvin JR, Franks TJ, et al. From the archives of the AFIP: pulmonary vasculature: hypertension and infarction. Radiographics 2000;20: 491–524.

45. Egermayer P, Peacock AJ. Is pulmonary embolism a common cause of chronic pulmonary hypertension? Limitations of the embolic hypothesis. Eur Respir J 2000;15:440–8.

46. McNeil K, Dunning J. Chronic thromboembolic pulmonary hypertension (CTEPH). Heart 2007;93: 1152–8.

47. Kim NH. Assessment of operability in chronic thromboembolic pulmonary hypertension. Proc Am Thorac Soc 2006;3:584–8.

48. Madani MM, Jamieson SW. Technical advances of pulmonary endarterectomy for chronic thromboembolic pulmonary hypertension. Semin Thorac Cardiovasc Surg 2006;18:243–9.

49. Puis L, Vandezande E, Vercaemst L, et al. Pulmonary thromboendarterectomy for chronic

thromboembolic pulmonary hypertension. Perfusion 2005;20:101–8.

50. Jamieson SW, Kapelanski DP. Pulmonary endarterectomy. Curr Probl Surg 2000;37:165–252.

51. Hoeper MM, Kramm T, Wilkens H, et al. Bosentan therapy for inoperable chronic thromboembolic pulmonary hypertension. Chest 2005;128:2363–7.

52. Prince MR, Alderson PO, Sostman HD. Chronic pulmonary embolism: combining MR angiography with functional assessment. Radiology 2004;232:325–6.

53. Kreitner KF, Kunz RP, Ley S, et al. Chronic thromboembolic pulmonary hypertension—assessment by magnetic resonance imaging. Eur Radiol 2007;17: 11–21.

Functional MR Imaging of the Lung

Shin Matsuoka, MD, PhD[a], Andetta R. Hunsaker, MD[b],
Ritu R. Gill, MBBS[b], Francine L. Jacobson, MD, MPH[b],
Yoshiharu Ohno, MD, PhD[c], Samuel Patz, PhD[a,d],
Hiroto Hatabu, MD, PhD[b,d],*

KEYWORDS

• MR • Lung • Function • Perfusion • Ventilation

Functional information of the lung is indispensable in the diagnosis and treatment of various lung diseases. In general, pulmonary function testing (PFT) has been used to measure global pulmonary function; however, it can provide little regional information in the lung. Pulmonary imaging techniques, including lung scintigraphy and positron emission tomography (PET), have played important roles in measuring aspects of regional pulmonary physiology. These imaging techniques have the disadvantage of using ionizing radiation, which is of concern because of the potential for cancer induction.

MR imaging may be preferable for investigating pulmonary physiology because of its lack of reliance on ionizing radiation. In its infancy, pulmonary MR imaging had drawbacks attributable to susceptibility artifacts caused by multiple air–tissue interfaces, the low proton density of the lung, and motion artifacts attributable to cardiac pulsation and respiration.[1–3] The development of new MR techniques has overcome many of these problems, however, allowing both static and dynamic MR lung imaging and providing quantitative information of pulmonary function, including perfusion, ventilation, and respiratory motion. The information provided by these new MR imaging methods is useful in research and in clinical applications in various lung diseases.

PULMONARY PERFUSION MR IMAGING

Pulmonary perfusion can be assessed by two different MR techniques. The first technique is known as dynamic contrast-enhanced MR perfusion imaging, whereby multiple images are acquired rapidly as intravascular contrast travels through the pulmonary circulation. The method consists of an intravenous bolus injection of a gadolinium-based paramagnetic contrast agent in conjunction with a gradient-echo pulse sequence with ultrashort repetition time (TR) and echo time (TE).[4] Under these conditions, pulmonary perfusion images can be obtained within a matter of seconds and can be evaluated qualitatively and quantitatively. The quantitative parameters, including transit time, blood volume, and blood flow, are derived from the time–intensity curve. Because of limitations associated with administration of gadolinium, repeat scanning is not possible during a single scan session. The second technique is known as arterial spin labeling. This technique involves labeling arterial water in a selected spatial region with the use of selective radio frequency pulses and using the labeled water as an endogenous contrast agent.[5]

The usefulness of these pulmonary perfusion MR imaging techniques has been shown in normal subjects and in various lung diseases.[6–17] Initially,

This work was supported by Grant No. R21CA116271-02.

[a] Department of Radiology, Brigham and Women's Hospital, 75 Francis Street, Boston, MA 02115, USA

[b] Department of Radiology, Brigham and Women's Hospital, Harvard Medical School, 75 Francis Street, Boston, MA 02115, USA

[c] Department of Radiology, Kobe University Graduate School of Medicine, 7-5-2 Kusunoki-cho, Chuo-ku, Kobe 650-0017, Japan

[d] Center for Pulmonary Functional Imaging, Brigham and Women's Hospital, 221 Longwood Avenue, Boston, MA 02115, USA

* Corresponding author. Department of Radiology, Brigham and Women's Hospital, Harvard Medical School, 75 Francis Street, Boston, MA 02115.

E-mail address: hhatabu@partners.org (H. Hatabu).

Magn Reson Imaging Clin N Am 16 (2008) 275–289
doi:10.1016/j.mric.2008.03.006
1064-9689/08/$ – see front matter © 2008 Elsevier Inc. All rights reserved.

mri.theclinics.com

perfusion MR imaging was used primarily for pulmonary vascular disorders, such as pulmonary embolism. Many patients suspected of pulmonary embolism undergo multislice CT (MSCT) angiography as the first imaging modality, however. More recently, evaluation of tumor angiogenesis has received attention, and dynamic contrast-enhanced MR perfusion imaging may be a useful imaging modality in evaluation of this process. Tumor angiogenesis has been recognized as an important factor in tumor growth and prognosis (**Figs. 1–3**). Typically during malignant tumor growth, blood supply more than normal level is required to support the viability of malignant cells. Angiogenic factors from the malignant cells, such as vascular endothelial growth factor, are released, causing increases in the microvascular density of malignant tumors.[18–25] The increased extent of microvascular density leads to increase in perfusion and permeability of the tumor capillaries, and is associated with strong enhancement of a malignant tumor on contrast-enhanced dynamic CT and MR imaging.[26–29] Fujimoto and colleagues[28] evaluated the correlation between histologic tumor angiogenesis and perfusion parameters obtained from dynamic contrast-enhanced MR perfusion imaging in 94 lung cancers. They found that the maximum enhancement ratio and slope value were positively correlated, and the time at maximum enhancement was negatively correlated with microvessel counts. They also demonstrated that patients who had a higher slope value had a significantly shorter overall survival than did those who had a lower slope value. Perfusion MR parameters could therefore serve as biomarkers of angiogenesis and prognosis for malignant tumors. Antiangiogenic drugs are being developed for the treatment of malignant tumors,

and an accurate and noninvasive assessment to evaluate the change of tumor angiogenesis after treatment is necessary. For the evaluation of tumor angiogenesis, dynamic contrast-enhanced MR imaging may be superior to CT and PET because dynamic CT requires repeated radiation exposure, and PET has proven inadequate in the direct assessment of the tumor microvasculature.[30] In addition, more recently, diffusion-weighted MR imaging might be useful in evaluating pulmonary nodules by differentiating benign and malignant lesions.[31] This additional information will be an added benefit of MR imaging for the evaluation of pulmonary nodules. Non–contrast-enhanced perfusion MR imaging, such as arterial spin labeling, has also been applied to evaluate the tumor angiogenesis in various organs;[32–34] however, no published reports regarding lung cancer and angiogenesis are as yet available.

The usefulness of dynamic contrast-enhanced perfusion MR imaging for the prediction of postoperative lung function in patients who have lung cancer has been reported,[35] and dynamic contrast-enhanced perfusion MR imaging provides more accurate prediction of the postoperative lung function than qualitative CT and perfusion single photon emission computerized tomography (SPECT).[35]

Dynamic contrast-enhanced MR perfusion imaging is also used for the evaluation of pulmonary hypertension (**Fig. 4**). Objective assessment of severity of pulmonary hypertension is important because of its poor prognosis. Echocardiography is routinely used for the evaluation of pulmonary hypertension, but limitations exist. For example, the sensitivity and specificity of echocardiographic assessment of pulmonary arterial pressure are

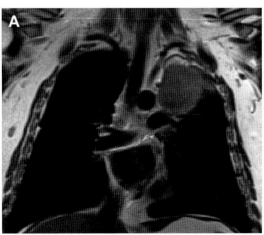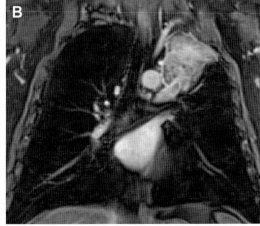

Fig. 1. (*A*) Coronal T2-weighted HASTE image scanned 3T MR scanner system shows lung cancer in the left upper lobe. (*B*) 3D contrast-enhanced gradient-echo MR image demonstrates heterogeneous enhancement of the mass.

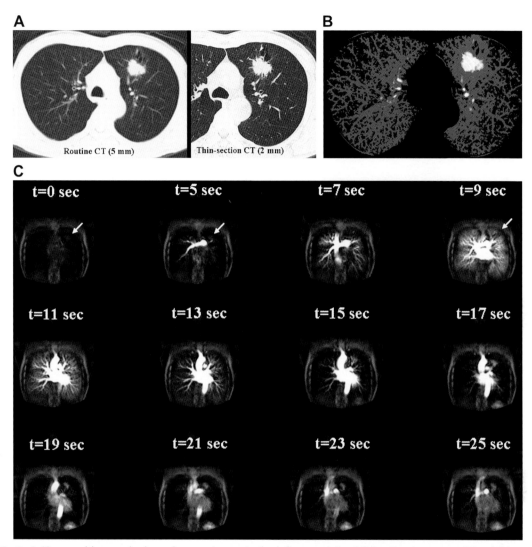

Fig. 2. A 63-year-old man who has adenocarcinoma in the left upper lobe. (*A*) Routine transverse CT and thin-section CT show low attenuation areas in both lungs. Carcinoma is visible within the left upper lobe. (*B*) On quantitative CT, functional lung is shown in red, pulmonary emphysema in black, and lung cancer in white. (*C*) Dynamic perfusion MR imaging shows heterogeneous but well-enhanced pulmonary parenchyma in both lungs, but not within the lung cancer (*arrow*) between 5 seconds and 13 seconds. Lung carcinoma enhancement is seen after 13 seconds. (*From* Ohno Y, Koyama H, Nogami M, et al. Postoperative lung function in lung cancer patients: comparative analysis of predictive capability of MRI, CT, and SPECT. AJR Am J Roentgenol 2007;189(2):404; with permission.)

poor in patients who have severe emphysema.[36] Ohno and colleagues[37] demonstrated good correlation between parameters of MR perfusion imaging and pulmonary vascular resistance or mean pulmonary arterial pressure measured with right-heart catheterization. Although MR assessment of severity of pulmonary hypertension can be performed by phase contrast flow measurements at the pulmonary trunk and by morphologic evaluation of right ventricle,[38,39] quantitative assessment of regional pulmonary perfusion

parameters from dynamic contrast-enhanced perfusion MR images in patients who have pulmonary hypertension may offer the opportunity for noninvasive physiologic and pathophysiologic evaluation of the lungs with relatively high spatial resolution but without radiation exposure.

HYPERPOLARIZED NOBLE GAS MR IMAGING

The principal reason the signal-to-noise ratio (SNR) of traditional proton MR imaging in the

A   **B**

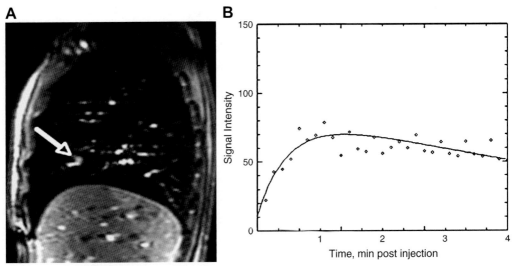

Fig. 3. (*A*) Dynamic sagittal spoiled gradient echo image shows intense enhancement of a pulmonary nodule (*arrow*). (*B*) Example of model-based full parametric analysis fitting of signal intensity versus time curve of the nodule following bolus injection of gadolinium diethylenetrianine-pentaacid. (*From* Kino A, Takahashi M, Ashiku SK, et al. Optimal breathing protocol for dynamic contrast-enhanced MRI of solitary pulmonary nodules at 3T. Eur J Radiol 2007;64(3);399; with permission.)

lung is poor is because most of the lung (~80%) is composed of gas spaces where the concentration of water molecules is ~1000 times less than in tissue. A typical voxel located in the parenchyma contains ~20% of the number of protons compared with nonpulmonary tissue, resulting in an immediate reduction in SNR by a factor of 5. A solution to this problem, the use of hyperpolarized noble gases ^{3}He or ^{129}Xe, was demonstrated in 1994.[40] Using optical pumping techniques, ^{3}He and ^{129}Xe can be polarized to ~50% polarization. This level of polarization is ~100,000 times higher than what is provided by a typical 1.5T MR imaging scanner. In practice, a laser polarizer is used to magnetize a quantity of gas (typically ~300 to ~1000 mL). After the polarized gas is prepared, it is brought to the subject in the scanner where it is inhaled. Because of the large polarization, even with the relatively low density of a gas, the observed SNR is comparable to that of traditional proton MR imaging in other soft tissues. One important consideration for MR imaging pulse sequences is that during the TR time period, when longitudinal magnetization recovery takes place, for hyperpolarized noble gases this recovery is negligible compared with the non-equilibrium magnetization produced by the laser polarization. The pulse sequences used can thus only use small flip angles; otherwise the magnetization will be exhausted in a few excitations of the nuclei. This finding also implies that the observed signal does not depend on TR and therefore one can use short values of TR to reduce the imaging time.

To date, the vast majority of hyperpolarized noble gas MR imaging has been performed with ^{3}He rather than ^{129}Xe, because of the relative ease of polarizing ^{3}He compared with ^{129}Xe. This practice is beginning to change, however, as a new generation of ^{129}Xe polarizers has recently become available.[41,42] ^{3}He has negligible solubility in tissue and therefore, after inhalation, remains in the bronchial tree and alveolar gas spaces. Hyperpolarized helium is thus used solely for measuring properties of the gas spaces in the lung, including ventilatory information obtained from images reflecting the static concentration of ^{3}He following an inhalation and breath-hold maneuver, and dynamic movies of breathing. Also measured is the apparent diffusion coefficient (ADC), which is related to the root mean square displacement of the diffusing gas molecules. When gaseous molecules experience diffusion restriction, such as alveolar wall boundaries, ADC is reduced. One thus expects an increase in ADC for emphysematous disease. Finally, because of the known dependence of T1 on oxygen concentration, measurement of this relaxation rate can provide regional measurements of the partial pressure of oxygen (Po_2) in the lung.

In comparison to ^{3}He, ^{129}Xe not only enters the pulmonary gas spaces but also diffuses into the septal tissue where it is easily distinguished from ^{129}Xe in the gas phase because of a ~200 ppm chemical shift in its frequency. ^{129}Xe thus can provide information not only about the gas phase but also about gas exchange, including alveolar surface area,[43-46] septal thickness,[47] and blood flow transit times.[48,49]

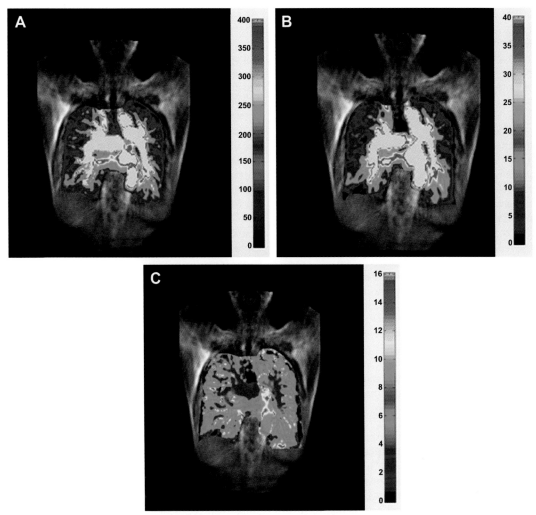

Fig. 4. Quantitative pulmonary perfusion parameter maps on one of 10 slices in a 42-year-old female who has primary pulmonary hypertension. (*A*) Pulmonary blood flow (PBF) map clearly shows decreased PBF in both lungs. Mean regional PBF in this slice was 43.9 ± 4.9 mL/100 mL/min. (*B*) Pulmonary blood volume (PBV) map clearly shows decreased PBV in both lungs. Mean regional PBF in this slice was 5.8 ± 2.5 mL/100 mL. (*C*) Mean transit time (MTT) map clearly shows prolonged MTT in both lungs. Mean regional MTT in this slice was 6.9 ± 1.2 seconds. (*From* Ohno Y, Hatabu H, Murase K, et al. Primary pulmonary hypertension: 3D dynamic perfusion MRI for quantitative analysis of regional pulmonary perfusion. AJR Am J Roentgenol 2007;188(1):52; with permission.)

Ventilation MR Imaging

Several studies have shown that the size and extent of ventilation defects demonstrated by hyperpolarized gas MR imaging correlates well with spirometry.[50–52] In addition, recent studies have shown that hyperpolarized gas MR imaging has much higher sensitivity to detect ventilation abnormalities than either spirometry or scintigraphy.[52] Hyperpolarized gas MR imaging has been evaluated in several clinical studies. In patients who have asthma, hyperpolarized gas MR ventilation imaging has shown the ability to detect airway obstruction before and after inhalation of methacholine.[53,54] Several studies comparing quantitative CT evaluation to hyperpolarized ³He MR imaging have shown similar sensitivity and specificity for the detection of obstructive lung lesions in patients who have bronchiolitis obliterans as a complication of lung transplantation.[55,56] Static ventilation MR imaging provides limited information, however, because only the affected lung lesions attributable to emphysema or airway obstruction are shown.

Ventilation MR imaging during free-breathing "dynamic ventilation" imaging allows the visualization of the full respiratory cycle. ³He hyperpolarized MR imaging with high temporal resolution shows the dynamic distribution of ventilation during continuous breathing after inhalation of ^{3}He hyperpolarized gas and can demonstrate dynamic airflow abnormalities.[57,58] Notably, the distribution and severity of air trapping can be evaluated directly with dynamic ventilation MR imaging,[59] whereas several quantitative CT studies evaluating the degree of air trapping rely on the assessment of regional differences in lung attenuation as an indirect measure of airway disease.[60–63] In patients who have cystic fibrosis,[64,65] qualitative or semiqualitative air trapping can be evaluated with dynamic hyperpolarized gas MR ventilation imaging. In patients who have chronic obstructive pulmonary disease (COPD), delayed outflow of ^{3}He gas has been reported, which is believed to reflect the presence of air trapping.[58,59] There are few reported quantitative dynamic hyperpolarized gas MR ventilation studies that were designed to assess air trapping, however.[66] The evaluation of air trapping caused by small airway obstruction in patients who have COPD is important because it correlates with airflow limitations that define the severely of COPD. Dynamic ventilation MR imaging may potentially play a role in imaging small airway disease as, in the last few years, great attention has been paid to therapeutic agents that specifically address airflow obstruction in COPD.[67,68] The efficacy of various medications might be assessed using dynamic ventilation MR imaging because it allows the direct identification of specific airways responsible for airflow limitation without requiring radiation. Dynamic ventilation MR imaging may play an increasingly important role in quantitative evaluation of small airway obstruction in various obstructive lung diseases.

Diffusion-Weighted Imaging of Lung Microstructure Through Measurement of Apparent Diffusion Coefficient

Diffusion-weighted MR imaging can be used to measure the diffusion coefficient of the hyperpolarized gas within the lung airspaces. In normal subjects, the gas is highly restricted by the walls of the alveoli and terminal bronchioles. In contrast, as alveolar tissue degenerates in emphysema, the gas is less restricted and can diffuse over greater lengths resulting in greater signal loss. A regional ADC value that increases with the increasing size of the alveolar airspaces can be used to evaluate airspace size. Indeed, in patients who have emphysema, the ADC value of ^{3}He has been found to be significantly increased when compared with normal subjects.[69–72] Good correlations between the global and regional ADC as measured

by hyperpolarized gas MR imaging and alveolar size as measured histologically have been reported.[73–75] Furthermore, regional ADC maps in patients who have COPD demonstrate increased severity of emphysema in the apical versus the basal lung regions compared with a more diffuse increase in regional ADC in patients who have α1-antitrypsin deficiency.[70] Quantitative ADC values are also strongly correlated with spirometry, including forced expiratory volume at one second (FEV$_1$) and ratio of FEV$_1$ to forced vital capacity (FEV$_1$/FVC). Several studies have shown the sensitivity of the mean ADC for detecting microstructural changes in the lungs in patients who have emphysema,[69,70] asymptomatic smokers,[76] and aging never-smokers.[77] Furthermore, the ADC measurements have been shown to be potentially more sensitive than high-resolution CT using the RA950 index (relative area of lung attenuation below −950 HU) for early detection of emphysematous changes in asymptomatic smokers.[67] In addition, quantitative ADC measurements may provide information regarding longitudinal change in emphysema as shown in animal models,[73,75] and for monitoring individual regional disease progression in response to drug therapies without using radiation.

It is well known that aging leads to changes in lung structure and function, and enlargement of airspace is not rare in the elderly.[78] In fact, ADC values in lungs of healthy never-smokers show a statistically significant increase with age.[77] Early detection of airspace enlargement therefore might not invariably indicate pathologic emphysema; it could represent a degenerative airspace enlargement. Additionally, no studies are available assessing the longitudinal change using hyperpolarized gas MR imaging in patients who have emphysema, so it would be necessary to clarify whether diffusion-weighted hyperpolarized gas MR imaging can differentiate emphysema from normal degenerative airspace enlargement. Considering the heterogeneity of airway dimension in patients who have COPD, increases in ADC values might not only reflect enlargement of airspaces but also could be seen in patients who have bronchiolectasis. Currently, these different pathologic conditions cannot be differentiated on diffusion-weighted MR imaging in COPD. Another drawback of ADC maps is that the data for calculating these maps can only be derived in ventilated lung areas.

Intrapulmonary Measurement of Po$_2$

Measurement of intrapulmonary Po$_2$ can be achieved by using the paramagnetic effect of oxygen on hyperpolarized ^{3}He. In the presence of oxygen, the longitudinal relaxation of ^{3}He is hastened.[79] The application of radio frequency pulses also leads to depolarization of ^{3}He, however. Experimental and human studies have demonstrated that the oxygen-induced signal decay rate is linearly proportional to the concentration of alveolar oxygen.[80] The paramagnetic effects of O_2 have been demonstrated to provide quantitative measurements of P_{O_2}[81,82] that can then be used to calculate ventilation-to-perfusion ratios (V_A/Q).[83] With MR imaging, this V_A/Q mismatch also can be assessed using dynamic contrast MR perfusion imaging in conjunction with MR ventilation images. The regional P_{O_2} can then be used to infer V_A/Q using mass–balance relationships for alveolar CO_2 and O_2 gas exchange. The ability to perform regional V_A/Q mapping may provide valuable information that can be used to assess ventilation and perfusion response in various lung disorders, such as pulmonary embolism and COPD.

Hyperpolarized ^{129}Xe gas MR Imaging

The first MR ventilation images were obtained using hyperpolarized ^{129}Xe in 1994;[40] however, many more studies with hyperpolarized gas MR imaging have been performed using ^{3}He, even though ^{129}Xe has a much higher natural abundance and is less expensive, because ^{3}He is easier to polarize. Hyperpolarized ^{3}He and ^{129}Xe gases have different physiologic properties. Helium is basically insoluble in tissue, thereby remaining in the lung airspaces during a breath hold. Xenon, however, is soluble in blood with a partition coefficient of ~ 0.1.[84] ^{129}Xe can thus be used not only to measure ventilation and ADC in the gas spaces, but may also allow assessment of gas exchange between alveoli and capillaries, and provides information regarding the diffusion capacity of

the lung.[41,44–46,49,85,86] One straightforward example uses a chemical shift saturation recovery method to measure alveolar surface area and is shown in **Fig. 5** [42–44] Here, a 90° selective radio frequency (RF) pulse is applied at an initial time t = 0 to destroy the dissolved-state (eg, tissue) ^{129}Xe magnetization. The pulse sequence then includes a time delay during which magnetized ^{129}Xe atoms diffuse from the alveolar gas spaces into the septal tissue, after which the dissolved state magnetization is interrogated with a second selective 90° RF pulse. Two quantities are measured: the initial gas phase magnetization, Mgas (t = 0), and the dissolved phase magnetization as a function of diffusion time, Mdiss(t). The fraction F = Mdiss(t)/ Mgas(t = 0) is proportional to the alveolar surface area per unit volume of gas (S/V) (see **Fig. 5**; **Fig. 6**). This quantity is a primary measure of emphysema and represents a noninvasive measure of lung function. Another technique, called xenon transfer contrast (XTC)[45,46] modified for a single-breath protocol [42] has recently demonstrated images of the quantity F(t = 62 milliseconds) in healthy human subjects (**Fig. 7**). Relative values of F represent relative values of S/V. In the XTC method, two image pairs are used. The first pair is used to measure the loss of signal between two sequential gradient-echo images attributable to loss of ^{129}Xe magnetization from the imaging process itself (ie, the RF pulses), and second, from the presence of oxygen in the lung, which decreases T1. Between the second pair of images (ie, images B and C) the gas phase signal is reduced by the application of numerous 180° selective RF pulses applied to the dissolved phase frequencies. Between each RF pulse, there is a small delay during which gas exchange takes place, reducing the gas phase ^{129}Xe magnetization by $\sim 2\%$. The application of numerous pulses builds up the decay in the gas phase magnetization to an easily measurable value. In addition to

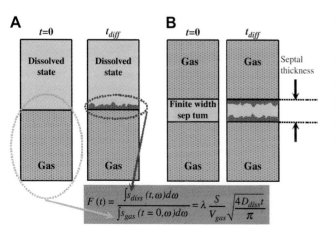

$$F(t) = \frac{\int s_{diss}(t,\omega)d\omega}{\int s_{gas}(t=0,\omega)d\omega} = \lambda \frac{S}{V_{gas}} \sqrt{\frac{4D_{diss}t}{\pi}}$$

Fig. 5. Chemical shift saturation recovery method. (*A*) Idealized one-dimensional semi-infinite phases. (*B*) A more realistic model with a finite width septum. Net diffusion from gas to dissolved phase after time tdiff is shown in purple. (*From* Patz S, Hersman FW, Muradian I, et al. Hyperpolarized (129)Xe MRI: A viable functional lung imaging modality? Eur J Radiol 2007;64(3): 340; with permission.)

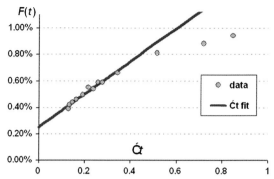

Fig. 6. Experimentally measured *F(t)* shown with blue dots as a function of √t. Lung volume was fixed at total lung capacity (TLC). Also shown is a fit to the early time data (*red line*). (*From* Patz S, Hersman FW, Muradian I, et al. Hyperpolarized (129)Xe MRI: A viable functional lung imaging modality? Eur J Radiol 2007;64(3):340; with permission.)

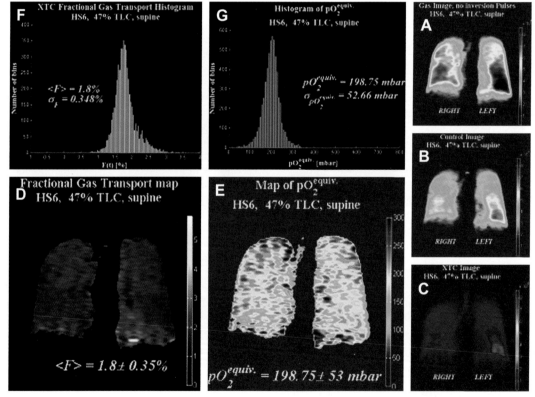

Fig. 7. Single-breath (SB)–XTC raw and processed data. Coronal projection images were acquired from subject HS6 in the supine position after 1 L of 86% enriched [129]Xe was inhaled (47% TLC). (*A–C*) Example of the three serially acquired SB-XTC gradient echo images and the information obtained from them. (*A*) First image shows [129]Xe ventilation; (*B*) second "control" image acquired after image (*A*) and then an XTC exchange sensitization (RF pulses off resonance) such that the only attenuation between images (*A*) and (*B*) is due to RF depletion and T1 decay from Po2; and (*C*) third XTC image acquired after image (*B*) and an XTC exchange sensitization (RF pulses applied on resonance) such that the attenuation between images (*B*) and (*C*) is due to RF depletion, T1 decay from Po2, and [129]Xe interphase diffusion. Voxels in image (*C*) have been scaled up by the attenuation factor measured between (*A*) and (*B*) such that the attenuation observed between (*B*) and (*C*) is solely due to interphase diffusion. Also shown are (*D*), the resulting FXTC, and (*E*) Po2-equiv maps, and their respective histograms (*F*) and (*G*). (*From* Patz S, Hersman FW, Muradian I, et al. Hyperpolarized (129)Xe MRI: A viable functional lung imaging modality? Eur J Radiol 2007;64(3):341; with permission.)

measuring a quantity related to the alveolar surface area (ie, S/V) others have demonstrated the ability to measure septal thickness in animals [47,49] and humans.[48] In a recent study, evaluation of emphysema severity and progression was shown.[73]

Regarding measuring the ADC of ^{129}Xe, it is important to note that ^{129}Xe has a much lower diffusivity than ^{3}He. The lower diffusion coefficient of ^{129}Xe can be used for diffusion-weighted imaging applications designed to more suitable for measurement of alveolar and small airway dimensions.[87–89]

Hyperpolarized ^{129}Xe gas is also sensitive to intrapulmonary oxygen partial pressures; however, the measurement of P_{O_2} by observation of ^{129}Xe signal decay is more complex than that for ^{3}He because of an additional signal loss mechanism attributable to interphase diffusion of ^{129}Xe from alveolar gas spaces to septal tissue.[42] This results in measurements of an equivalent P_{O_2} that accounts for both traditional T1 decay from P_{O_2} and that from interphase diffusion (see **Fig. 7**).

OXYGEN-ENHANCED MR IMAGING

Visualization of ventilation is also feasible using oxygen-enhanced MR imaging. Oxygen modulates the signal intensity of blood and other fluids through two different mechanisms: (1) the paramagnetic property of deoxyhemoglobin, and (2) the paramagnetic property of molecular oxygen itself.[90,91] Deoxyhemoglobin is compartmentalized in red blood cells; water protons of tissue do not have access to coordination sites.[92] Deoxyhemoglobin in red blood cells therefore has a T2* shortening effect with little T1 shortening effect.[92,93] Blood oxygenation level–dependent contrast is based on this effect of deoxyhemoglobin.[94–96] This mechanism has been widely used to evaluate regional blood flow and tissue oxygenation. When oxygen is exchanged between air in the alveoli and blood in the capillary beds, the oxygen not only couples with hemoglobin but also dissolves as molecular oxygen in the blood.[97] Because O_2 has the paramagnetic property, the dissolved molecular oxygen then shortens the T1 relaxation time of the pulmonary venous blood. The shortening of T1 relaxation time caused by 100% oxygen inhalation leads to visualization of ventilation by MR imaging as an increase in signal intensity (**Fig. 8**). The T1 effect that results from a higher proportion of oxygen-bound hemoglobin during the breathing of 100% oxygen is very small, because the concentration of dissolved oxygen in arterial blood increases much more than the amount of oxygen bound to hemoglobin. The concentration of oxygen in the blood depends on the partial pressure of oxygen in the alveoli. Concentration of dissolved oxygen in arterial blood increases by five times after inhalation of 100% oxygen.[97]

To visualize ventilation effectively, the oxygen-enhanced MR ventilation sequence is performed as follows: (1) single-shot rapid acquisition with relaxation enhancement or half-Fourier single-shot turbo spin-echo (HASTE) sequences, (2) as short a TE as possible, (3) a centrically reordered phase-encoding scheme on HASTE sequence, and (4) respiratory triggering or shorter data acquisition time than the respiratory cycle to reduce motion artifacts.[98]

Several experimental studies have shown the relation between physiologic change and the result of oxygen-enhanced MR imaging. The relationship between T1 and oxygen concentration was studied by using a pig model, and strong linear correlation between arterial blood oxygen pressure (Pa_{O_2}) and relativity of pulmonary parenchyma (1/T1) was found.[99] Pa_{O_2} was also closely related to pulmonary venous oxygen pressure and therefore to oxygen pressure in the pulmonary capillary blood. This linear relationship between Pa_{O_2} and 1/T1 suggests the feasibility of quantitative measurement of regional pulmonary ventilation and oxygen transfer.[100] The ability of oxygen-enhanced MR imaging to detect regional ventilation abnormalities was proved in a pig model of airway obstruction,[101] and the ability of oxygen-enhanced MR imaging to detect regional ventilation–perfusion abnormalities was also reported in a pig model of pulmonary embolism, and the mismatch between ventilation and perfusion was demonstrated successfully.[102]

Several researchers have reported promising results with oxygen-enhanced MR imaging for evaluation of normal ventilation,[99,103–105] diseases with ventilation abnormalities including lung cancer,[106] cystic fibrosis,[107] pulmonary embolism,[9] interstitial pneumonia,[108] pulmonary emphysema,[109] and COPD.[110] In these clinical studies, regional oxygen enhancement was quantitatively or semiquantitatively evaluated and correlated with the parameters of PFTs. Regional morphologic and functional abnormalities were assessed with scintigraphy or quantitative CT. Ohno and colleagues[111] reported that oxygen-enhanced MR revealed regional changes in ventilation that reflected regional lung function. The maximum mean relative enhancement ratio showed a good correlation with the diffusion capacity for carbon monoxide ($r^2 = 0.83$), whereas the mean slope of relative enhancement was strongly correlated with FEV_1 ($r^2 = 0.74$). In addition, they showed

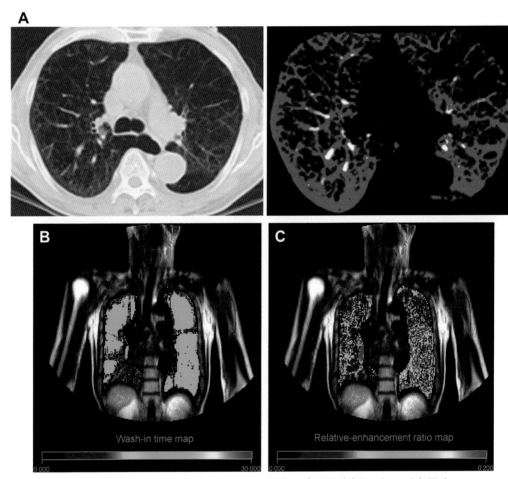

Fig. 8. A 76-year-old smoking subject who had Brinkman index of 1480. (*A*) Routine axial CT demonstrates multiple low attenuation areas because of pulmonary emphysema in both lungs. Heterogeneously functional lung is shown in red and pulmonary emphysema in black on quantitative axial CT. (*B*) Coronal wash-in time map calculated from dynamic oxygen-enhanced MR images obtained by using centrically reordered inversion-recovery HASTE sequence demonstrates heterogeneous and markedly prolonged regional wash-in time in both lungs. Mean wash-in time was 53.0 seconds. (*C*) Coronal relative-enhancement map calculated from the same dynamic oxygen-enhanced MR data shows heterogeneously and markedly reduced relative enhancement ratio in the both lungs. Mean relative enhancement ratio was 0.08. (*From* Ohno Y, Koyama H, Nogami M, et al. Dynamic oxygen-enhanced MRI versus quantitative CT: pulmonary functional loss assessment and clinical stage classification of smoking-related COPD. AJR Am J Roentgenol 2008;190(2):W97; with permission.)

significant correlation between maximum mean relative enhancement and HRCT emphysema scores ($r^2 = 0.38$). These findings might prove useful for classifying the phenotype of COPD because each parameter could evaluate emphysema and airway disease separately.

Although the usefulness of hyperpolarized noble gas MR technique has been proved, oxygen-enhanced MR imaging is inexpensive and readily available with conventional clinical proton MR scanners without any modification. In addition, the underlying physiology for oxygen-enhanced MR imaging is different from that for hyperpolarized noble gas; thus oxygen-enhanced MR

imaging might provide regional information based on ventilation, perfusion, and oxygen transfer from alveoli to the capillary bed.

RESPIRATORY DYNAMICS

Image-based assessment of the respiratory lung motion has been explored for the evaluation of the physiologic aspects of respiratory function in normal patients and for the diagnosis and treatment of disease states. MR imaging has been used to assess anatomic structure variations resulting from respiration with reasonable spatial and temporal resolution. The advantage of MR imaging over other imaging modalities, such as fluoroscopy and CT, is that MR is free from radiation exposure.

Severe hyperinflation of the lung in COPD alters diaphragmatic movement with subsequent reduction of the mechanical properties of respiratory muscle function. The evaluation of diaphragmatic movement alteration is important because treatments, such as lung volume reduction surgery (LVRS), are believed to improve lung function by facilitating breathing mechanics and increasing elastic recoil.[112] Two-dimensional or three-dimensional dynamic MR imaging can provide information regarding diaphragmatic motion.[113–117] In contrast to normal subjects, patients who have emphysema frequently show reduced, irregular, or asynchronous motion of the diaphragm, with a significant decrease in the maximum amplitude and the length of apposition of the diaphragm.[118] In some patients who have paradoxical movement of the diaphragm, the ventral portion of the diaphragm moves caudally while the dorsal part moves cranially.[119] Paradoxical diaphragmatic motion also correlates with hyperinflation.[120] After LVRS, patients show improvement in abnormal diaphragm movement and mobility.[119] Recently, our group showed that, with the use of a 3T whole-body scanner using 128-channel coils, dynamic three-dimensional MR images with high spatial and temporal resolution were capable of demonstrating lung motion with acceptable image quality for automated postprocessing. MR imaging may play a role in the future for the assessment of diaphragm movement.

SUMMARY

With recent development of MR techniques, MR imaging is playing an increasingly important role for the evaluation of pulmonary function.

Dynamic contrast-enhanced MR perfusion imaging is suitable for the evaluation of angiogenesis of pulmonary solitary nodules.

^{129}Xe MR imaging is potentially a robust technique for the evaluation of various pulmonary functions and may replace ^{3}He.

As new MR imaging techniques become more widely available, further investigations for the pulmonary functional MR imaging are expected.

REFERENCES

1. Hatabu H, Chen Q, Stock KW, et al. Fast magnetic resonance imaging of the lung. Eur J Radiol 1999; 29(2):114–32.

2. Hatabu H, Alsop DC, Listerud J, et al. T2* and proton density measurement of normal human lung parenchyma using submillisecond echo time gradient echo magnetic resonance imaging. Eur J Radiol 1999;29(3):245–52.

3. Bergin CJ, Glover GM, Pauly J. Magnetic resonance imaging of lung parenchyma. J Thorac Imaging 1993;8(1):12–7.

4. Hatabu H, Gaa J, Kim D, et al. Pulmonary perfusion: qualitative assessment with dynamic contrast-enhanced MRI using ultra-short TE and inversion recovery turbo FLASH. Magn Reson Med 1996; 36(4):503–8.

5. Edelman RR, Siewert B, Adamis M, et al. Signal targeting with alternating radiofrequency (STAR) sequences: application to MR angiography. Magn Reson Med 1994;31(2):233–8.

6. Ogasawara N, Suga K, Karino Y, et al. Perfusion characteristics of radiation-injured lung on Gd-DTPA-enhanced dynamic magnetic resonance imaging. Invest Radiol 2002;37(8):448–57.

7. Amundsen T, Kvaerness J, Jones RA, et al. Pulmonary embolism: detection with MR perfusion imaging of lung—a feasibility study. Radiology 1997;203(1):181–5.

8. Amundsen T, Torheim G, Waage A, et al. Perfusion magnetic resonance imaging of the lung: characterization of pneumonia and chronic obstructive pulmonary disease. A feasibility study. J Magn Reson Imaging 2000;12(2):224–31.

9. Nakagawa T, Sakuma H, Murashima S, et al. Pulmonary ventilation-perfusion MR imaging in clinical patients. J Magn Reson Imaging 2001;14(4): 419–24.

10. Matsuoka S, Uchiyama K, Shima H, et al. Detectability of pulmonary perfusion defect and influence of breath holding on contrast-enhanced thick-slice 2D and on 3D MR pulmonary perfusion images. J Magn Reson Imaging 2001;14(5):580–5.

11. Ohno Y, Hatabu H, Takenaka D, et al. Solitary pulmonary nodules: potential role of dynamic MR imaging in management initial experience. Radiology 2002;224:503–11.

12. Schaefer JF, Vollmar J, Schick F, et al. Solitary pulmonary nodules: dynamic contrast-enhanced MR imaging–perfusion differences in malignant and benign lesions. Radiology 2004;232(2):544–53.

13. Kono R, Fujimoto K, Terasaki H, et al. Dynamic MRI of solitary pulmonary nodules: comparison of enhancement patterns of malignant and benign small peripheral lung lesions. AJR Am J Roentgenol. 2007;188(1):26–36.

14. Hittmair K, Eckersberger F, Klepetko W, et al. Evaluation of solitary pulmonary nodules with dynamic contrast-enhanced MR imaging: a promising technique. Magn Reson Imaging 1995;13: 923–33.

15. Tozaki M, Ichiba N, Fukuda K. Dynamic magnetic resonance imaging of solitary pulmonary nodules: utility of kinetic patterns in differential diagnosis. J Comput Assist Tomogr 2005;29(1):13–9.

16. Hunter GJ, Hamberg LM, Choi N, et al. Dynamic T1-weighted magnetic resonance imaging and positron emission tomography in patients with lung cancer—correlating vascular physiology with glucose metabolism. Clin Cancer Res 1998;4(4):949–55.

17. Schaefer JF, Schneider V, Vollmar J, et al. Solitary pulmonary nodules: association between signal characteristics in dynamic contrast enhanced MRI and tumor angiogenesis. Lung Cancer 2006;53(1):39–49.

18. Mattern J, Koomagi R, Volm M. Coexpression of VEGF and bFGF in human epidermoid lung carcinomas in associated with increase vessel density. Anticancer Res 1997;17(3C):2249–52.

19. Mattern J, Koomagi R, Volm M. Association of vascular endothelial growth factor expression with intratumoral microvessel density and tumor cell proliferation in human epidermoid lung carcinoma. Br J Cancer 1996;73(7):931–4.

20. Imoto H, Osaki T, Taga S, et al. Vascular endothelial growth factor expression in non-small cell lung cancer: prognostic significance in squamous cell carcinoma. J Thorac Cardiovasc Surg 1998;115(5):1007–14.

21. Ohta Y, Endo Y, Tanaka M, et al. Significance of vascular endothelial growth factor messenger RNA expression in primary lung cancer. Clin Cancer Res 1996;2(8):1411–6.

22. Shibusa T, Shijubo N, Abe S. Tumor angiogenesis and vascular endothelial growth factor expression in stage I lung adenocarcinoma. Clin Cancer Res 1998;4(6):1483–7.

23. Takanami I, Tanaka F, Hashizume T, et al. Vascular endothelial growth factor and its receptor correlate with angiogenesis and survival in pulmonary adenocarcinoma. Anticancer Res 1997;17(4A):2811–4.

24. Fontanini G, Vignati S, Boldrini L, et al. Vascular endothelial growth factor in associated with neovascularization and influences progression of non-small cell lung carcinoma. Clin Cancer Res 1997;3(6):861–5.

25. Fontanini G, Vignati S, Lucchi M, et al. Neoangiogenesis and p53 protein in lung cancer: their prognostic role and their relation with vascular endothelial growth factor (VEGF) expression. Br J Cancer 1997;75(9):1295–301.

26. Yamashita K, Matsnobe S, Tsuda T, et al. Solitary pulmonary nodules: preliminary study of evaluation with incremental dynamic CT. Radiology 1995;194(2):399–405.

27. Swensen SJ, Brown LR, Colby TV, et al. Lung nodule enhancement at CT: prospective findings. Radiology 1996;201(2):447–55.

28. Fujimoto K, Abe T, Müller NL, et al. Small peripheral pulmonary carcinomas evaluated with dynamic MR imaging: correlation with tumor vascularity and prognosis. Radiology 2003;227(3):786–93.

29. Tateishi U, Kusumoto M, Nishihara H, et al. Contrast-enhanced dynamic computed tomography for the evaluation of tumor angiogenesis in patients with lung carcinoma. Cancer 2002;95(4):835–42.

30. Barrett T, Brechbiel M, Bernardo M, et al. MRI of tumor angiogenesis. J Magn Reson Imaging 2007;26(2):235–49.

31. Matoba M, Tonami H, Kondou T, et al. Lung carcinoma: diffusion-weighted MR imaging—preliminary evaluation with apparent diffusion coefficient. Radiology 2007;243(2):570–7.

32. Kimura H, Takeuchi H, Koshimoto Y, et al. Perfusion imaging of meningioma by using continuous arterial spin-labeling: comparison with dynamic susceptibility-weighted contrast-enhanced MR images and histopathologic features. AJNR Am J Neuroradiol 2006;27(1):85–93.

33. Moffat BA, Chen M, Kariaapper MS, et al. Inhibition of vascular endothelial growth factor (VEGF)-a causes a paradoxical increase in tumor blood flow and up-regulation of VEGF-D. Clin Cancer Res 2006;12(5):1525–32.

34. De Bazelaire C, Rofsky NM, Duhamel G, et al. Arterial spin labeling blood flow magnetic resonance imaging for the characterization of metastatic renal cell carcinoma. Acad Radiol 2005;12(3):347–57.

35. Ohno Y, Koyama H, Nogami M, et al. Postoperative lung function in lung cancer patients: comparative analysis of predictive capability of MRI, CT, and SPECT. AJR Am J Roentgenol 2007;189(2):400–8.

36. Fisher MR, Criner GJ, Fishman AP, et al. Estimating pulmonary artery pressures by echocardiography in patients with emphysema. Eur Respir J 2007;30(5):914–21.

37. Ohno Y, Hatabu H, Murase K, et al. Primary pulmonary hypertension: 3D dynamic perfusion MRI for quantitative analysis of regional pulmonary perfusion. AJR Am J Roentgenol 2007;188(1):48–56.

38. Vonk-Noordegraaf A, Marcus JT, Holverda S, et al. Early changes of cardiac structure and function in COPD patients with mild hypoxemia. Chest 2005;127(6):1898–903.

39. Marcus JT, Vonk Noordegraaf A, De Vries PM, et al. MRI evaluation of right ventricular pressure overload in chronic obstructive pulmonary disease. J Magn Reson Imaging 1998;8(5):999–1005.

40. Albert MS, Cates GD, Driehuys B, et al. Biological magnetic resonance imaging using laser-polarized ^{129}Xe. Nature 1994;370(6486):199–201.

41. Ruset IC, Ketel S, Hersman FW. Optical pumping system design for large production of hyperpolarized. Phys Rev Lett 2006;96(5): 053002.

42. Patz S, Hersman FW, Muradian I, et al. Hyperpolarized ^{129}Xe MRI: a viable functional lung imaging modality? Eur J Radiol 2007;64(3):335–44.

43. Patz S, Muradian I, Hrovat MI, et al. Human pulmonary imaging and spectroscopy with hyperpolarized ^{129}Xe at 0.2T. Acad Radiol, in press.

44. Butler JP, Mair RW, Hoffmann D, et al. Measuring surface-area-to-volume ratios in soft porous materials using laser-polarized xenon interphase exchange NMR. J Phys Condens Matter 2002;14: L297–304.

45. Ruppert K, Brookeman JR, Hagspiel KD, et al. Probing lung physiology with xenon polarization transfer contrast (XTC). Magn Reson Med 2000; 44(3):349–57.

46. Ruppert K, Mata JF, Brookeman JR, et al. Exploring lung function with hyperpolarized ^{129}Xe nuclear magnetic resonance. Magn Reson Med 2004; 51(4):676–87.

47. Driehuys B, Cofer GP, Pollaro J, et al. Imaging alveolar-capillary gas transfer using hyperpolarized ^{129}Xe MRI. Proc Natl Acad Sci U S A 2006; 103(48):18278–83.

48. Patz S, Butler JP, Muradian I, et al. Human pulmonary physiology with hyperpolarized ^{129}Xe. Chicago (IL): RSNA; 2007.

49. Månsson S, Wolber J, Driehuys B, et al. Characterization of diffusing capacity and perfusion of the rat lung in a lipopolysaccharide disease model using hyperpolarized ^{129}Xe. Magn Reson Med 2003; 50(6):1170–9.

50. MacFall JR, Charles HC, Black RD, et al. Human lung air spaces potential for MR imaging with hyperpolarized He-3. Radiology 1996;200(2): 553–8.

51. Kauczor HU, Hofmann D, Kreitner KF, et al. Normal and abnormal pulmonary ventilation: visualization at hyperpolarized He-3 MR imaging. Radiology 1996;201(2):564–8.

52. de Lange EE, Mugler JP III, Brookeman JR, et al. Lung air spaces: MR imaging evaluation with hyperpolarized ^{3}He gas. Radiology 1999;210(3): 851–7.

53. Samee S, Altes T, Powers P, et al. Imaging the lungs in asthmatic patients by using hyperpolarized helium-3 magnetic resonance: assessment of response to methacholine and exercise challenge. J Allergy Clin Immunol 2003;111(6):1205–11.

54. de Lange EE, Altes TA, Patrie JT, et al. The variability of regional airflow obstruction within the lungs of patients with asthma: assessment with hyperpolarized helium-3 magnetic resonance imaging. J Allergy Clin Immunol 2007;119(5):1072–8.

55. Gast KK, Viallon M, Eberle B, et al. MRI in lung transplant recipients using hyperpolarized ^{3}He: comparison with CT. J Magn Reson Imaging 2002;15(3):268–74.

56. Zaporozhan J, Ley S, Gast KK, et al. Functional analysis in single lung transplant recipients: a comparative study of high-resolution CT, ^{3}He-MRI, and pulmonary function tests. Chest 2004; 125(1):173–81.

57. Salerno M, Altes TA, Brookeman JR, et al. Dynamic spiral MRI of pulmonary gas flow using hyperpolarized ^{3}He: preliminary studies in healthy and diseased lungs. Magn Reson Med 2001;46(4): 667–77.

58. Wild JM, Paley MN, Kasuboski L, et al. Dynamic radial projection MRI of inhaled hyperpolarized ^{3}He gas. Magn Reson Med 2003;49(6):991–7.

59. Gast KK, Puderbach MU, Rodriguez I, et al. Dynamic ventilation ^{3}He-magnetic resonance imaging with lung motion correction: gas flow distribution analysis. Invest Radiol 2002;37(3):126–34.

60. Eda S, Kubo K, Fujimoto K, et al. The relations between expiratory chest CT using helical CT and pulmonary function tests in emphysema. Am J Respir Crit Care Med 1997;155(4):1290–4.

61. O'Donnell RA, Peebles C, Ward JA, et al. Relationship between peripheral airway dysfunction, airway obstruction, and neutrophilic inflammation in COPD. Thorax 2004;59(10):837–42.

62. Matsuoka S, Kurihara Y, Yagihashi K, et al. Quantitative assessment of peripheral airway obstruction on paired expiratory/inspiratory thin-section CT in COPD with emphysema. J Comput Assist Tomogr 2007;31(3):384–9.

63. Matsuoka S, Kurihara Y, Yagihashi K, et al. Quantitative assessment of air trapping in chronic obstructive pulmonary disease using inspiratory and expiratory volumetric MDCT. AJR Am J Roentgenol 2008;190(3):762–9.

64. McMahon CJ, Dodd JD, Hill C, et al. Hyperpolarized 3helium magnetic resonance ventilation imaging of the lung in cystic fibrosis: comparison with high resolution CT and spirometry. Eur Radiol 2006;16(11):2483–90.

65. Koumellis P, van Beek EJ, Woodhouse N, et al. Quantitative analysis of regional airways obstruction using dynamic hyperpolarized ^{3}He MRI-preliminary results in children with cystic fibrosis. J Magn Reson Imaging 2005;22(3):420–6.

66. Swift A, Wild JM, Paley MNJ, et al. Hyperpolarized ^{3}He MRI of normal and abnormal ventilation using a dynamic radial projection sequence. Eur Radiol 2003;13(Suppl 1):161.

67. Burge PS, Calverley PM, Jones PW. Randomized double blind, placebo controlled trial of fluticasone propionate in patients with moderate to severe

chronic obstructive pulmonary disease: the ISOLDE trial. BMJ 2000;320(7245):1297–303.

68. Goldin JG, Tashkin DP, Kleerup EC, et al. Comparative effects of hydrofluoroalkane and chlorofluorocarbon beclomethasone dipropionate inhalation on small airways: assessment with functional helical thin-section computed tomography. J Allergy Clin Immunol 1999;104(6):S258–67.

69. Saam BT, Yablonskiy DA, Kodibagkar VD, et al. MR imaging of diffusion of ^{3}He gas in healthy and diseased lungs. Magn Reson Med 2000;44(2):174–9.

70. Salerno M, de Lange EE, Altes TA, et al. Emphysema: hyperpolarized helium 3 diffusion MR imaging of the lungs compared with spirometric indexes—initial experience. Radiology 2002; 222(1):252–60.

71. Swift AJ, Wild JM, Fichele S, et al. Emphysematous changes and normal variation in smokers and COPD patients using diffusion ^{3}He MRI. Eur J Radiol 2005;54(3):352–8.

72. Woods JC, Yablonskiy DA, Choong CK, et al. Long-range diffusion of hyperpolarized ^{3}He in explanted normal and emphysematous human lungs via magnetization tagging. J Appl Phys 2005;99(5):1992–7.

73. Mata JF, Altes TA, Cai J, et al. Evaluation of emphysema severity and progression in a rabbit model: comparison of hyperpolarized ^{3}He and ^{129}Xe diffusion MRI with lung morphometry. J Appl Phys 2007;102(3):1273–80.

74. Peces-Barba G, Ruiz-Cabello J, Cremillieux Y, et al. Helium-3 MRI diffusion coefficient: correlation to morphometry in a model of mild emphysema. Eur Respir J 2003;22(1):14–9.

75. Tanoli TS, Woods JC, Conradi MS, et al. In vivo lung morphometry with hyperpolarized ^{3}He diffusion MRI in canines with induced emphysema: disease progression and comparison with computed tomography. J Appl Phys 2007;102(1):477–84.

76. Fain SB, Panth SR, Evans MD, et al. ^{3}He MRI detects early emphysematous changes in asymptomatic smokers. Radiology 2006;239(3):875–83.

77. Fain SB, Altes TA, Panth SR, et al. Detection of age-dependent changes in healthy adult lungs with diffusion-weighted ^{3}He MRI. Acad Radiol 2005; 12(11):1385–93.

78. Gillooly M, Lamb D. Airspace size in lungs of lifelong non-smokers effect of age and sex. Thorax 1993;48(1):39–43.

79. Saam B, Happer W, Middleton H. Nuclear relaxation of ^{3}He in the presence of O_2. Phys Rev A 1995;52(1):862–5.

80. Eberle B, Weiler N, Markstaller K, et al. Analysis of intrapulmonary O_2 concentration by MR imaging of inhaled hyperpolarized ^{3}He. J Appl Phys 1999; 87(6):2043–52.

81. Deninger AJ, Eberle B, Bermuth J, et al. Assessment of a single-acquisition imaging sequence for oxygen-sensitive (3)He-MRI. Magn Reson Med 2002;47(1):105–14.

82. Fischer M, Spector Z, Ishii M, et al. Single-acquisition sequence for the measurement of oxygen partial pressure by hyperpolarized gas MRI. Magn Reson Med 2004;52(4):766–73.

83. Rizi RR, Baumgardner JE, Ishii M, et al. Determination of regional VA/Q by hyperpolarized ^{3}He MRI. Magn Reson Med 2004;52(1):65–72.

84. Eger EL, Larson CP. Anaesthetic solubility in blood and tissues. Br J Anaesth 1964;36:140–9.

85. Mugler JP 3rd, Driehuys B, Brookeman JR, et al. MR imaging and spectroscopy using hyperpolarized ^{129}Xe gas: preliminary human results. Magn Reson Med 1997;37(6):809–15.

86. Abdeen N, Cross A, Cron G, et al. Measurement of xenon diffusing capacity in the rat lung by hyperpolarized ^{129}Xe MRI and dynamic spectroscopy in a single breath-hold. Magn Reson Med 2006; 56(2):255–64.

87. Mugler JP, Mata JF, Wang H- TJ, et al. The apparent diffusion coefficient of Xe-129 in the lung: preliminary human results. Proceedings of the 11th International Society of Magnetic Resonance in Medicine 2004;11:769.

88. Sindile A, Muradian I, Hrovat M, et al. Human pulmonary diffusion weighted imaging at 0.2T with hyperpolarized ^{129}Xe. American Physical Society March Meeting 2007;269.

89. Chen X, Moller H, Chawla M, et al. Spatially resolved measurements of hyperpolarized gas properties in the lung in vivo. Part I: diffusion coefficient. Magn Reson Med 1999;42(4):721–8.

90. Young IR, Clarke GJ, Bailes DR, et al. Enhancement of relaxation rate with paramagnetic contrast agents in NMR imaging. J Comput Tomogr 1981; 5(6):543–6.

91. Pauling L, Coryell CD. The magnetic properties and structure of the hemochromogens and related substances. Proc Natl Acad Sci U S A 1936;22(3): 159–63.

92. Brooks RA, Di Chiro G. Magnetic resonance imaging of stationary blood: a review. Med Phys 1987; 14(6):903–13.

93. Thulborn KR, Waterton JC, Matthews PM, et al. Oxygenation dependence of the transverse relaxation time of water protons in whole blood at high field. Biochim Biophys Acta. 1982;714(2): 265–70.

94. Ogawa S, Lee TM, Nayak AS, et al. Oxygenation sensitive contrast in magnetic resonance image of rodent brain at high magnetic field. Magn Reson Med 1990;14(1):68–78.

95. Ogawa S, Lee TM, Kay AR, et al. Brain magnetic resonance imaging with contrast dependent on blood oxygenation. Proc Natl Acad Sci USA. 1990;87(24):9868–72.

96. Ogawa S, Tank DW, Menon R, et al. Intrinsic signal changes accompanying sensory stimulation: functional brain mapping with magnetic resonance imaging. Proc Natl Acad Sci U S A 1992;89(13):5951–5.

97. Tadamura E, Hatabu H, Li W, et al. Effect of oxygen inhalation on relaxation time in various tissues. J Magn Reson Imag 1997;7(1):220–5.

98. Ohno Y, Hatabu H. Basics concepts and clinical applications of oxygen-enhanced MR imaging. Eur J Radiol 2007;64(3):320–8.

99. Hatabu H, Tadamura E, Chen Q, et al. Pulmonary ventilation: dynamic MRI with inhalation of molecular oxygen. Eur J Radiol 2001;37(3):172–8.

100. Chen Q, Jakob PM, Griswold MA, et al. Oxygen-enhanced MR ventilation imaging of the lung. MAGMA 1998;7(3):153–61.

101. Chen Q, Levin DL, Kim D, et al. Pulmonary disorder: ventilation-perfusion MR imaging with animal models. Radiology 1999;213(3):871–9.

102. Edelman RR, Hatabu H, Tadamura E, et al. Noninvasive assessment of regional ventilation in the human lung using oxygen-enhanced magnetic resonance imaging. Nat Med 1996;2(11): 1236–9.

103. Loffler R, Muller CJ, Peller M, et al. Optimization and evaluation of the signal intensity change in multisection oxygen-enhanced MR lung imaging. Magn Reson Med 2000;43(6):860–6.

104. Mai VM, Chen Q, Bankier AA, et al. Multiple inversion recovery MR subtraction imaging of human ventilation from inhalation of room air and pure oxygen. Magn Reson Med 2000;43(6):913–6.

105. Ohno Y, Hatabu H, Takenaka D, et al. Oxygen-enhanced MR ventilation imaging of the lung: preliminary clinical experience in 25 subjects. AJR Am J Roentgenol 2001;177(1):185–94.

106. Ohno Y, Hatabu H, Higashino T, et al. Oxygen-enhanced MR imaging: correlation with postsurgical lung function in patients with lung cancer. Radiology 2005;236(2):704–11.

107. Jakob PM, Wang T, Schultz G, et al. Assessment of human pulmonary function using oxygen-enhanced T(1) imaging in patients with cystic fibrosis. Magn Reson Med 2004;51(5):1009–16.

108. Muller CJ, Schwaiblmair M, Scheidler J, et al. Pulmonary diffusing capacity: assessment with oxygen-enhanced lung MR imaging preliminary findings. Radiology 2002;222(2):499–506.

109. Ohno Y, Hatabu H, Takenaka D, et al. Dynamic oxygen-enhanced MRI reflects diffusing capacity of the lung. Magn Reson Med 2002;47(6):1139–44.

110. Ohno Y, Hatabu H, Higashino T, et al. Oxygen-enhanced MR imaging: correlation with postsurgical ling function in patients with lung cancer. Radiology 2005;236(2):704–11.

111. Ohno Y, Sugimura K, Hatabu H. Clinical oxygen-enhanced magnetic resonance imaging of the lung. Top Magn Reson Imaging 2003;14(3):237–43.

112. Henderson AC, Ingenito EP, Salcedo ES, et al. Dynamic lung mechanics in late-stage emphysema before and after lung volume reduction surgery. Respir Physiolo Neurobiol 2007;155(3):234–42.

113. Shimizu S, Shirato H, Aoyama H, et al. High-speed magnetic resonance imaging for four-dimensional treatment planning of conformal radiotherapy of moving body tumors. Int J Radiat Oncol Biol Phys 2000;48(2):471–4.

114. Gee J, Sundaram T, Hasegawa I, et al. Characterization of regional pulmonary mechanics from serial magnetic resonance imaging data. Acad Radiol 2003;10(10):1147–52.

115. Kiryu S, Loring SH, Mori Y, et al. Quantitative analysis of the velocity and synchronicity of diaphragmatic motion: dynamic MRI in different postures. Magn Reson Imaging 2006;24(10):1325–32.

116. Paiva M, Verbanck S, Estenne M, et al. Mechanical implications of in vivo human diaphragm shape. J Appl Phys 1992;72(4):1407–12.

117. Gauthier AP, Verbanck S, Estenne M, et al. 3-dimensional reconstruction of the in-vivo human diaphragm shape at different lung-volumes. J Appl Phys 1994;76(2):495–506.

118. Suga K, Tsukuda T, Awaya H, et al. Impaired respiratory mechanics in pulmonary emphysema: evaluation with dynamic breathing MRI. J Magn Reson Imaging 1999;10(4):510–20.

119. Iwasawa T, Yoshiike Y, Saito K, et al. Paradoxical motion of the hemidiaphragm in patients with emphysema. J Thorac Imaging 2000;15(3):191–5.

120. Iwasawa T, Kagei S, Gotoh T, et al. Magnetic resonance analysis of abnormal diaphragmatic motion in patients with emphysema. Eur Respir J 2002; 19(2):225–31.

MR for the Evaluation of Obstructive Pulmonary Disease

Julia Ley-Zaporozhan, MD[a,b],*, Michael Puderbach, MD[b],
Hans-Ulrich Kauczor, MD[c,d]

KEYWORDS

- Obstructive lung disease • Emphysema • Imaging
- MR imaging

Obstructive lung diseases include chronic bronchitis, chronic obstructive pulmonary disease (COPD), emphysema, asthma, and cystic fibrosis (CF). They are all characterized by airflow limitation that is either reversible or irreversible and a variable degree of inflammation. The manifestations of obstructive lung disease are not limited to the tracheobronchial tree but also affect the parenchyma by hyperinflation and destruction and the vasculature by hypoxic vasoconstriction.

For severity assessment of obstructive lung diseases lung function tests are used. Pulmonary function tests only provide a global measure, however, without any regional information, and certainly do not provide any detail about lung structure. Although extremely useful, pulmonary function tests are known to be relatively insensitive to early stages and small changes of manifest disease. Furthermore, pulmonary function tests depend on the effort and compliance of the patient and are difficult for young children to perform.

In contrast to pulmonary function tests, radiologic imaging techniques might allow for differentiation of the different components of obstructive lung disease on a regional basis. CT has proved quite valuable for some time in this field, with emphasis on structural imaging of lung parenchyma and airways. MR imaging has the potential to provide regional information about the lung without the use of ionizing radiation, but is hampered by several challenges: (1) the low amount of tissue relates to a small number of protons leading to low signal, and (2) countless air–tissue interfaces cause substantial susceptibility artifacts along with respiratory and cardiac motion.

In several lung diseases, such as tumors, the amount of protons or the blood volume is actually increased and motion is reduced, which provides better preconditions for MR imaging. In obstructive pulmonary disease, however, there are no facilitating disease-related effects because there is loss of tissue and reduced blood volume attributable to hypoxic vasoconstriction and the degree of hyperinflation has a negative correlation with the MR signal. The depiction of the airways by MR imaging is certainly limited to the central bronchi. Fortunately, MR imaging has significant potential beyond the mere visualization of structure by providing comprehensive information about function (ie, perfusion, hemodynamics, ventilation, and respiratory mechanics). In this article the current knowledge about the potential of MR imaging in obstructive pulmonary disease is presented.

TECHNICAL PREREQUISITES

The most frequently used sequences in MR imaging of obstructive lung disease are acquired in

[a] Department of Pediatric Radiology, University Hospital Heidelberg, Im Neuenheimer Feld 153, 69120 Heidelberg, Germany
[b] Department of Radiology (E010), German Cancer Research Center, Im Neuenheimer Feld 280, 69120 Heidelberg, Germany
[c] Department of Diagnostic Radiology, University Hospital Heidelberg, Im Neuenheimer Feld 110, 69120 Heidelberg, Germany
[d] German Cancer Research Center, Im Neuenheimer Feld 400, 69120 Heidelberg, Germany
* Corresponding author. Department of Pediatric Radiology, University Hospital Heidelberg, Im Neuenheimer Feld 153, 69120 Heidelberg, Germany.
E-mail address: julia.leyzaporozhan@gmail.com (J. Ley-Zaporozhan).

Magn Reson Imaging Clin N Am 16 (2008) 291–308
doi:10.1016/j.mric.2008.02.014
1064-9689/08/$ – see front matter © 2008 Elsevier Inc. All rights reserved.

a breath hold. For fast T2-weighted imaging, single shot techniques with partial Fourier acquisition (HASTE) or ultrashort echo time (TE) (UTSE) are recommended. The T2-weighted HASTE sequence in coronal or axial orientation allows for the depiction of pulmonary infiltrates, inflammatory bronchial wall thickening, and mucus collections. T1-weighted three-dimensional (3D) gradient echo sequences, such as volume interpolated gradient echo sequence (VIBE), are suitable for the assessment of the mediastinum and common nodular lesions. The intravenous application of contrast material markedly improves the diagnostic yield of T1-weighted sequences by a clearer depiction of vessels, hilar structures, and solid pathologies. A major goal in inflammatory obstructive airway disease is to differentiate inflammation within the wall from muscular hypertrophy, edema, and mucus collection, which cannot be achieved by CT, but can be addressed by the use of T1- and T2-weighted images and contrast enhancement.

Respiration is the result of the complex interaction between chest wall and diaphragm motion, and it can be visualized by 2D or 3D dynamic MR techniques.[1–3] For data acquisition time-resolved techniques are used, which can be based on fast low angle shot or stready-state free precession sequences. This allows for a high temporal resolution down to 100 milliseconds per frame.

Obstructive pulmonary disease is associated with ventilation defects, which can be directly visualized by MR imaging. Several different techniques are available, with oxygen enhancement and inhalation of hyperpolarized noble gases being the most prominent. Oxygen-enhanced MR imaging requires no special scanner hardware, is easy to use, and the costs for oxygen are low. The use of high oxygen concentrations (15 L/min) may be risky in patients who have severe COPD, however. [3]He MR imaging is based on the inhalation of hyperpolarized [3]He gas. It allows for direct evaluation of the distribution of the tracer gas after a breath hold (static) or during continuous breathing (dynamic) along with airspace dimensions. The latter is done by diffusion-weighted MR imaging. Areas with ventilation defects caused by airway obstruction and emphysema represent the only limitation because they cannot be assessed because of lack of the tracer gas entering these areas. There is thus almost no information about these affected lung regions. Overall, the high cost of the noble gas [3]He, the process of laser-induced hyperpolarization, and the need for non-proton imaging remain the major drawbacks of this technology, limiting its use in broader clinical applications.

Because of the reflex of hypoxic vasoconstriction, ventilation defects in obstructive pulmonary disease largely correspond to perfusion defects in the same areas. The assessment of pulmonary perfusion makes sense, especially because perfusion MR imaging is much easier and more straightforward than ventilation MR imaging. The basic principle of contrast-enhanced perfusion MR imaging is a dynamic acquisition during and after an intravenous bolus injection of a paramagnetic contrast agent. Perfusion MR imaging of the lung requires a high temporal resolution to visualize the peak enhancement of the lung parenchyma. Consequently, contrast-enhanced perfusion MR imaging uses T1-weighted gradient echo MR imaging with ultrashort repetition time and TE, such as fast low angle shot. With the introduction of parallel imaging techniques, 3D perfusion imaging with a high spatial and temporal resolution and an improved anatomic coverage and z-axis resolution can be acquired.[4–6] These data sets are also well suited for high-quality multiplanar reformats. Because of high spatial resolution detailed analysis of pulmonary perfusion and precise anatomic localization of the perfusion defects on a lobar and even segmental level can be performed. Quantitative values for pulmonary perfusion can be obtained by applying the principles of indicator dilution techniques. The quantitative indices, such as mean transit time (MTT), pulmonary blood volume (PBV), and blood flow (PBF), are derived from the time intensity curve, defined by the dynamic series of perfusion MR images.

Widespread perfusion defects can result in changes of pulmonary blood flow and pressure finally leading to right heart strain. Assessment of right ventricular function using MR imaging by can be done either by phase contrast flow measurements in the pulmonary trunk or by short axis cine-acquisition of the right ventricle.[7,8] Early changes of the complex geometry of the right ventricular wall and chamber volume can thus be accurately measured.

CHRONIC OBSTRUCTIVE PULMONARY DISEASE AND EMPHYSEMA

COPD is the fourth most common cause of death among adults.[9] COPD is characterized by airflow limitation that is not fully reversible. The airflow limitation is usually progressive and associated with an abnormal inflammatory response of the lung to noxious particles or gases. It is caused by a mixture of airway obstruction (obstructive bronchiolitis) and parenchymal destruction (emphysema), the relative contributions of which are variable.[9] Chronic bronchitis, or the presence of cough and sputum production for at least 3 months in each of 2 consecutive years, remains a clinically and epidemiologically useful term. Pulmonary emphysema is a pathologic term and is defined by the American Thoracic Society as an abnormal permanent enlargement of the air spaces distal to the terminal bronchiole, accompanied by the destruction of their walls. In a simplified way, obstructive airflow limitation leads to air trapping with subsequent hyperinflation and later destruction of the lung parenchyma. For severity assessment of COPD lung function tests, such as forced expiration volume in one second (FEV_1), FEV_1/FVC (forced vital capacity), and diffusing capacity for carbon monoxide, are used. These are global measures of all changes occurring in COPD, however. Chronic hyperinflation affects diaphragmatic geometry with subsequent dysfunction attributable to dissociation of the breathing mechanics. The disease also affects the pulmonary arteries: intimal thickening, smooth muscle hypertrophy, and inflammation were described, finally leading to vascular remodeling.[10] The direct vascular changes and hyperinflation lead to the precapillary type of pulmonary hypertension.[11]

A precise characterization of each component of the disease is desirable for therapy decisions and monitoring. In contrast to spirometry, radiologic imaging might allow for regional assessment of the compartments involved (ie, airways, parenchyma, and vasculature). CT has long been used in this field and emphasizes structural imaging of lung parenchyma and airways. Proton MR imaging of the lung is a major challenge because the lung is probably the most difficult organ to be studied by MR imaging. Especially in emphysema, the loss of tissue and reduced blood volume because of hypoxic vasoconstriction and the degree of hyperinflation has a negative correlation with the MR signal.[12] The strength of the MR technique in COPD is the assessment of functions, such as perfusion, ventilation, and respiratory dynamics.[13]

Parenchyma

The use MR imaging for depiction of pulmonary structure in COPD will always be compared with CT. By physics, MR imaging can never outperform CT when it comes to visualization of bronchial dilation, wall thickening, or emphysematous destruction. The extent of hyperinflation and hypoxic vasoconstriction is directly associated with the loss of signal.[12] Until now MR imaging of the pulmonary parenchyma has only been successfully applied to diseases with an increase of tissue and signal. Although emphysematous destruction can hardly be diagnosed by a loss of signal, it is much easier to detect hyperinflation just by the size or volume of the thorax (**Fig. 1**). In a recent study it was shown that the change of parenchymal signal intensity measured by MR imaging at inspiration and expiration correlates with FEV_1 (r = 0.508) and might warrant further studies as a predictor of airflow obstruction.[14]

Airways

Several pathologic studies have shown that a major site of airway obstruction in patients who have

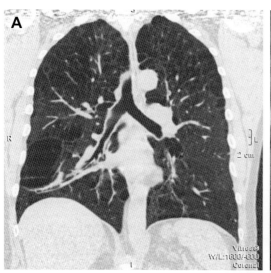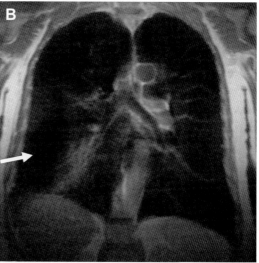

Fig. 1. Coronal CT reformat (*A*) and corresponding coronal T2-weighted (HASTE) image (*B*) of 55-year-old male patient who had severe emphysema. Severe emphysema with right lung predominance and scar tissue of the right lower lobe on CT correspond to a loss of signal MR imaging (*arrow*) reflecting destruction of the parenchyma and pulmonary hypovascularity.

COPD is in airways smaller than 2 mm internal diameter.[15] The 2 mm airways are located between the 4th and the 14th generation of the tracheobronchial tree. Airflow limitation is closely associated with the severity of luminal occlusion by inflammatory exudates and thickening of the airway walls because of remodeling. Severe peripheral airflow obstruction can also affect the proximal airways from subsegmental bronchi to the trachea.

For assessment of tracheal instability MR cine acquisitions during continuous respiration or forced expiration are recommended.[16] The depiction of airway dimensions and size of the airway walls by MR imaging under physiologic conditions is limited to the central bronchi. For depiction of the bronchiectasis high spatial resolution is essential. By using a 3D VIBE with a voxel size of approximately $0.9 \times 0.88 \times 2.5$ mm^3 a sensitivity of 79% and a specificity of 98% regarding the visual depiction of bronchiectasis was shown compared with CT.[17]

Respiratory Dynamics

Hyperinflation of the lung severely affects diaphragmatic geometry with subsequent reduction of the mechanical properties, whereas the effects on the mechanical advantage of the neck and rib cage muscles are less pronounced.[18] The common clinical measurements of COPD do not provide insights into how structural alterations in the lung lead to dysfunction in the breathing

mechanics, yet treatments such as lung volume reduction surgery (LVRS) are believed to improve lung function by facilitating breathing mechanics and increasing elastic recoil.[19]

In contrast to normal subjects who have regular, synchronous diaphragm and chest wall motion, dynamic MR imaging in patients who have emphysema frequently showed reduced (**Fig. 2**), irregular, or asynchronous motion, with a significant decrease in the maximum amplitude and the length of apposition of the diaphragm.[20] In some patients the ventral portion of the hemidiaphragm moved downward at MR imaging while the dorsal part moved upward like a seesaw.[21] The paradoxical diaphragmatic motion correlated with hyperinflation, although severe hyperinflation tended to restrict both normal and paradoxical diaphragmatic motion.[22] After LVRS, patients showed improvements in diaphragm and chest wall configuration and mobility at MR imaging.[20]

Ventilation

Because sufficient gas exchange depends on matched perfusion and ventilation, assessment of regional ventilation is important for the diagnosis and evaluation of pulmonary emphysema. Currently the most established method for imaging regional lung ventilation are nuclear medicine studies using krypton-81 m, xenon-133, radiolabeled aerosol, and technetium-99 m–labeled diethylenetriaminepentaacetic acid. The usefulness of nuclear medicine in pulmonary diseases has

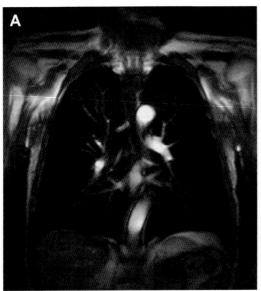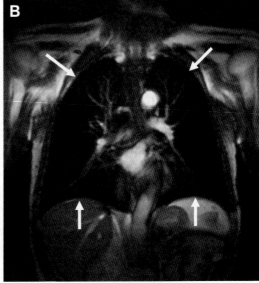

Fig. 2. A 66-year-old male patient who had COPD (FEV$_1$ = 1 L/s; 33% predicted). Coronal MR taken from a dynamic series acquired during forced expiration reflecting maximum inspiration (*A*) and maximum expiration (*B*) shows reduced motion of the diaphragm and thoracic wall (*arrows*).

been well documented. These techniques are hampered, however, by low spatial resolution and the necessity of inhalation of a radioactive tracer.

Recently, several investigators reported that oxygen-enhanced MR imaging could demonstrate regional ventilation.[23–25] The paramagnetic effect of molecular oxygen promotes longitudinal relaxation of nearby protons. Because oxygen is rapidly taken up into the blood, the exact location of the detected signal increase and the subsequent interpretation of its changes are still unclear. It seems obvious that the ventilatory component to the measured signal is actually small, whereas the contribution of dissolved oxygen in the interstitium and especially the blood seems to be much more predominant.

The technique of oxygen-enhanced MR imaging has been successfully applied in volunteers; the translation into clinical examination, however, is difficult. Only a few studies have successfully applied oxygen-enhanced MR imaging to patients who have pulmonary diseases in a clinical setting.

In some basic measurements it was shown that the T1 times of the lung parenchyma are significantly shorter in patients who have emphysema than in volunteers.[26] In a preliminary study an inhomogeneous and weak signal intensity increase after application of oxygen was observed, compared with healthy volunteers.[27] Ohno and colleagues[28] found that oxygen-enhanced MR showed that regional changes in ventilation reflected regional lung function. The maximum mean relative enhancement ratio correlated with the diffusion capacity for carbon monoxide ($r^2 = 0.83$), whereas the mean slope of relative enhancement was strongly correlated with the FEV$_1$ ($r^2 = 0.74$) and the maximum mean relative enhancement with the high-resolution CT (HRCT) emphysema score ($r^2 = 0.38$). Recent works also suggests that the simple administration of pure oxygen induces the pulmonary arteries to dilate

resulting in an increase of pulmonary blood volume and a consecutive increase in signal intensity.[29]

Over the past decade hyperpolarized noble gas MR imaging using ^{3}He and ^{129}Xe was developed to improve imaging of pulmonary ventilation. ^{3}He has become the most widely used gas for these studies because ^{3}He provides higher signal-to-noise ratios than ^{129}Xe.[30]

Airflow obstruction leads to a reduced level of ^{3}He in the distal lung regions allowing for sensitive detection of ventilation abnormalities (**Fig. 3**).[31] In healthy smokers who have normal lung function even subtle ventilation defects were visualized demonstrating the high sensitivity of the technique.[32] The volume of ventilated lung areas on ^{3}He MR imaging correlated well with vital capacity ($r = 0.9$) and the amount of non-emphysematous volume on CT ($r = 0.7$) in patients who had severe emphysema following single lung transplantation.[33] Ventilation defects correlated well with the parenchymal destruction assessed by HRCT in patients who had severe emphysema following single lung transplantation.[34] Quantification of ventilatory impairment can be achieved by automatic segmentation of the lung allowing for precise pre- and post-therapeutic comparison of ventilation.[35]

^{3}He MR imaging with high temporal resolution shows the dynamic distribution of ventilation during continuous breathing after inhalation of a single breath of ^{3}He gas being capable of demonstrating airflow abnormalities.[36,37] Homogeneous and fast distribution is regarded as normal, whereas patients who have COPD or emphysema show irregular and delayed patterns with redistribution and air trapping.[37,38]

The apparent diffusion coefficient (ADC) is a sensitive measure for the airspace size. Patients who have COPD showed increased airspace dimensions compared with nonsmokers.[39] ADC images were homogeneous in healthy volunteers, but demonstrated regional variations in patients who

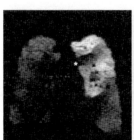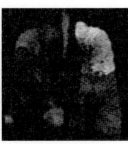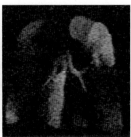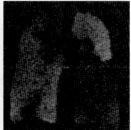

Fig. 3. MR ventilation images using hyperpolarized ^{3}He gas of a 65-year-old patient who had COPD: good ventilation of the left upper lobe with only one focal defect (*asterisk*) and large wedge-shaped ventilation defects in all remaining lung areas.

had emphysema. It was possible to distinguish emphysematous from normal lung.[40,41] The mean ADC for patients who had emphysema (0.452 cm^2/cm) was significantly larger (P<.002) than for volunteers (0.225 cm^2/cm).[41]

Pulmonary Perfusion

Gas exchange in the lungs is maintained by a balance between ventilation and perfusion. In patients who have COPD, ventilation is impaired because of airway obstruction and parenchymal destruction. In regions with reduced ventilation, hypoxic vasoconstriction occurs, leading to reduction of local pulmonary blood flow. The reduction of the pulmonary vascular bed is related to the severity of parenchymal destruction;[42] however, the distribution of perfusion does not necessarily match parenchymal destruction.[43,44] Conventional radionuclide perfusion scintigraphy has been used to assess these abnormalities, but it has substantial limitations with respect to spatial and temporal resolution. A superior technique is single photon emission computed tomography, which is rarely used because it is time consuming and not routinely applied.

MR perfusion allows for a high diagnostic accuracy in detecting perfusion abnormalities.[5,45] Furthermore, MR perfusion ratios correlate well with radionuclide perfusion scintigraphy ratios.[46,47] Lobar and segmental analysis of the perfusion defects can be achieved (**Fig. 4**).[43]

The perfusion abnormalities in COPD differ clearly from those caused by vascular obstruction. Although in embolic obstruction wedge-shaped perfusion defects occur, a generally low degree of contrast enhancement is found in patients who have COPD and emphysema.[48,49] Furthermore, the peak signal intensity is reduced. These features allow for easy visual differentiation.

In patients who have COPD the quantitative evaluation of 3D perfusion showed that the mean PBF, PBV, and MTT were significantly decreased, and these changes showed a heterogeneous distribution.[50] It has been noted that patients who have emphysema have hypoxia along with destruction of lung parenchyma and fewer alveolar capillaries, which cause pulmonary arterial resistance and, secondarily, pressure to increase. PBF was therefore decreased. In addition, the heterogeneous destruction of lung parenchyma caused the decrease in PBV. MTT is determined by the ratio between PBV and PBF. The results suggested that MTT is significantly decreased, reflecting a larger degree of decrease in PBV compared with PBF, and the heterogeneous changes of regional PBV and MTT were larger than those of PBF. Accurate quantitative measurements of such changes in the regional pattern of PBF are important to understand physiology and pathophysiology of the lung in obstructive disease (**Fig. 5**).

Hemodynamics

Although pulmonary hypertension and cor pulmonale are common sequelae of COPD, the direct mechanism remains unclear.[10] In patients who have COPD the pulmonary vessels show a reduced or no capacity for vessel dilatation because of a defect in synthesis or release of nitric oxide. Before the onset of clinical symptoms patients exhibit

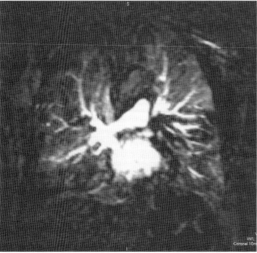
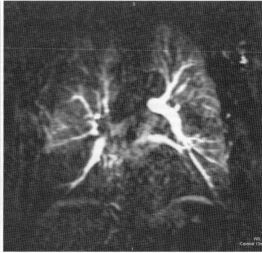

Fig. 4. A 58-year-old male patient who had severe paraseptal emphysema shows a typical subpleural distribution of lung perfusion defects at contrast-enhanced MR imaging.

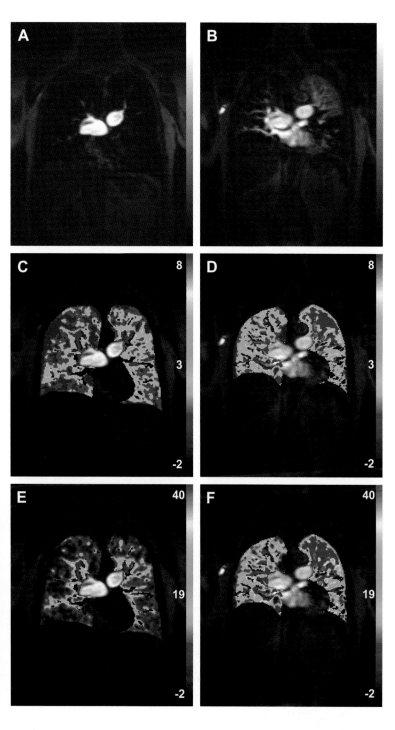

Fig. 5. Coronal contrast-enhanced MR perfusion of 65-year-old male patient who had COPD shows diminished perfusion at end-inspiration (*A*) with a distinct increase in perfusion, particularly in the left upper lung, at end-expiration (*B*). The corresponding parameter maps of the quantitative analysis of MR perfusion show the maximal concentration within the lung (*C* and *D*) and the distribution of the pulmonary blood volume (*E* and *F*).

signs of vascular bed obstruction and elevated pulmonary artery pressure, including main pulmonary artery dilatation. Pulmonary hypertension is most often mild to moderate (mean pulmonary artery pressure in the range 20 to 35 mm Hg) but may worsen markedly during acute exacerbations, sleep, and exercise. Assessment of the pulmonary arterial pressure is necessary in patients who have

COPD for at least two reasons: such patients have a poor prognosis, and they need adequate treatment that might include pulmonary vasodilators.

It has been demonstrated by several studies that the level of pulmonary hypertension has a prognostic impact in patients who have COPD. In one of these studies, the 5-year survival rates were 50% in patients who had mild

(20–30 mm Hg), 30% in those who had moderate to severe (30–50 mm Hg), and 0% in the small group (n = 15) of patients who had severe pulmonary hypertension (>50 mm Hg). Severe pulmonary hypertension thus bears a poor prognosis, and this also has been observed in patients who have COPD receiving long-term oxygen therapy.[51]

Before the onset of clinical symptoms, patients exhibit signs of vascular bed obstruction and elevated pulmonary artery pressure, including pulmonary artery dilatation, whereas right ventricular performance is usually maintained. Evaluation of the right ventricle and pulmonary blood flow by echocardiography is difficult in patients who have emphysema because the acoustic window is limited. MR imaging has been successfully used for imaging the right ventricle for some time, and a loose correlation between increased right ventricular mass and the severity of emphysema has been found.[52]

In patients who have COPD with hypoxemia, increased right ventricular volumes, decreased right ventricular function, and impaired left ventricular diastolic function were found.[53] In a study by Vonk Noordegraaff and colleagues[54] the right ventricular mass and ejection fraction in 25 clinically stable, normoxic patients who had COPD with emphysema were analyzed. It was found that the position of the heart is rotated and shifted to a more vertical position in the thoracic cavity because of hyperinflation of the lungs and increase of the retrosternal space. The right ventricular wall mass was significantly higher (68 g) in the patient group compared with healthy volunteers (59 g). The right ventricular ejection fraction was not changed (53%). In another study from the same group structural and functional cardiac changes in patients who had COPD with normal Pao_2 and without signs of right ventricular failure were evaluated. Compared with healthy volunteers there were no indications of pulmonary hypertension. The end-systolic and end-diastolic volumes of the right ventricle were significantly reduced but the ejection fraction was not changed. The right ventricular mass was significantly elevated, whereas the left ventricular myocardial mass was not changed. The authors conclude that concentric right ventricular hypertrophy is the earliest sign of right ventricular pressure increase in patients who have COPD. This structural adaptation of the heart does not alter right and left ventricular systolic function.[8]

Because this is the only study so far in patients who have mild emphysema, no strong conclusions can be drawn from this first description of the early adaptation mechanisms of the right ventricle in patients who have normoxemia or mild hypoxemia,

and the consequences of any structural changes on right and left ventricular function remain unclear.

ASTHMA

Asthma is a chronic inflammatory disorder that predominantly involves the peripheral airways, leading to variable and reversible airflow obstruction.[55–57] The relationship between the degree of inflammation and severity of clinical symptoms is not completely clear. Asymptomatic patients who have a normal pulmonary function test can have obvious airway inflammation. The accurate determination of disease severity is therefore sometimes difficult.[58]

Lung function testing plays a central role in the diagnosis and management of asthma. The drawback of this technique is that it cannot determine the regional differences of disease lung involvement. At the same time radiologic techniques play a limited role in the routine clinical diagnosis and management of patients who have asthma. Chest radiographs sometimes show signs of hyperinflation during an acute disease exacerbation, but usually there are no abnormalities in an uncomplicated clinical asthma situation.[59] HRCT provides detailed images of the lung structure and bronchial walls. Air trapping can be demonstrated. Correlation with asthma severity has been variable, however.[60–63] More direct information on regional airflow is provided using ventilation scintigraphy. In patients who have asthma an uneven distribution of the inhaled radionuclide gas has been demonstrated.[64] Nevertheless, this technique is used infrequently in managing asthma.

Even at HRCT the morphologic changes in the lungs of patients who have asthma are not distinct. The sensitivity and specificity of proton MR imaging for morphologic changes is thus very low. Most MR imaging studies in asthma have used hyperpolarized [3]He MR imaging.

In a preliminary study, hyperpolarized [3]He MR imaging was performed in 10 patients who had asthma and 10 healthy subjects. Whereas 7 patients who had asthma had ventilation defects distributed throughout the lungs, the lungs of volunteers were normal. These ventilation defects were more numerous and larger in the 2 patients who had symptomatic asthma who had abnormal spirometry. Ventilation defects studied over time demonstrated no change in appearance over 30 to 60 minutes, but some might resolve and new ones might occur for a time period of 3 weeks.[65]

[3]He MR imaging after a challenge using methacholine or a standard exercise test revealed

a significant increase in the number of ventilation defects, which nicely correlated with the decrease in FEV$_1$.[66] The authors hypothesized that the variability and speed of changes in ventilation and the complete lack of signal in many areas represent the results from airway closure.

In a larger study of 58 patients who had asthma and 18 volunteers the regional changes of airflow obstruction correlated reasonably well with the measures of asthma severity and spirometry. In the group of patients who had moderate to severe persistent asthma, there were more and larger defects than in the group that had mild-intermittent and mild-persistent disease.[67] ^{3}He MR imaging also provided additional spatial information of the distribution of the ventilation changes.

In a recent study the distribution of ventilation changes in patients who had asthma, including the distribution after repeated bronchoconstriction, was studied. The authors found that many of the ventilation defects persisted or recurred in the same location with time or repeated bronchoconstriction, suggesting that the regional changes of airflow obstruction are relatively fixed within the lung.[68]

In parallel to the experience in patients who had COPD fixed ventilation defects in asthma lead to hypoxic vasoconstriction. The subsequent perfusion defects are easily depicted by perfusion MR imaging (**Fig. 6**). It is a matter of current research whether transient ventilation defects might also be associated with perfusion defects visible at perfusion MR imaging. Most likely only a temporal analysis of perfusion detects subtle changes of the meant transit time of the contrast agent in these areas.

BRONCHOPULMONARY DYSPLASIA

Bronchopulmonary dysplasia (BPD), or chronic lung disease (CLD) of prematurity, occurs in babies who have been subjected to mechanical ventilation with oxygen as neonates. In more recent years, BPD is seen in premature infants who have undergone more technically advanced ventilation at lower mean airway pressures and oxygen concentrations, but who underwent prolonged ventilation often because of severe prematurity. Although in most children who have mild to moderate BPD radiographic findings and abnormalities of pulmonary function may be subtle and improve with age,[69] less fortunate children suffer long-term pulmonary complications, including poor respiratory function, reduced exercise tolerance, and reactive airways disease.

Imaging in these patients is performed using chest radiography and HRCT. Chest radiography studies may show characteristic findings,[70] but often show only minor abnormalities in children affected by BPD despite significant ventilatory dysfunction. CT is the modality of choice to image BPD-related lung changes and demonstrates abnormalities in all patients who have a clinical diagnosis of BPD.[71]

The most frequent patterns of lung disease include hyperlucent areas (hyperexpansion, air trapping, and emphysema), linear opacities, triangular subpleural opacities, air trapping, and mosaic perfusion. Bronchiectasis is not obvious. An increased number of subpleural opacities and limited linear opacities were associated with low functional residual capacity and longer duration of neonatal oxygen exposure, whereas the number of triangular subpleural opacities also correlated with the

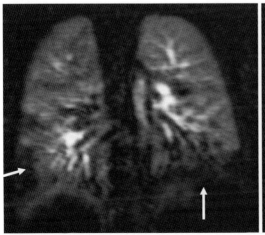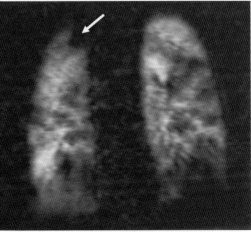

Fig. 6. Coronal contrast-enhanced MR perfusion images of a 12-year-old male patient who had asthma demonstrate focal perfusion defects in both lungs (*arrows*) and reduced perfusion in the basal lung areas on the left. No pathologic changes of lung structure were found at 1 mm multislice CT.

duration of mechanical ventilation.[72] These observations recently led to the proposal of a new scoring system for BPD.[73]

Few data regarding MR imaging of the lung findings in BPD are available, although MR imaging seems to have an obvious potential to provide detailed images of the affected airways and lungs. Not surprisingly, pulmonary perfusion demonstrated by MR imaging shows defects in the affected areas (**Fig. 7**).

CYSTIC FIBROSIS

CF is an autosomal recessive disorder caused by gene mutations of the long arm of chromosome 7. This gene codes for the cystic fibrosis transmembrane regulator protein (CFTR), which functions as an anion channel. The impaired CFTR function causes aberrations of volume and ion composition of airway surface fluid, leading to viscous secretions with the consequence of bacterial colonization, chronic lung infection, airway obstruction, and consecutive destruction of the lung parenchyma.[74] Despite improved understanding of the underlying pathophysiology and the introduction of new therapies, CF remains one of the most life-shortening inherited diseases in the white population. The median survival of patients who have CF has increased to more than 35 years of age.

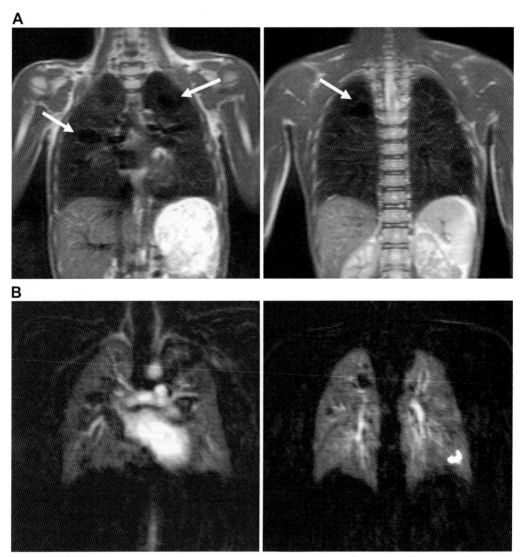

Fig. 7. T2-weighted (HASTE) images (*A*) and corresponding MR perfusion (*B*) acquired during free breathing in a 8-year-old female patient who had BPD show focal bullous changes in both lungs (*arrows*) and focal perfusion defects in the same regions.

Although CF affects most body systems, most morbidity and mortality in patients who have CF is attributable to chronic progressive lung disease. The standard radiologic tools for monitoring of lung disease in patients who have CF are chest radiography and HRCT, evaluated using different scoring systems.[75] HRCT provides submillimeter resolution images of lung structure and has been proposed as a possible outcome measure for CF lung disease.[76,77] CT and HRCT have been shown to be more sensitive to early CF lung disease than pulmonary function testing, likely because of the regional nature of the information obtained. Despite the promising early studies related to the use of CT and HRCT scanning in CF, a major drawback remains the radiation exposure associated with CT and HRCT.[78,79] Radiation safety concerns may ultimately limit the usefulness of CT and HRCT in CF lung disease for applications in which repeated and follow-up CT scans are required.

Pulmonary function tests remain one of the primary outcome measures in CF lung disease. A decrease of FEV_1 was shown to be the most important prognostic factor for the course of the disease and the most significant predictor of mortality in a study of 673 patients who had CF.[80] A more sensitive radiation-free test that is not effort dependent and can be performed by young children would be highly desirable for the assessment of CF lung disease.

MR imaging of the chest has already been proposed as a potential imaging alternative in patients who have CF since the late 1980s. At least until recently, however, MR imaging technology was not capable of producing comparable results to CT or an adequate clinical evaluation. Recently, new strategies have been implemented, ready to overcome the inherent difficulties of MR imaging of the lung.[81] With the introduction of parallel imaging in clinical practice, faster image acquisition is possible, enabling substantial improvement in temporal or spatial resolution.[23,82] Although spatial resolution is lower than with CT and HRCT, MR imaging has the advantages to evaluate different aspects of tissue and improve lesion characterization by different contrasts in T1-weighted and T2-weighted images and enhancement after contrast media administration.

Currently, MR imaging research in CF lung disease lags behind CT. The following sections describe the common findings of CF lung disease on conventional proton MR imaging and discuss some of the newer MR imaging techniques that provide additional functional information about the lung.

Structural Changes

Using common proton MR imaging sequences, it is possible to visualize the structural changes of CF lung disease, including bronchial wall thickening, mucus plugging, bronchiectasis, air–fluid levels, consolidation, and segmental/lobar destruction, albeit with lower spatial and temporal resolution than with CT.[83] Although not yet proved, it seems likely that the lower spatial and temporal resolution of MR imaging will mean that MR imaging will be less sensitive than CT to specific imaging features, such as distal bronchiectasis. This lower resolution does not necessarily mean that MR imaging will provide less useful information about CF, however, because sensitivity to these imaging features may not be critical for the assessment of the overall burden of disease.[74]

Bronchial wall thickening

The visualization of bronchial wall thickening depends on bronchial size, bronchial wall thickness, and bronchial wall signal. In MR imaging studies of normal lung, only the central airways down to the level of the lobar bronchi are routinely visualized, and some segmental bronchi can be identified. This is in contrast to CT, in which the sixth to eighth generation bronchi are easily identified. In patients who have CF, however, bronchial wall thickening of small airways enhances their detection by MR imaging so that small airways with thick walls can be visualized in the lung periphery (**Fig. 8**A, B).[83] The T2-weighted signal of the thickened bronchial walls in CF varies from high intensity to low intensity. Because water and edema produce a high T2-weighted signal, it would not be surprising if the high bronchial wall signal is attributable to edema, which is most likely caused by active inflammation. This phenomenon is not observable in CT. A T1-weighted sequence allows for evaluation of the contrast enhancement of the bronchial wall. In CF, different patterns of bronchial wall contrast enhancement have been observed. In some lung regions, bronchi demonstrate a striking enhancement, whereas in other regions a weak contrast enhancement is observed. This phenomenon may also be related to inflammatory activity within the bronchial wall, but further studies are required to improve our understanding of these findings (**Fig. 9**).

Mucus plugging

Mucus plugging is well visualized by MR imaging because of the high T2-weighted signal of its fluid content (see **Fig. 8**A, B). Mucus plugging in central large bronchi and peripheral small bronchi can be visualized on MR imaging. In central mucus plugging, there is a high T2-weighted signal filling the

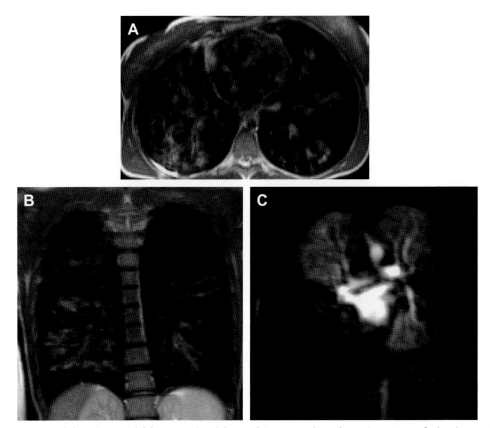

Fig. 8. Transverse (*A*) and coronal (*B*) T2-weighted (HASTE) image and a subtraction MR perfusion image (*C*) of a 16-year-old female patient who had CF. In images (*A*) and (*B*) bronchial wall thickening, bronchiectasis, and peripheral mucus plugging are demonstrated. Image (*C*) shows a loss of perfusion in both lower lobes.

bronchus within its course. Peripheral mucus plugging shows a grapelike appearance of small T2-weighted high intensity areas, similar to the "tree-in-bud" phenomenon in small airway inflammation on CT. Mucus plugging does not show any contrast enhancement. Mucus and bronchial wall thickening can thus be differentiated by the combination of T2-weighted and contrast-enhanced sequences. At CT, these two pathologic entities cannot be reliably distinguished because the CT attenuation of mucus and soft tissue are similar.

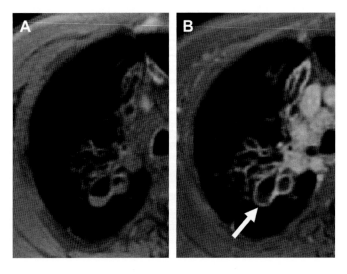

Fig. 9. T1 weighted (VIBE) images of a 43-year-old patient who had CF (*A*) pre- and (*B*) postcontrast. The contrast-enhanced images demonstrate extensive bronchial wall enhancement and permit differentiation of a thickened wall from intrabronchial secretions, with intrabronchial fluid showing an air-fluid level (*arrow*).

Depending on the stage of disease, patients who have CF have an increased risk for hemoptysis. The localization of the origin of bleeding can be crucial for the outcome of the patient. With CT, mucus and blood are similar in attenuation and cannot be distinguished. On MR imaging, using the combination of T1- and T2-weighted and contrast-enhanced sequences, mucus and fresh blood can be distinguished. Mucus has a high T2-weighted and low T1-weighted signal, whereas fresh blood has a low T2-weighted and T1-weighted signal.

Bronchiectasis
The MR imaging appearance of bronchiectasis depends on bronchial level, bronchial diameter, wall thickness, wall signal, and the signal within the bronchial lumen. Central bronchiectasis is well visualized on MR imaging independent of wall thickening or wall signal because of the anatomically thicker wall of the central bronchi. Peripheral bronchi, starting at the third to fourth generation, are poorly visualized by MR imaging except when they are pathologic with bronchial wall thickening or mucus plugging.

Air–fluid levels
Air–fluid levels indicate active infection and occur in saccular or varicose bronchiectasis. Bronchial air–fluid levels can be visualized by MR imaging because of the high T2-weighted signal from the fluid. Discriminating between a bronchus with an air–fluid level and one with a partial mucus plug or a severely thickened wall can be difficult. Nevertheless, by evaluating the signal characteristics on T1-weighted, T2-weighted, and contrast-enhanced sequences, air–fluid levels can frequently be differentiated (see **Fig. 9**).

Consolidation
Consolidation in CF is mainly caused by alveolar filling with inflammatory fluid. The visualization of consolidation at MR imaging is based on the high T2-weighted signal from the inflammatory fluid. Comparable to CT, MR imaging is able to visualize air bronchograms as low signal areas following the course of the bronchi within the consolidation.[84,85] With disease progression, complete destruction of lung segments or a complete lung lobe can occur and these destructed lung areas have a similar appearance on MR imaging as CT.

Mosaic pattern
On CT, a mosaic pattern of lung attenuation is a common finding in patients who have CF. This pattern can be observed on inspiratory scans as areas of relative hyperlucency, which can be because of air trapping or regional hypoperfusion (mosaic perfusion). These two entities can be distinguished on expiratory HRCT images because regions of air trapping do not change significantly in volume and thus change little in measured CT attenuation. Conversely, in areas of hypoperfusion without air trapping, the lung attenuation increases with expiration.

On MR imaging, the phenomenon of air trapping is not typically apparent because even normal lung parenchyma has a very low signal, and an increase of the air content does not cause a detectable decrease in lung parenchymal signal. An approach to overcome this limitation might be the measurement of T1 relaxation times.[26] Mosaic perfusion also is not typically apparent on routine MR images, but MR perfusion imaging has the potential to overcome this limitation.[86]

Ventilation

In a study of five patients who had CF and five healthy volunteers, the lungs of the patients who had CF had an inhomogeneous appearance following the inhalation of high oxygen concentrations suggesting inhomogeneous lung ventilation, presumably due to inhomogeneous lung ventilation.[87] Because oxygen is soluble in blood, the oxygen-enhanced MR images depict a combination of ventilation and perfusion.[88] One of the difficulties with this method is that there is a relatively low difference in signal from the lung parenchyma with 21% versus 100% inspired oxygen concentration resulting in a relatively low signal-to-noise level in the resulting MR oxygen-enhanced images.

Most studies investigating the use of hyperpolarized helium MR imaging in CF have used static spin density imaging. Static spin density imaging, often referred to as ventilation imaging, is performed during a breath hold following the inhalation of the hyperpolarized ³He gas.[89] Well-ventilated areas of the lung receive more helium gas and thus appear brighter than poorly ventilated areas of the lung on the MR images. Typically, the entire lung volume can be imaged in a 4- to 20-second breath hold, but the in-plane spatial resolution is typically in the order of 3 mm and thus lower than with CT. Because children have smaller lungs than adults, the breath hold duration is shorter for children, and hyperpolarized helium MR imaging has been successfully performed in children as young as 4 years of age without sedation.[90]

The first report of hyperpolarized helium MR imaging in CF found extensive abnormalities of ventilation on static spin density images in four subjects who had moderate to severe pulmonary CF and abnormal FEV$_1$% predicted.[81]

Also using static spin density imaging, a study of 31 subjects (16 healthy volunteers and 15 patients who had CF) found the patients who had CF had a significantly higher number of ventilation defects on helium MR imaging than the normal subjects.[91] Even the 4 subjects who had CF with a normal FEV$_1$% predicted had significantly higher ventilation defect score than the normal subjects, suggesting hyperpolarized gas MR imaging may be more sensitive to ventilation abnormalities than spirometry. Moderate correlations between the ventilation defect score and spirometry were found. In this study, 8 patients who had CF underwent a therapeutic intervention first with nebulized albuterol followed by DNase and chest physical therapy. Repeated ^{3}He MR imaging after therapy showed changes in the ventilation defect score. This study thus demonstrated the feasibility of using hyperpolarized ^{3}He MR as an outcome measure in the evaluation of airway clearance techniques.

A recent study of 18 children who had CF (aged 5 to 17 years) confirmed that hyperpolarized ^{3}He MR imaging can be performed by children who have CF and found moderate to weak correlations between static spin density hyperpolarized helium MR imaging and spirometry or chest radiography.[92] It was the opinion of the authors that the weak correlations were the result of a greater sensitivity of hyperpolarized ^{3}He MR imaging to ventilatory abnormalities than spirometry or chest radiography. Another recent study compared static spin density helium MR imaging with CT in eight adults who had CF and found a strong correlation between the MR imaging percent ventilation and the Bhalla[75] score from CT.[93] Furthermore, the correlations between hyperpolarized helium MR imaging and spirometry were stronger than those between CT and spirometry. This study thus suggests that hyperpolarized helium MR imaging may represent a safe alternative to CT for the evaluation of CF lung disease.

Pulmonary Perfusion

In CF, regional ventilatory defects cause changes in regional lung perfusion because of the reflex of hypoxic vasoconstriction or tissue destruction. Various MR imaging methods have been used to assess lung perfusion, including methods that rely on the endogenous signal from blood[94] and others that require the administration of intravenous contrast.[5,95,96]

Using a contrast-enhanced 3D MR imaging acquisition in 11 children who had CF, it was found that MR imaging perfusion defects correlated with the degree of tissue destruction (**Fig. 8C**).[86] It is plausible that reversibility of perfusion defects after a therapeutic intervention might serve as an indicator for response to therapy and might differentiate between regions with reversible and irreversible disease.

Hemodynamics

Parenchymal destruction can lead to dilatation and flow augmentation of bronchial arteries. Because bronchial arteries are part of the systemic circulation, they do not contribute to blood oxygenation. A higher flow in the bronchial arteries leads to a shunt volume, which can be assessed by MR imaging–based flow measurements. Decreased peak blood flow velocities in the right and left pulmonary arteries were found in 10 patients who had CF as compared with 15 healthy volunteers. This may represent early development of pulmonary hypertension in this patient group.[43] The clinical significance of the systemic arterial shunt volume is not yet known.

SUMMARY

MR imaging is a promising modality to comprehensively assess the different aspects of obstructive pulmonary disease.

Although the spatial resolution of MR imaging is lower than that of CT, the strength of MR imaging is to image the characteristic changes of the lung parenchyma and their functional precursors and consequences at the level of perfusion, ventilation, and respiratory dynamics.

MR imaging is a highly sensitive and effort-independent test for obstructive lung disease that might be used as a first-line diagnostic test in CF during follow-up and as a complement to CT for sensitive detection, phenotype-driven characterization, and therapy monitoring in COPD.

REFERENCES

1. Cluzel P, Similowski T, Chartrand-Lefebvre C, et al. Diaphragm and chest wall: assessment of the inspiratory pump with MR imaging—preliminary observations. Radiology 2000;215:574–83.
2. Plathow C, Fink C, Ley S, et al. Measurement of diaphragmatic length during the breathing cycle by dynamic MRI: comparison between healthy adults and patients with an intrathoracic tumor. Eur Radiol 2004; 14:1392–9.
3. Plathow C, Schoebinger M, Fink C, et al. Evaluation of lung volumetry using dynamic three-dimensional

magnetic resonance imaging. Invest Radiol 2005; 40:173–9.

4. Fink C, Ley S, Kroeker R, et al. Time-resolved contrast-enhanced three-dimensional magnetic resonance angiography of the chest: combination of parallel imaging with view sharing (TREAT). Invest Radiol 2005;40:40–8.

5. Fink C, Puderbach M, Bock M, et al. Regional lung perfusion: assessment with partially parallel three-dimensional MR imaging. Radiology 2004;231: 175–84.

6. Ley S, Fink C, Puderbach M, et al. [Contrast-enhanced 3D MR perfusion of the lung: application of parallel imaging technique in healthy subjects]. Rofo 2004;176:330–4 [in German].

7. Gatehouse PD, Keegan J, Crowe LA, et al. Applications of phase-contrast flow and velocity imaging in cardiovascular MRI. Eur Radiol 2005;15:2172–84.

8. Vonk-Noordegraaf A, Marcus JT, Holverda S, et al. Early changes of cardiac structure and function in COPD patients with mild hypoxemia. Chest 2005; 127:1898–903.

9. Rabe KF, Hurd S, Anzueto A, et al. Global strategy for the diagnosis, management, and prevention of chronic obstructive pulmonary disease: GOLD executive summary. Am J Respir Crit Care Med 2007; 176(6):532–55.

10. Szilasi M, Dolinay T, Nemes Z, et al. Pathology of chronic obstructive pulmonary disease. Pathol Oncol Res 2006;12:52–60.

11. Rosenkranz S. Pulmonary hypertension: current diagnosis and treatment. Clin Res Cardiol 2007;96: 527–41.

12. Bankier AA, O'Donnell CR, Mai VM, et al. Impact of lung volume on MR signal intensity changes of the lung parenchyma. J Magn Reson Imaging 2004; 20:961–6.

13. Ley-Zaporozhan J, Ley S, Kauczor HU. Proton MRI in COPD. COPD 2007;4:55–65.

14. Iwasawa T, Takahashi H, Ogura T, et al. Correlation of lung parenchymal MR signal intensity with pulmonary function tests and quantitative computed tomography (CT) evaluation: a pilot study. J Magn Reson Imaging 2007;26:1530–6.

15. Hogg JC, Chu F, Utokaparch S, et al. The nature of small-airway obstruction in chronic obstructive pulmonary disease. N Engl J Med 2004;350: 2645–53.

16. Heussel CP, Ley S, Biedermann A, et al. Respiratory luminal change of the pharynx and trachea in normal subjects and COPD patients: assessment by cine-MRI. Eur Radiol 2004;14:2188–97.

17. Biederer J, Both M, Graessner J, et al. Lung morphology: fast MR imaging assessment with a volumetric interpolated breath-hold technique: initial experience with patients. Radiology 2003;226: 242–9.

18. Decramer M. Hyperinflation and respiratory muscle interaction. Eur Respir J 1997;10:934–41.

19. Henderson AC, Ingenito EP, Salcedo ES, et al. Dynamic lung mechanics in late-stage emphysema before and after lung volume reduction surgery. Respir Physiol Neurobiol 2007;155:234–42.

20. Suga K, Tsukuda T, Awaya H, et al. Impaired respiratory mechanics in pulmonary emphysema: evaluation with dynamic breathing MRI. J Magn Reson Imaging 1999;10:510–20.

21. Iwasawa T, Yoshiike Y, Saito K, et al. Paradoxical motion of the hemidiaphragm in patients with emphysema. J Thorac Imaging 2000;15:191–5.

22. Iwasawa T, Kagei S, Gotoh T, et al. Magnetic resonance analysis of abnormal diaphragmatic motion in patients with emphysema. Eur Respir J 2002;19: 225–31.

23. Edelman RR, Hatabu H, Tadamura E, et al. Noninvasive assessment of regional ventilation in the human lung using oxygen-enhanced magnetic resonance imaging. Nat Med 1996;2:1236–9.

24. Loffler R, Muller CJ, Peller M, et al. Optimization and evaluation of the signal intensity change in multisection oxygen-enhanced MR lung imaging. Magn Reson Med 2000;43:860–6.

25. Ohno Y, Chen Q, Hatabu H. Oxygen-enhanced magnetic resonance ventilation imaging of lung. Eur J Radiol 2001;37:164–71.

26. Stadler A, Jakob PM, Griswold M, et al. T1 mapping of the entire lung parenchyma: influence of the respiratory phase in healthy individuals. J Magn Reson Imaging 2005;21:759–64.

27. Muller CJ, Schwaiblmair M, Scheidler J, et al. Pulmonary diffusing capacity: assessment with oxygen-enhanced lung MR imaging preliminary findings. Radiology 2002;222:499–506.

28. Ohno Y, Sugimura K, Hatabu H. Clinical oxygen-enhanced magnetic resonance imaging of the lung Top. Magn Reson Imaging 2003;14:237–43.

29. Ley S, Puderbach M, Risse F, et al. Impact of oxygen inhalation on the pulmonary circulation: assessment by magnetic resonance (MR)-perfusion and MR-flow measurements. Invest Radiol 2007;42: 283–90.

30. van Beek EJ, Wild JM, Kauczor HU, et al. Functional MRI of the lung using hyperpolarized 3-helium gas. J Magn Reson Imaging 2004;20:540–54.

31. Kauczor HU, Hofmann D, Kreitner KF, et al. Normal and abnormal pulmonary ventilation: visualization at hyperpolarized He-3 MR imaging. Radiology 1996;201:564–8.

32. Guenther D, Eberle B, Hast J, et al. (3)He MRI in healthy volunteers: preliminary correlation with smoking history and lung volumes. NMR Biomed 2000;13:182–9.

33. Zaporozhan J, Ley S, Gast KK, et al. Functional analysis in single-lung transplant recipients: a comparative

study of high-resolution CT, 3He-MRI, and pulmonary function tests. Chest 2004;125:173–81.

34. Gast KK, Viallon M, Eberle B, et al. MRI in lung transplant recipients using hyperpolarized 3He: comparison with CT. J Magn Reson Imaging 2002;15:268–74.

35. Ray N, Acton ST, Altes T, et al. Merging parametric active contours within homogeneous image regions for MRI-based lung segmentation. IEEE Trans Med Imaging 2003;22:189–99.

36. Salerno M, Altes TA, Brookeman JR, et al. Dynamic spiral MRI of pulmonary gas flow using hyperpolarized (3)He: preliminary studies in healthy and diseased lungs. Magn Reson Med 2001;46:667–77.

37. Wild JM, Paley MN, Kasuboski L, et al. Dynamic radial projection MRI of inhaled hyperpolarized 3He gas. Magn Reson Med 2003;49:991–7.

38. Gast KK, Puderbach MU, Rodriguez I, et al. Distribution of ventilation in lung transplant recipients: evaluation by dynamic 3He-MRI with lung motion correction. Invest Radiol 2003;38:341–8.

39. Swift AJ, Wild JM, Fichele S, et al. Emphysematous changes and normal variation in smokers and COPD patients using diffusion 3He MRI. Eur J Radiol 2005;54:352–8.

40. Ley S, Zaporozhan J, Morbach A, et al. Functional evaluation of emphysema using diffusion-weighted 3Helium-magnetic resonance imaging, high-resolution computed tomography, and lung function tests. Invest Radiol 2004;39:427–34.

41. Salerno M, de Lange EE, Altes TA, et al. Emphysema: hyperpolarized helium 3 diffusion MR imaging of the lungs compared with spirometric indexes–initial experience. Radiology 2002;222:252–60.

42. Thabut G, Dauriat G, Stern JB, et al. Pulmonary hemodynamics in advanced COPD candidates for lung volume reduction surgery or lung transplantation. Chest 2005;127:1531–6.

43. Ley S, Puderbach M, Fink C, et al. Assessment of hemodynamic changes in the systemic and pulmonary arterial circulation in patients with cystic fibrosis using phase-contrast MRI. Eur Radiol 2005;15:1575–80.

44. Sandek K, Bratel T, Lagerstrand L, et al. Relationship between lung function, ventilation-perfusion inequality and extent of emphysema as assessed by high-resolution computed tomography. Respir Med 2002;96:934–43.

45. Sergiacomi G, Sodani G, Fabiano S, et al. MRI lung perfusion 2D dynamic breath-hold technique in patients with severe emphysema. In Vivo 2003;17:319–24.

46. Molinari F, Fink C, Risse F, et al. Assessment of differential pulmonary blood flow using perfusion magnetic resonance imaging: comparison with radionuclide perfusion scintigraphy. Invest Radiol 2006;41:624–30.

47. Ohno Y, Hatabu H, Takenaka D, et al. Dynamic MR imaging: value of differentiating subtypes of peripheral small adenocarcinoma of the lung. Eur J Radiol 2004;52:144–50.

48. Amundsen T, Torheim G, Kvistad KA, et al. Perfusion abnormalities in pulmonary embolism studied with perfusion MRI and ventilation-perfusion scintigraphy: an intra-modality and inter-modality agreement study. J Magn Reson Imaging 2002;15:386–94.

49. Morino S, Toba T, Araki M, et al. Noninvasive assessment of pulmonary emphysema using dynamic contrast-enhanced magnetic resonance imaging. Exp Lung Res 2006;32:55–67.

50. Ohno Y, Hatabu H, Murase K, et al. Quantitative assessment of regional pulmonary perfusion in the entire lung using three-dimensional ultrafast dynamic contrast-enhanced magnetic resonance imaging: Preliminary experience in 40 subjects. J Magn Reson Imaging 2004;20:353–65.

51. Weitzenblum E, Chaouat A. Severe pulmonary hypertension in COPD: is it a distinct disease? Chest 2005;127:1480–2.

52. Boxt LM. MR imaging of pulmonary hypertension and right ventricular dysfunction. Magn Reson Imaging Clin N Am 1996;4:307–25.

53. Budev MM, Arroliga AC, Wiedemann HP, et al. Cor pulmonale: an overview. Semin Respir Crit Care Med 2003;24:233–44.

54. Vonk Noordegraaf A, Marcus JT, Roseboom B, et al. The effect of right ventricular hypertrophy on left ventricular ejection fraction in pulmonary emphysema. Chest 1997;112:640–5.

55. Hamid Q, Song Y, Kotsimbos TC, et al. Inflammation of small airways in asthma. J Allergy Clin Immunol 1997;100:44–51.

56. Hogg JC, editor. Asthma and COPD: basic mechanisms and clinical management. London: Academic Press; 2002.

57. James A, Carroll N. Transbronchial biopsy as a tool to evaluate small-airways disease in asthma. Cons Eur Respir J 2002;20:249–51.

58. Heaney LG, Robinson DS. Severe asthma treatment: need for characterising patients. Lancet 2005;365:974–6.

59. Petheram IS, Kerr IH, Collins JV. Value of chest radiographs in severe acute asthma. Clin Radiol 1981;32:281–2.

60. Gono H, Fujimoto K, Kawakami S, et al. Evaluation of airway wall thickness and air trapping by HRCT in asymptomatic asthma. Eur Respir J 2003;22:965–71.

61. Mitsunobu F, Ashida K, Hosaki Y, et al. Decreased computed tomographic lung density during exacerbation of asthma. Eur Respir J 2003;22:106–12.

62. Mitsunobu F, Mifune T, Ashida K, et al. Influence of age and disease severity on high resolution CT lung densitometry in asthma. Thorax 2001;56:851–6.

63. Paganin F, Seneterre E, Chanez P, et al. Computed tomography of the lungs in asthma: influence of disease severity and etiology. Am J Respir Crit Care Med 1996;153:110–4.

64. Vernon P, Burton GH, Seed WA. Lung scan abnormalities in asthma and their correlation with lung function. Eur J Nucl Med 1986;12:16–20.

65. Altes TA, Powers PL, Knight-Scott J, et al. Hyperpolarized 3He MR lung ventilation imaging in asthmatics: preliminary findings. J Magn Reson Imaging 2001;13:378–84.

66. Samee S, Altes T, Powers P, et al. Imaging the lungs in asthmatic patients by using hyperpolarized helium-3 magnetic resonance: assessment of response to methacholine and exercise challenge. J Allergy Clin Immunol 2003;111:1205–11.

67. de Lange EE, Altes TA, Patrie JT, et al. Evaluation of asthma with hyperpolarized helium-3 MRI: correlation with clinical severity and spirometry. Chest 2006;130:1055–62.

68. de Lange EE, Altes TA, Patrie JT, et al. The variability of regional airflow obstruction within the lungs of patients with asthma: assessment with hyperpolarized helium-3 magnetic resonance imaging. J Allergy Clin Immunol 2007;119:1072–8.

69. Hakulinen AL, Jarvenpaa AL, Turpeinen M, et al. Diffusing capacity of the lung in school-aged children born very preterm, with and without bronchopulmonary dysplasia. Pediatr Pulmonol 1996;21:353–60.

70. Griscom NT, Wheeler WB, Sweezey NB, et al. Bronchopulmonary dysplasia: radiographic appearance in middle childhood. Radiology 1989;171:811–4.

71. Aukland SM, Halvorsen T, Fosse KR, et al. High-resolution CT of the chest in children and young adults who were born prematurely: findings in a population-based study. AJR Am J Roentgenol 2006;187:1012–8.

72. Mahut B, De Blic J, Emond S, et al. Chest computed tomography findings in bronchopulmonary dysplasia and correlation with lung function. Arch Dis Child Fetal Neonatal Ed 2007;92:F459–64.

73. Ochiai M, Hikino S, Yabuuchi H, et al. A new scoring system for computed tomography of the chest for assessing the clinical status of bronchopulmonary dysplasia. J Pediatr 2008;152:90–5, 5 e1-3.

74. Puderbach M, Eichinger M, Haeselbarth J, et al. Assessment of morphological MRI for pulmonary changes in cystic fibrosis (CF) patients: comparison to thin-section CT and chest x-ray. Invest Radiol 2007;42:715–25.

75. Bhalla M, Turcios N, Aponte V, et al. Cystic fibrosis: scoring system with thin-section CT. Radiology 1991;179:783–8.

76. Brody AS, Molina PL, Klein JS, et al. High-resolution computed tomography of the chest in children with cystic fibrosis: support for use as an outcome surrogate. Pediatr Radiol 1999;29:731–5.

77. Robinson TE. High-resolution CT scanning: potential outcome measure. Curr Opin Pulm Med 2004;10:537–41.

78. Brenner DJ. Estimating cancer risks from pediatric CT: going from the qualitative to the quantitative. Pediatr Radiol 2002;32:228–33 [discussion: 42–4].

79. Huda W, Vance A. Patient radiation doses from adult and pediatric CT. AJR Am J Roentgenol 2007;188:540–6.

80. Kerem E, Reisman J, Corey M, et al. Prediction of mortality in patients with cystic fibrosis. N Engl J Med 1992;326:1187–91.

81. Donnelly LF, MacFall JR, McAdams HP, et al. Cystic fibrosis: combined hyperpolarized 3He-enhanced and conventional proton MR imaging in the lung—preliminary observations. Radiology 1999;212:885–9.

82. Swift AJ, Woodhouse N, Fichele S, et al. Rapid lung volumetry using ultrafast dynamic magnetic resonance imaging during forced vital capacity maneuver: correlation with spirometry. Invest Radiol 2007;42:37–41.

83. Puderbach M, Eichinger M, Gahr J, et al. Proton MRI appearance of cystic fibrosis: comparison to CT. Eur Radiol 2007;17:716–24.

84. Eibel R, Herzog P, Dietrich O, et al. Pulmonary abnormalities in immunocompromised patients: comparative detection with parallel acquisition MR imaging and thin-section helical CT. Radiology 2006;241:880–91.

85. Rupprecht T, Bowing B, Kuth R, et al. Steady-state free precession projection MRI as a potential alternative to the conventional chest x-ray in pediatric patients with suspected pneumonia. Eur Radiol 2002;12:2752–6.

86. Eichinger M, Puderbach M, Fink C, et al. Contrast-enhanced 3D MRI of lung perfusion in children with cystic fibrosis—initial results. Eur Radiol 2006;16:2147–52.

87. Jakob PM, Wang T, Schultz G, et al. Assessment of human pulmonary function using oxygen-enhanced T(1) imaging in patients with cystic fibrosis. Magn Reson Med 2004;51:1009–16.

88. Keilholz S, Knight-Scott J, Mata J, et al. The contributions of ventilation and perfusion in O2-enhanced MRI. Seattle (WA): International Society of Magnetic Resonance in Medicine (ISMRM); 2006.

89. Altes TA, Rehm PK, Harrell F, et al. Ventilation imaging of the lung: comparison of hyperpolarized helium-3 MR imaging with Xe-133 scintigraphy. Acad Radiol 2004;11:729–34.

90. Altes TA, Mata J, Froh D, et al. Abnormalities of lung structure in children with bronchopulmonary dysplasia as assessed by diffusion hyperpolarized helium-3 MRI. Seattle (WA): International Society of Magnetic Resonance in Medicine (ISMRM); 2006.

91. Mentore K, Froh DK, de Lange EE, et al. Hyperpolarized HHe 3 MRI of the lung in cystic fibrosis: assessment at baseline and after bronchodilator and airway clearance treatment. Acad Radiol 2005;12: 1423–9.

92. van Beek EJ, Hill C, Woodhouse N, et al. Assessment of lung disease in children with cystic fibrosis using hyperpolarized 3-Helium MRI: comparison with Shwachman score, Chrispin-Norman score and spirometry. Eur Radiol 2007;17:1018–24.

93. McMahon CJ, Dodd JD, Hill C, et al. Hyperpolarized 3helium magnetic resonance ventilation imaging of the lung in cystic fibrosis: comparison with high resolution CT and spirometry. Eur Radiol 2006;16: 2483–90.

94. Mai VM, Berr SS. MR perfusion imaging of pulmonary parenchyma using pulsed arterial spin labeling techniques: FAIRER and FAIR. J Magn Reson Imaging 1999;9:483–7.

95. Hatabu H, Gaa J, Kim D, et al. Pulmonary perfusion: qualitative assessment with dynamic contrast-enhanced MRI using ultra-short TE and inversion recovery turbo FLASH. Magn Reson Med 1996;36: 503–8.

96. Levin DL, Hatabu H. MR evaluation of pulmonary blood flow. J Thorac Imaging 2004;19:241–9.

MR Imaging in Diagnosis and Staging of Pulmonary Carcinoma

Alla Godelman, MD[a,b,*], Linda B. Haramati, MD[a,b]

KEYWORDS

- MR imaging • Lung cancer staging
- Carcinoma • Pulmonary

Lung cancer is the most common cause of cancer-related death for men and women in the United States. According to the National Cancer Institute, the estimated total number of newly diagnosed cases of lung cancer in the United States in 2007 was 213,380 and the number of lung cancer–related deaths in 2007 was 160,390. The incidence of lung cancer in men has declined from 102 cases per 100,000 in 1984 to 78.5 in 2003. The lung cancer–related death rate in men has declined between 1991 and 2003. In women, the incidence and death rate reached a plateau in 2003. Between 1987 and 2003, more women died from lung cancer than from breast cancer.[1]

Cigarette smoking is the most important risk factor for the development of lung cancer. The risk is related to the duration and quantity of smoking. Other risk factors for developing lung cancer include exposure to second-hand smoke and occupational and environmental exposure to carcinogens, such as asbestos, arsenic, chromium, and nickel. Exposure to radon has been associated with an increased risk for developing lung carcinoma. Genetic susceptibility and the presence of interstitial lung disease also can contribute to the development of lung cancer.[2]

The major histologic types of lung cancer include squamous cell carcinoma, adenocarcinoma, large cell carcinoma, and small cell undifferentiated carcinoma. These four types of lung cancer comprise approximately 90% of lung cancer in the United States.[2] Adenocarcinoma currently is the most common subtype of lung cancer. The increase in incidence of adenocarcinoma in recent years has been attributed to the change in composition of cigarettes and the subsequent change in the dosage of inhaled carcinogens and their distribution in the lung parenchyma.[2]

LUNG CANCER STAGING

From the perspective of clinical management, lung cancer is divided into two categories: small cell lung cancer (SCLC) and non-SCLC (NSCLC). SCLC is a high-grade aggressive cancer that accounts for approximately 20% of lung cancers. SCLC is staged as limited disease that is managed with chemotherapy and radiation and as extensive disease that is managed with chemotherapy alone. In limited disease, the tumor is confined to one hemithorax within a single radiation port. Surgically operable limited stage SCLC is rare. Median survival is approximately 18 months for limited disease and approximately 9 months for extensive disease.[3,4]

The majority of lung cancers fall under the category of NSCLC and are classified using a TNM staging system (**Table 1**). The primary tumor is described with the "T" stage and is described as T1 if it does not exceed 3 cm and does not invade proximal to the lobar bronchus. T2 tumors exceed 3 cm or involve the mainstem bronchus at least 2 cm distal to the carina, invade the visceral pleura, or associated with atelectasis/obstructing pneumonitis extending to the hilum (**Fig. 1**). T3 tumors invade any of the following: the chest wall,

[a] Albert Einstein College of Medicine, 1300 Morris Park Avenue, Bronx, NY 10461, USA
[b] Division of Cardiothoracic Imaging, Department of Radiology, Montefiore Medical Center, 111 East 210th Street, Bronx, NY 10467-2401, USA
* Corresponding author. Division of Cardiothoracic Imaging, Department of Radiology, Montefiore Medical Center, 111 East 210th Street, Bronx, NY 10467-2401.
E-mail address: agodelma@yahoo.com (A. Godelman).

Magn Reson Imaging Clin N Am 16 (2008) 309–317
doi:10.1016/j.mric.2008.02.013
1064-9689/08/$ – see front matter © 2008 Elsevier Inc. All rights reserved.

Table 1
TNM staging for non-small cell lung cancer

Stage	T	N	M
IA	1	0	0
IB	2	0	0
IIA	1	1	0
IIB	2	1	0
	3	0	0
IIIA	1	2	0
	2	2	0
	3	1–2	0
IIIB	1–4	3	0
	4	0–3	0
IV	1–4	0–3	1

mediastinum, heart, great vessels, trachea, carina, esophagus, or vertebral body (**Fig. 2**). Tumors also are described as T4 in the presence of a malignant pleural or pericardial effusion or satellite tumor nodules within an ipsilateral lobe of the lung.

The "N" stage describes the nodal involvement. N0 represents no nodal disease. Metastases to the ipsilateral peribronchial or hilar lymph nodes are described as N1. Metastases to the ipsilateral mediastinal or subcarinal lymph nodes are described as N2. Metastases to the contralateral mediastinal and hilar lymph nodes and metastases to the scalene or supraclavicular lymph nodes are described as N3.

The "M" stage refers to distant metastatic disease. When distant metastases are present, the stage is described as M1.[5]

The correct staging of lung cancer is paramount in establishing an appropriate treatment protocol and predicting the survival of patients. Patients who have stage I and II disease can benefit from surgery and have a 5-year survival rate of 50% and 30%, respectively. Patients who have stage III disease are treated, for the most part, with a combination of chemotherapy and radiation.

diaphragm, mediastinal pleura, or parietal pericardium. Tumors also are classified as T3 if they involve the mainstem bronchus less than 2 cm distal to the carina or if they are associated with atelectasis/obstructive pneumonitis of the entire lung. T4 tumors invade any of the following:

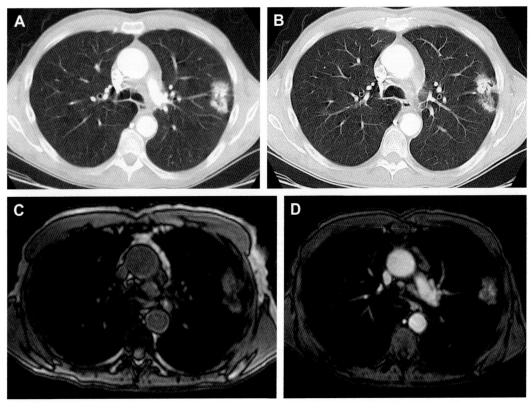

Fig. 1. A 63-year-old man who had adenocarcinoma. (*A, B*) Axial contrast-enhanced CT images with lung windows demonstrate a peripheral left upper-lobe mass with air bronchograms and pleural tags. The mass is well demonstrated on axial precontrast (*C*) and postcontrast (*D*) T1-weighted MR images.

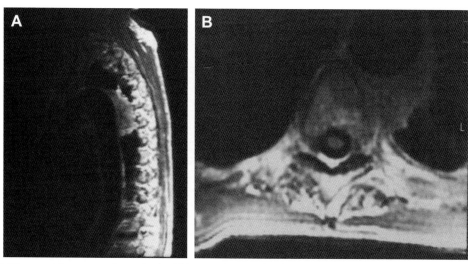

Fig. 2. A 70-year-old man, smoker, who had history of severe back pain radiating along the left T5 dermatome. Sagital (*A*) and axial (*B*) T1-weighted MR images demonstrate a left lung mass abutting the aorta and invading the vertebral body. The mass was diagnosed as large cell carcinoma at biopsy.

The 5-year survival rate is 17% for stage IIIA and 5% for stage IIIB. Patients who have stage IV disease are managed with supportive care with or without chemotherapy.[4]

Imaging plays an essential role in accurate staging of lung cancer. According to the most recent recommendations from the American College of Radiology and the American College of Chest Physicians (ACCP), a CT of the chest should be performed in patients who have known or suspected lung carcinoma who are eligible for treatment.[4,6] The ACCP also includes chest radiographs and CT in a recommended surveillance protocol for patients being treated with curative intent therapy.[7] CT is widely available, fast, offers excellent spatial resolution and, with current generation scanners, is able to provide high-quality multiplanar reconstructions. The major disadvantage of CT is radiation exposure. Radiation exposure is of concern especially in patients who undergo regular CT examinations as part of surveillance.

MR imaging is not a first-line imaging modality for lung cancer. In current clinical practice, MR imaging is reserved mostly for the evaluation of superior sulcus tumors and extrathoracic metastases. Advantages of MR imaging compared to CT include superior soft tissue contrast resolution and lack of ionizing radiation. MR imaging of the chest presents unique challenges. The low proton density of the lung parenchyma leads to low signal-to-noise ratio. Interfaces between air-filled alveoli and lung tissue create significant susceptibility artifacts. Cardiac pulsation and respiratory motion result in signal loss.[8] MR imaging is more vulnerable to motion artifacts than CT because of

relatively long acquisition times. With the introduction of new equipment and software in recent years, efforts have been made to develop MR imaging sequences and technique to help overcome these difficulties and establish MR imaging as a valid alternative to CT in imaging of lung cancer.

PULMONARY NODULES

The rate of unnecessary resection of benign solitary pulmonary nodules can be as high as 30%.[9] The role of imaging is to try to provide a noninvasive way of differentiating benign from malignant nodules. CT currently is the modality used most commonly for diagnosis and follow-up of pulmonary nodules. The presence of fat or specific benign patterns of calcifications within a nodule suggests a hamartoma or granuloma. As discussed previously, the main concern with CT is radiation exposure. Positron emission tomography with fluorodeoxyglucose (FDG-PET) is used for evaluation of indeterminate nodules. The disadvantages of FDG-PET in evaluating pulmonary nodules are low specificity and high cost.[9]

Because of the limitations discussed previously, MR imaging is not used routinely for the evaluation of pulmonary nodules (**Fig. 3**). An additional disadvantage of MR imaging in evaluating pulmonary nodules is its inability to detect calcifications within a nodule accurately. Small heavily calcified pulmonary nodules can be difficult to identify on MR imaging.

MR imaging scanners with field strengths higher than 1.5 T allow for improved signal-to-noise ratio and better temporal and spatial resolution. Yi and

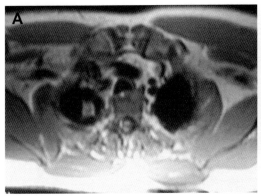
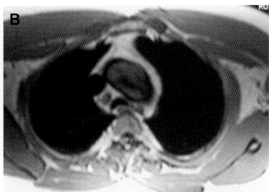

Fig. 3. A 52-year-old man underwent MR imaging angiogram of the thoracic aorta. (*A*) Axial T1-weighted image demonstrates an incidentally noted irregularly marginated nodule in the right lung apex. (*B*) Axial T1-weighted MR imaging demonstrates a right paratracheal lymph node. A nodule was diagnosed as adenocarcinoma on biopsy. The lymph node contained adenocarcinoma.

colleagues[10] studied 112 patients who had pathologically proved NSCLC and showed that 3-T MRI with T1-weighted 3-D turbo field-echo and T2-weighted triple inversion black blood turbo spin-echo (TSE) sequences can depict noncalcified pulmonary nodules larger than 5 mm nearly as well as CT. Detection rate for 3- to 5-mm nodules was 40%. Yi and colleagues[10] also commented on the accuracy of these techniques in describing the morphologic features of the nodules. The accuracy for depicting spiculated and lobulated margins in the study was 97% and 95% to 96% for depicting cavities within the nodules. Schroeder and colleagues[11] compared multirow detector CT and 2-D HASTE (fast single shot turbo spin echo sequence) 1.5-T MR imaging in the detection of pulmonary nodules in 30 patients who had pulmonary metastases. Compared to CT, the sensitivity of MR imaging in the study was 73% for nodules less than 3 mm, 86.3% for 3- to 5-mm nodules, 95.7% for 6- to 10-mm nodules, and 100% for nodules larger than 10 mm.

Benign and malignant pulmonary nodules have different morphologic and kinetic characteristics on dynamic MR imaging. Ohno and colleagues[12] used 1.5-T dynamic MR imaging to evaluate the pattern of enhancement of benign, malignant, and infectious nodules in 58 patients who had noncalcified solitary pulmonary nodules less than 3 mm. Based on the mean maximum relative enhancement ratio and mean slope of enhancement of the nodules, the investigators were able to differentiate the nodules that required further evaluation or treatment (malignant nodules and active infection) from nodules that did not (hamartoma or tuberculoma). There was an overlap, however, between the enhancement characteristics of malignant nodules and active infection because

both processes are associated with increased blood flow, perfusion, and capillary permeability (**Fig. 4**).

Schaefer and colleagues[13] analyzed 51 patients who had noncalcified solitary pulmonary nodules 6 to 40 mm in size. Dynamic contrast-enhanced MR images were performed using a 1.0-T magnet. The analysis of maximum enhancement peak and slope of enhancement of nodules demonstrated that contrast washout is highly specific for malignancy. One of the limitations of the study was that it excluded patients who had a history of recent infection or immunodeficiency. Donmez and colleagues[9] studied contrast enhancement features of noncalcified pulmonary nodules on 3-D volumetric gradient-recalled echo MR images in 40 patients who had nodules ranging from 7 to 40 mm. Images were performed on a 1.5-T magnet. This group described four different time-signal intensity curves, which can be used to differentiate between lung cancer, round atelectasis, and tuberculoma. Almost all malignant lesions in this study demonstrated early increasing enhancement with rapid washout. This study did not include patients who had laboratory findings of active infection or immunodeficiency.

PRIMARY AND RECURRENT TUMOR

In evaluating lung cancer, it is important to establish the full extent of the tumor and to differentiate the primary tumor from the surrounding postobstructive pneumonitis. Coronal and sagital MR images are useful in determining the extent of the tumor and relation of the tumor to the carina, aortopulmonary window, and pulmonary vessels.[14] T2-weighted and contrast-enhanced MR images can help differentiate tumor from adjacent

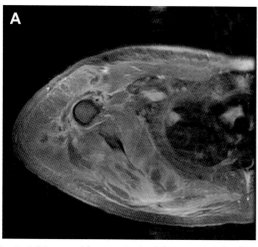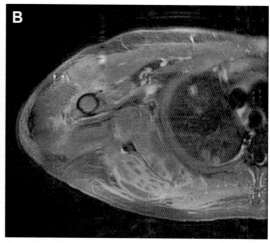

Fig. 4. A 36-year-old man who had fever and right shoulder pain. (*A, B*) Axial contrast-enhanced T1-weighted MR images of the right shoulder demonstrate soft tissue edema, inflammation, and multiple fluid collections in the musculature of the right shoulder consistent with cellulitis, myositis, and multiple abcesses. There are multiple right upper-lobe nodules, diagnosed as septic emboli.

postobstructive changes. High soft tissue contrast makes MR imaging a good modality for the evaluation of chest wall involvement. The use of dedicated surface coils improves the quality of images.

MR imaging is an excellent choice for the evaluation of superior sulcus tumors, especially when involvement of the brachial plexus and subclavian vessels is of concern (**Fig. 5**). MR imaging is excellent in demonstrating tumor extension into the neural foramina and epidural space. Rapoport and colleagues[15] used 1.5-T MR imaging to evaluate 32 patients who had symptoms referable to the brachial plexus. In 12 patients whose symptoms were the result of neoplasm, MR imaging was able to accurately identify the mass and its relationship to the brachial plexus. Proximal brachial plexus involvement was best evaluated on the axial images. Evaluation of the mid and distal brachial plexus was best evaluated on the sagittal images. The study also demonstrated the superiority of MR imaging to CT in demonstrating the extent of brachial plexus lesions; however, only axial CT images were used at the time.[15]

Pleural effusions are easily seen on CT and MR imaging. Dynamic MR imaging and CT imaging during inspiration and expiration can be used to assess the mobility of tumors contiguous with the pleura in order to differentiate between adherence to the pleura and infiltration of the pleural by tumor. False-positive results from benign fibrous adhesions can be seen with CT and MR imaging.[16]

Because of its superior soft tissue contrast resolution, MR imaging is better than CT in documenting involvement of the pericardium. MR imaging also is useful in evaluating for aortic invasion. Obliteration of the mediastinal fat planes, compression, encasement, or involvement of mediastinal vessels are better demonstrated on MR imaging than on CT.[14] Webb and colleagues[17] compared CT and MR imaging in staging of NSCLC in 170 patients. With respect to the diagnosis of mediastinal invasion, MR imaging was found significantly more accurate than CT. Takahashi and colleagues[18] examined contrast-enhanced helical CT images and gadolinium-enhanced 1.5-T MR images in patients who had lung carcinoma and suspected pulmonary vein and left atrium invasion. They found that gadolinium-enhanced MR images of 11 sites in 8 patients who underwent surgical resection correlated better with surgical findings than CT (**Figs. 6 and 7**).

Both and colleagues[19] examined diagnostic capabilities of three MR imaging sequences in 20 patients who had lung cancer. Coronal T1-weighted 3-D gradient-echo volumetric interpolated breath-hold (VIBE), coronal cardiac-triggered T2 HASTE, and respiration-triggered T2-weighted TSE (T2-TSE) sequences performed on 1.5-T magnet were evaluated. Contrast-enhanced images from a single detector row spiral CT were used as a reference. VIBE sequence was superior to other sequences in evaluating the mediastinal lymph nodes and small pulmonary lesions. Invasion of large vessels and other mediastinal structures was well demonstrated on VIBE. HASTE sequence was better than VIBE in demarcation of atelectasis adjacent to primary tumor. HASTE also is advantageous in evaluating

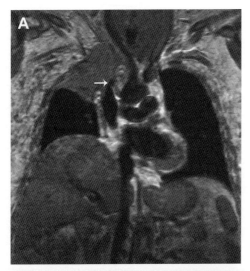

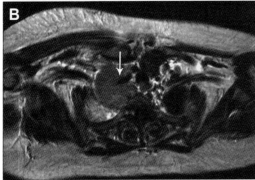

Fig. 5. A 63-year-old woman who had squamous cell lung carcinoma and superior vena cava syndrome. (A) Coronal contrast-enhanced T1-weighted MR image demonstrates a right upper-lobe mass, associated with right upper-lobe collapse, invading the mediastinum and causing marked narrowing of the superior vena cava (*arrow*). (B) Axial contrast-enhanced T1-weighted MR image demonstrates the mass extending through the superior sulcus and encasing the right subclavian artery (*arrow*). The high signal intensity in the soft tissues of the right chest wall is indicative of edema related to the superior vena cava syndrome.

patients in respiratory distress, as it is less susceptible to motion and breathing artifacts. T2-TSE was superior to other sequences in separating tumor from adjacent atelectasis in some patients.[19]

One of the challenges of lung cancer surveillance is differentiation between recurrent tumor and post-treatment fibrosis. Recurrent tumor has high signal intensity on T2-weighted images and can be differentiated from post-treatment fibrosis. Inflammatory changes, however, also have high T2 signal–producing false-positive results.[14]

LYMPH NODES

Accurate lymph node staging can make a difference between a resectable and a nonresectable cancer. The role of imaging is to offer a noninvasive way of differentiating benign reactive lymph nodes from metastatic disease (**Fig. 8**).

At the present time, the evaluation for lymph node metastases on CT and MR imaging is based primarily on the short-axis diameter of a lymph node with 10 mm a cutoff for normal. Normal-size lymph nodes, however, can be found on histologic evaluation to harbor disease. FDG-PET uses the difference in metabolic activity between healthy and diseased tissues to document lymph node metastases and has a high negative predictive value. Inflammatory and infectious lymph nodes, however, also pick up radioactive tracer leading to a decreased positive predictive value of FDG-PET in lymph node staging. Additionally, FDG-PET can give false-negative results in patients who have metastatic lymph nodes from bronchoalveolar cell carcinoma.

Characteristics of a normal lymph node on MR imaging include the presence of the fatty hilum, regular contour, and homogeneous signal intensity.[20] Calcifications within a lymph node, which can be used as a sign of benignity on CT, are inconspicuous on MR imaging.

Use of contrast-enhanced MR imaging lymphography is intended to help differentiate metastatic lymph nodes from benign nodes. Gadolinium-enhanced MR imaging is equal or superior to other imaging modalities in demonstrating extranodal spread of tumor and central necrosis.[21] Differences in enhancement profiles between malignant and benign lymph nodes suggest the usefulness of dynamic MR imaging.[22] Ohno and colleagues[23] performed qualitative and quantitative analysis of signal intensity of 802 lymph nodes in 110 patients who had NSCLC using short inversion time inversion recovery TSE MR imaging (STIR TSE MR). Quantitative analysis was performed by comparing the signal intensity of a lymph node to the signal intensity of a 0.9% saline phantom to produce a lymph node–to–saline ratio. Qualitative analysis was performed by assigning each lymph node a visual score based on comparison of signal intensity of the lymph node to the signal intensity of the mediastinal fat, muscle, and primary lesion. Patients in the study also underwent contrast-enhanced examinations with multidetector row CT. Lymph nodes on CT were evaluated with respect to size. When correlating the imaging results with pathology, the investigators concluded that qualitative and quantitative analyses with STIR TSE MR have significantly

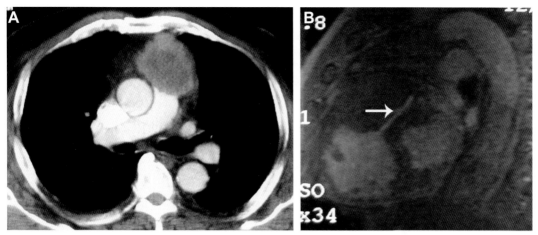

Fig. 6. A 75-year-old man who had chest pain and pulmonic stenosis on cardiac catheterization. Biopsy revealed epidermoid carcinoma of the lung. (*A*) Axial contrast-enhanced CT demonstrates a mass invading the main pulmonary artery. (*B*) Sagital contrast-enhanced MR demonstrates invasion of the right ventricle by the tumor. There is marked narrowing of the right ventricular outflow tract (*arrow*).

higher sensitivity and accuracy than contrast-enhanced CT in differentiating metastatic lymph nodes from lymph nodes without metastases. There was no significant difference between the quantitative and qualitative analysis with STIR TSE MR.[23]

Superparamagnetic nanoparticles show promise in demonstrating micrometastases in normal-size lymph nodes. Superparamagnetic particles accumulate in the phagocytic cells and cause a signal loss in the functional lymph nodes whereas the signal of nonphagocytic metastatic lymph nodes is unaffected.[24] Unfortunately, this contrast medium shows decreased specificity in the evaluation of lymph nodes in the chest and mediastinum. There is decreased uptake of contrast material in inflammatory nodes generating false-positive results. Gradient-echo sequences, which are used for nodal evaluation, exacerbate motion artifacts.[25] Another disadvantage of the superparamagnetic nanoparticle contrast medium is the need for two scans, one before the administration of contrast and one 24 hours after the administration of contrast.

Other MR imaging contrast agents, such as liposome encapsulated T1-type contrast agents and cell surface–specific agents, are being investigated.[21]

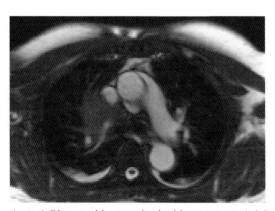

Fig. 7. A 79-year-old man who had lung cancer. Axial postcontrast T1-weighted MR imaging demonstrates a right hilar mass invading the mediastinum. (*Courtesy of* Charles S. White, MD, Baltimore, MD.)

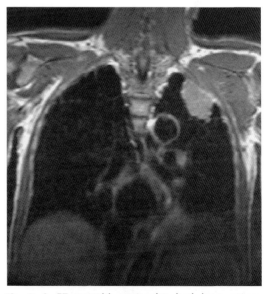

Fig. 8. A 57-year-old man who had lung cancer. Coronal T1-weighted MR image demonstrates a left upper-lobe mass and left hilar lymph nodes. (*Courtesy of* Charles S. White, MD, Baltimore, MD.)

DISTANT METASTASES

The most common sites of extrathoracic metastases in lung cancer are the adrenal glands, liver, brain, and skeletal system. Forty percent of patients who have NSCLC have distant metastases at presentation.[26]

According to most recent ACCP guidelines, patients who have known or suspected lung cancer should undergo a complete clinical evaluation, including thorough history, physical examination, and laboratory tests. Patients who have abnormal clinical evaluation should be imaged to evaluate for extrathoracic metastases.[4] Patients who have organ-specific symptoms should have imaging studies appropriate for that organ. ACCP recommends routine imaging for extrathoracic metastases in all patients who have stage IIIA and IIIB disease even if the clinical evaluation is negative.[4]

The adrenal glands and a portion of the liver routinely are visualized on the lower images from a CT of the chest. When adrenal nodules are present that do not meet criteria for adenoma on a routine CT scan, a dedicated washout CT study or an MR imaging can be performed for further evaluation.

MR imaging of the brain with contrast is a highly accurate examination for the evaluation of brain metastases. The skeletal system can be evaluated with a technetium-99m bone scan.

In recent years, FDG-PET has emerged as an alternative examination for evaluation of extrathoracic metastases. Because of high tracer uptake by normal brain tissue, FDG-PET is not used for evaluation of brain metastases. The specificity of PET for demonstrating adrenal metastases is 80% to 100%.[26] FDG-PET is at least as sensitive and is more specific than bone scan in demonstrating skeletal metastases in patients who have NSCLC. Osteoblastic lesions are seen better on bone scan.[26]

In comparing imaging studies in 90 patients who had lung cancer, Ohno and colleagues[27] found total-body MR imaging to be accurate and at least as effective as FDG-PET in assessing the M stage of patients who have lung cancer. Specifically, they found that total-body MR imaging was significantly more accurate than FDG-PET in evaluating head and neck and osseous metastases.

FUNCTIONAL ANALYSIS

Patients who have lung cancer often have concomitant conditions, such as chronic obstructive pulmonary disease (COPD). Patients who have severe COPD may not tolerate lung resection. Currently, a combination of spirometry and ventilation/perfusion scans is used to predict the postoperative lung function in this group of patients. Poor spatial resolution of ventilation/perfusion scans, however, makes it a suboptimal examination in this context. Alternative techniques, such as single photon emission CT (SPECT) and qualitative and quantitative CT imaging, have been suggested.

Müller and colleagues[28] studied the use of oxygen-enhanced lung MR imaging in evaluating the pulmonary diffusion capacity in 11 healthy volunteers and 17 patients who had various pulmonary diseases (idiopathic pulmonary fibrosis, allergic alveolitis, emphysema, adult respiratory distress syndrome, and pulmonary hypertension). The group concluded that the signal intensity slope during breathing of 100% oxygen allows evaluation of pulmonary diffusion capacity. Regional differences in diffusion also were observed. Ohno and colleagues[29] evaluated the value of oxygen-enhanced MR imaging in predicting postsurgical lung function in patients who had lung cancer. Thirty patients who had lung cancer underwent imaging with contrast-enhanced multidetector-row CT, oxygen-enhanced MR imaging, perfusion scintigraphy, and pre- and postsurgical pulmonary function testing. On MR imaging, regional and total functional lung volumes were assessed based on regional oxygen enhancement. Oxygen-enhanced MR imaging was found useful in predicting postsurgical lung function similar to quantitative CT.[29] Recently, Ohno and colleagues compared perfusion MR imaging, SPECT, and CT images in 150 patients who had lung cancer and concluded that dynamic contrast-enhanced perfusion MR imaging is more accurate in predicting postoperative lung function than are qualitative CT and perfusion SPECT and may be at least as accurate as quantitative CT.[30]

SUMMARY

- Lung cancer is the most common cause of cancer-related death for men and women in the United States. Accurate cancer staging is essential for determining appropriate management and predicting prognosis.
- CT, along with FDG-PET, currently is the main imaging modality for staging lung cancer. The development of new equipment and introduction of more advanced techniques and contrast media potentially can make MR imaging a valid ionizing-radiation-free alternative.

ACKNOWLEDGMENTS

The authors thank Vineet R. Jain, MD, and Seymour Sprayregen, MD, for thorough review of the manuscript. The authors thank Richard Zampolin, MD, for help in preparation of the figures.

REFERENCES

1. American Cancer Society. Cancer facts and figures. Available at: http://www.cancer.org.

2. Alberg AJ, Ford JG, Samet JM. Epidemiology of lung cancer: ACCP evidence-based clinical practice guidelines 2nd edition. Chest 2007;132(3):29S–55S.

3. Ginsberg MS, Grewal RK, Heelan RT. Lung cancer. Radiol Clin North Am 2007;45(1):21–43.

4. Silvesti GA, Gould MK, Margolis ML, et al. Noninvasive staging of non-small cell lung cancer: ACCP evidenced-based clinical practice guidelines (2nd edition). Chest 2007;132(3):178S–201S.

5. Mountain CF. Revisions in the international system for staging lung cancer. Chest 1997;111(6):1710–7.

6. McLoud TC, Westcott J, Davis SD, et al. Staging of bronchogenic carcinoma, non-small cell lung carcinoma. American college of radiology: ACR appropriateness criteria. Radiology 2000;(Suppl 215):611–9.

7. Rubins J, Unger M, Colice GL. Follow-up and surveillance of the lung cancer patient following curative intent therapy: ACCP evidence-based clinical practice guideline (2nd edition). Chest 2007;132(3):355S–67S.

8. Kauczor HU, Kreitner KF. Contrast-enhanced MRI of the lung. Eur J Radiol 2000;34(3):196–207.

9. Donmez FY, Yekeler E, Saeidi V, et al. Dynamic contrast enhancement patterns of solitary pulmonary nodules on 3D gradient-recalled echo MRI. AJR Am J Roentgenol 2007;189(6):1380–6.

10. Yi CA, Jeon TY, Lee KS, et al. 3-T MRI: usefulness for evaluating primary lung cancer and small nodules in lobes not containing primary tumors. AJR Am J Roentgenol 2007;189(2):386–92.

11. Schroeder T, Ruehm SG, Debatin JF, et al. Detection of pulmonary nodules using a 2D HASTE MR sequence: comparison with MDCT. AJR Am J Roentgenol 2005;185(4):979–84.

12. Ohno Y, Hatabu H, Takenaka D, et al. Solitary pulmonary nodules: potential role of dynamic MR imaging in management initial experience. Radiology 2002;224(2):503–11.

13. Schaefer JF, Vollmar J, Schick F, et al. Solitary pulmonary nodules: dynamic contrast-enhanced MR imaging–perfusion differences in malignant and benign lesions. Radiology 2004;232(2):544–53.

14. Bittner RC, Felix R. Magnetic resonance (MR) imaging of the chest: state-of-the-art. Eur Respir J 1998;11(6):1392–404.

15. Rapoport S, Blair DN, McCarthy SM, et al. Brachial plexus: correlation of MR imaging with CT and pathologic findings. Radiology 1988;167(1):161–5.

16. Schaefer-Prokop C, Prokop M. New imaging techniques in the treatment guidelines for lung cancer. Eur Respir J Suppl 2002;35:71S–83S.

17. Webb WR, Gatsonis C, Zerhouni EA, et al. CT and MR imaging in staging non-small cell bronchogenic carcinoma: report of the radiologic diagnostic oncology group. Radiology 1991;178(3):705–13.

18. Takahashi K, Furuse M, Hanaoka H, et al. Pulmonary vein and left atrial invasion by lung cancer: assessment by breath-hold gadolinium-enhanced three-dimensional MR angiography. J Comput Assist Tomogr 2000;24(4):557–61.

19. Both M, Schultze J, Reuter M, et al. Fast T1- and T2-weighted pulmonary MR-imaging in patients with bronchial carcinoma. Eur J Radiol 2005;53(3):478–88.

20. Luciani A, Itti E, Rahmouni A, et al. Lymph node imaging: basic principles. Eur J Radiol 2006;58(3):338–44.

21. Wunderbaldinger P. Problems and prospects of modern lymph node imaging. Eur J Radiol 2006;58(3):325–37.

22. Laissy JP, Gay-Depassier P, Soyer P, et al. Enlarged mediastinal lymph nodes in bronchogenic carcinoma: assessment with dynamic contrast-enhanced MR imaging. Work in progress. Radiology 1994;191(1):263–7.

23. Ohno Y, Hatabu H, Takenaka D, et al. Metastases in mediastinal and hilar lymph nodes in patients with non-small cell lung cancer: quantitative and qualitative assessment with STIR turbo spin-echo MR imaging. Radiology 2004;231(3):872–9.

24. Misselwitz B. MR contrast agents in lymph node imaging. Eur J Radiol 2006;58(3):375–82.

25. Saksena MA, Saokar A, Harisinghani MG. Lymphotropic nanoparticle enhanced MR imaging (LNMRI) technique for lymph node imaging. Eur J Radiol 2006;58(3):367–74.

26. Wynants J, Stroobants S, Dooms C, et al. Staging of lung cancer. Radiol Clin North Am 2007;45(4):609–25.

27. Ohno Y, Koyama H, Nogami M, et al. Whole-body MR imaging vs. FDG-PET: comparison of accuracy of M-stage diagnosis for lung cancer patients. J Magn Reson Imaging 2007;26(3):498–509.

28. Müller CJ, Schwaiblmair M, Scheidler J, et al. Pulmonary diffusing capacity: assessment with oxygen-enhanced lung MR imaging preliminary findings. Radiology 2002;222(2):499–506.

29. Ohno Y, Hatabu H, Higashino T, et al. Oxygen-enhanced MR imaging: correlation with postsurgical lung function in patients with lung cancer. Radiology 2005;236(2):704–11.

30. Ohno Y, Koyama H, Nogami M, et al. Postoperative lung function in lung cancer patients: comparative analysis of predictive capability of MRI, CT, and SPECT. AJR Am J Roentgenol 2007;189(2):400–8.

MR Imaging of Benign and Malignant Pleural Disease

Ritu R. Gill, MBBS[a], Victor H. Gerbaudo, PhD[a],
Francine L. Jacobson, MD, MPH[a],
Beatrice Trotman-Dickenson, MBBS[a], Shin Matsuoka, MD, PhD[b],
Andetta Hunsaker, MD[a], David J. Sugarbaker, MD[c],
Hiroto Hatabu, MD, PhD[a,d,*]

KEYWORDS

- MR • Pleura • Pleural malignancy
- Pleural thickening • Pleural plaques • Mesothelioma

The thin visceral and parietal pleura are barely perceptible in the absence of disease. Development of disease within the potential space between the visceral and parietal pleura results in radiologic visualization of pleural disease. Imaging, particularly MR imaging, CT, and fluorodeoxyglucose (F18) positron emission tomography (PET)–CT, plays an important role in the diagnosis and management of patients who have pleural disease. CT scanning is the primary tool used to investigate pleural disease identified at chest radiography, whereas MR imaging is used as a problem-solving tool in specific cases, such as inflammatory and infectious pleural diseases and primary and secondary pleural malignancies.[1,2] This article describes the MR imaging appearance of pleural diseases, including pleural effusions and empyema, and benign and malignant pleural tumors, with a special focus on mesothelioma.

ANATOMY

The term pleura encompasses the parietal pleura (lining the inner surface of the chest wall), the visceral pleura (lining the outer surface of the lung and invaginating into the lung in the form of fissures), and the intervening pleural space. Visceral and parietal pleural surfaces consist of a mesothelial layer and three connective tissue layers, with the visceral pleura being thicker than the parietal pleura. Together the visceral and parietal pleural layers and the lubricating liquid in the pleural space have a combined thickness of 0.2 to 0.4 mm; the width of the pleural space is 10 to 20 micrometers.

The normal parietal pleura are never visualized on chest radiography (CXR). The visceral pleura are only seen on CXRs when they invaginate the lung parenchyma to form fissures or junctional lines, or if a pneumothorax is present. The appearance of fissures on CT images depends on slice thickness and the planes of the fissures relative to the CT slice. Relatively thick slice thickness, down to approximately 5 mm, shows the fissures as avascular planes, appearing as avascular, curvilinear, ill-defined areas of low attenuation extending from the hilum to the chest wall.[3] High-resolution CT (HRCT) images, less than

This work was partially supported by NIH Grant # R21CA116271-02.

[a] Department of Radiology, Brigham and Women's Hospital, Harvard Medical School, 75 Francis Street, Boston, MA 02115, USA

[b] Department of Radiology, Brigham and Women's Hospital, 75 Francis Street, Boston, MA 02115, USA

[c] Division of Thoracic Surgery, Department of Surgery, Brigham and Women's Hospital, Harvard Medical School, 75 Francis Street, Boston, MA 02115, USA

[d] Center for Pulmonary Functional Imaging, Brigham and Women's Hospital, Harvard Medical School, 221 Longwood Avenue, Boston, MA 02115, USA

* Corresponding author. Department of Radiology and Center for Pulmonary Functional Imaging, Brigham and Women's Hospital, Harvard Medical School, 75 Francis Street, Boston, MA 02115.

E-mail address: hhatabu@partners.org (H. Hatabu).

Magn Reson Imaging Clin N Am 16 (2008) 319–339
doi:10.1016/j.mric.2008.03.004

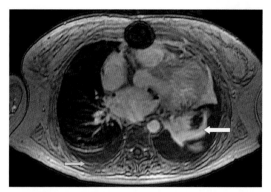

Fig. 1. Axial postcontrast 3D gradient echo sequence image in a postcardiac surgery patient showing nonenhancing transudative pleural effusions (*blue arrow*), with the enhancing consolidative opacity in the left lower lobe (*white arrow*) representing atelectasis.

2 mm in thickness, allow direct visualization of the linear pleural surface, but also the costal pleura, which appears as a 1- to 2-mm thick line referred to as the "intercostal stripe," representing the visceral pleura, normal physiologic pleural fluid, parietal pleura, endothoracic fascia, and the innermost intercostal muscles. The stripe extends to the lateral margins of the adjacent ribs and along the paravertebral margin. Normal pleura are not visualized with MR imaging.

PLEURAL EFFUSIONS

The normal pleural space contains 1 to 5 mL of lubricating pleural fluid. Pleural effusions occur when there is an imbalance of the normal physiologic processes that are necessary for the maintenance of the equilibrium that balances pleural fluid production and absorption. Exudative pleural effusions occur secondary to an increase in capillary permeability because of malignancy, infection, or thromboembolic disease. Transudative pleural effusions result from an increase in hydrostatic pressure or a decrease in colloid osmotic pressure.[4] On MR imaging, pleural fluid typically has low signal intensity on T1-weighted images and high signal intensity on T2-weighted images, reflecting its water content (**Fig. 1**) Pleural fluid is often heterogeneous, because motion within the effusion creates flow artifacts. Although the role of MR imaging is currently limited in the evaluation of pleural fluid, it remains superior for the characterization of the type of pleural fluid. Davis and colleagues[5] showed that the qualitative and

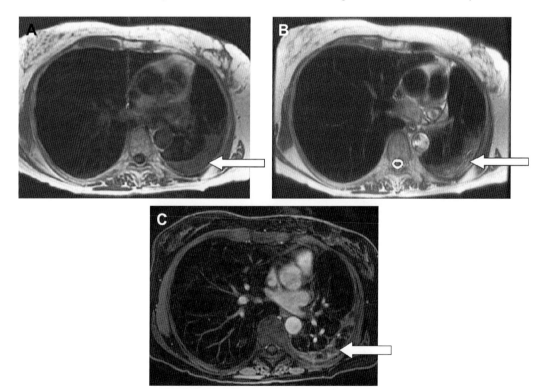

Fig. 2. Axial T1-weighted (*A*), T2-weighted (*B*), and postcontrast axial 3D gradient echo sequence images in a patient who has aspergillus empyema show a small exudative left pleural effusion with pleural nodularity, hypointense on T1-weighted imaging (*A*), hyperintense on T2-weighted imaging (*B*), with enhancement of the pleura on postcontrast images (*C*). Also note the septations (*white arrow*).

quantitative assessment of signal from pleural effusions differentiates transudative causes of pleural effusions from exudative causes. The exudates produced a higher signal than the transudates on T1-weighted and T2-weighted images, with T2-weighted images being more discriminatory.[5] Preliminary studies have suggested that single-shot, diffusion-weighted sequences may also be helpful in this regard, with high diffusion seen in transudates and low diffusion seen with exudates.[6] Three-plane scanning is helpful, with sagittal and axial images being most valuable in detecting subtle nodularity, particularly on contrast-enhanced three-dimensional (3D) gradient echo images. The assessment of pleural nodularity does not necessarily require intravenous contrast administration. On T2-weighted images, the high-signal pleural fluid and extrapleural fat act as inherent

contrast, outlining the low-signal parietal pleura and pleural nodularity, which allows for easy detection of septations compared with CT (**Fig. 2**).[7]

A chylothorax may have characteristics consistent with fat, including high signal intensity on T1-weighted and proton density images and lower signal intensity on T2-weighted images. Most chylothoraces appear as simple pleural effusions, even when large. Chylothorax and pneumothorax may be seen together, particularly in patients who have lymphangioleiomyomatosis.

Subacute or chronic hematomas in the pleural space are characteristically seen with high signal intensity on T1-weighted and T2-weighted images. The "concentric ring" sign describes the bright central signal intensity of methemoglobin related to T1 shortening effects, with the dark

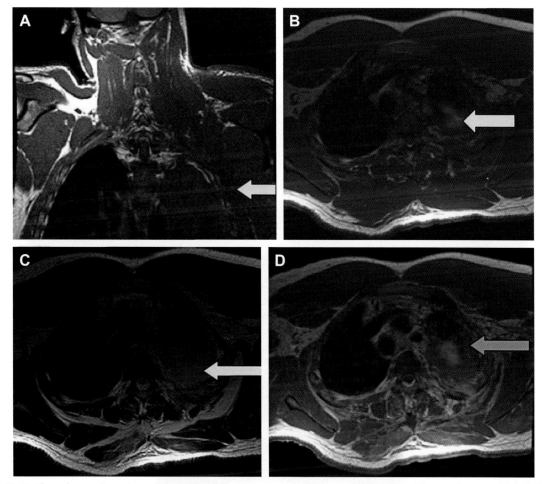

Fig. 3. Pleural space hematoma in a patient following trauma. (*A*) Coronal T1-weighted image shows multiple left rib fractures and chest wall hematoma (*arrow*). (*B*) Axial T1-weighted image shows hyperintense hematoma in the left upper pleura (*arrow*). (*C*) Left pleural space hematoma (*arrow*) is relatively hyperintense on T2-weighted imaging. (*D*) Axial contrast-enhanced T1-weighted image shows no enhancement of the left pleural process, with a dark rim of hemosiderin surrounding the hyperintense methemoglobin.

Table 1
Summary of MR appearance of pleural diseases

Pleural Abnormality	T1-Weighted	T2-Weighted	Postcontrast	Other Features
Transudate pleural effusion	Low	High	–	–
Exudative pleural effusion	Low	High	+	Septations, nodularity
Chylothorax	High	Low	–	Signal comparable to fat
Hemothorax	High	High	–	Concentric rim sign related to T1 shortening
Pleural plaques	Low	Low	–	Minimal to no enhancement following gadolinium
Localized fibrous tumor of the pleura	Low to intermediate	Low to intermediate	+	Pedunculated about diaphragm, myxoid degeneration
Lipoma	High	Moderate to high	–	Fat suppression sequence helpful
Liposarcoma	Low	High	Variable	Heterogeneous
Asbestos-related pleural thickening	Low	High	–	Round atelectasis

Abbreviations: +, enhancement present; –, no enhancement.

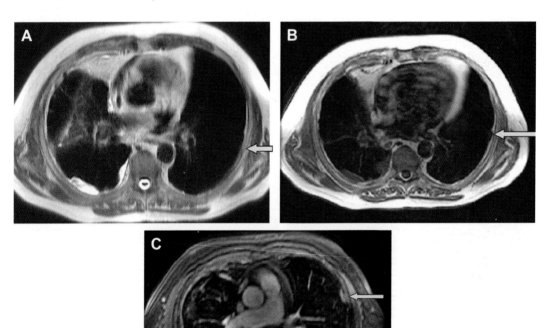

Fig. 4. Axial images in a patient who had asbestos exposure and right-sided mesothelioma with bilateral pleural plaques. (*A*) T1-weighted imaging shows that the pleural plaques are hypointense (*arrow*). (*B*) Axial T2-weighted image shows that the pleural plaque is profoundly hypointense (*arrow*). (*C*) Axial postcontrast 3D gradient echo axial image shows minimal enhancement (*arrow*).

outer ring representing hemosiderin (**Fig. 3**) (**Table 1**).[8,9]

PLEURAL DISEASES

Pleural thickening is readily detectable on CT and MR imaging. It is important to distinguish benign from malignant pleural disease and to determine the possible cause for pleural thickening. On cross-sectional imaging studies, pleural thickening may present as a focal or a diffuse abnormality (see **Table 1**).

Focal Pleural Abnormalities

Pleural plaques

Pleural plaques are the most common manifestation of asbestos exposure, with a latency period of 20 to 30 years. The plaques represent areas of dense hyaline collagen within the mesothelial layers of the pleura and predominantly involve the parietal pleura. Visceral plaques can occur but are relatively rare, and when present can simulate a parenchymal mass.[10] Pleural plaques are usually bilateral, with unilateral plaques seen in up to 25% of cases.[11]

Pleural plaques show low signal intensity on T1-weighted, T2-weighted, and proton density weighted (PDW) sequences, and enhance minimally, if at all, following gadolinium administration (**Fig. 4**). In a recent series of 21 patients, MR imaging was compared with CT for the diagnosis of asbestos-related pleural disease. MR imaging was superior for demonstrating diffuse pleural thickening, extrapleural fat hypertrophy, and pleural effusions, whereas CT was found to be better for detecting pleural calcification.[12]

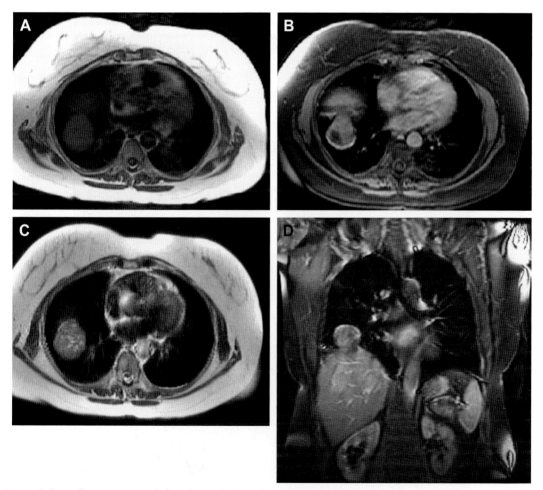

Fig. 5. Solitary fibrous tumor of the pleura. Pedunculated pleural-based mass arising from the diaphragmatic surface of the pleura on the right. (*A*) Axial T1-weighted image shows that the mass is hypointense. (*B*) Axial T2-weighted image also shows that the mass is predominantly hypointense with areas of high attenuation depicting myxoid degeneration. Axial (*C*) and coronal (*D*) postcontrast images showing heterogeneous enhancement of the lesion.

Solitary fibrous tumor of the pleura

Solitary fibrous tumor of the pleura (SFTP) are rare lesions, accounting for less than 5% of all pleural tumors.[13] These lesions originate from the mesenchymal cells of the pleura, with 80% arising from the visceral pleura. The mean age at presentation is 50 years, with a slight female predominance. SFTPs are typically solitary and slow growing. A correlation between tumor size and patient symptoms has been recognized, with masses

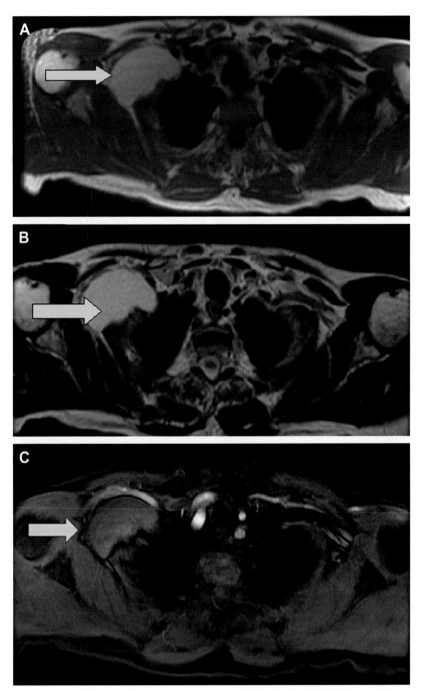

Fig. 6. Right lateral chest wall lipoma showing signal characteristics similar to fat. (*A*) Axial T1-weighted image shows homogeneous hyperintensity within the mass (*arrow*). (*B*) Axial T2-weighted image also shows homogeneous hyperintensity within the lesion (*arrow*). (*C*) Axial 3D gradient echo image shows no enhancement of the lesion (*arrow*).

measuring up to 10 cm tending to be asymptomatic, and masses greater than 16 cm presenting with pressure symptoms.[13] Approximately 4% of these tumors are associated with hypoglycemia, which is related to expression of insulinlike growth factor–II.

The imaging features of SFTP depend on lesion size. These tumors tend to be smooth or lobulated masses, abutting the diaphragm, and can mimic diaphragmatic eventration. Forty percent of cases may show a vascular pedicle attaching the tumor to the pleural surface, accounting for its mobility on chest radiographs and fluoroscopy.[14]

The MR imaging appearance of SFTP is consistent with the characteristics of fibrous tissue: lesions show low to intermediate signal on T1-weighted, T2-weighted, and PDW sequences. High signal on T2-weighted sequences can be seen in areas of necrosis and myxoid degeneration. After administration of gadolinium, intense homogeneous enhancement is typical and is an indicator of the tumor vascularity.[15] A rim of low signal surrounding the tumor on T2-weighted images may also be present (**Fig. 5**).

Lipomas and liposarcomas

Lipomas are rare benign pleural tumors.[1,16] Localized pleural lipomas are well-defined homogeneous masses, hyperintense on T1-weighted and moderately intense on T2-weighted images.[17] Additional fat suppression sequences are helpful when diagnostic doubt persists (**Fig. 6**). Liposarcomas are typically large, infiltrative, and often asymptomatic. There is no evidence to suggest they arise from pre-existing

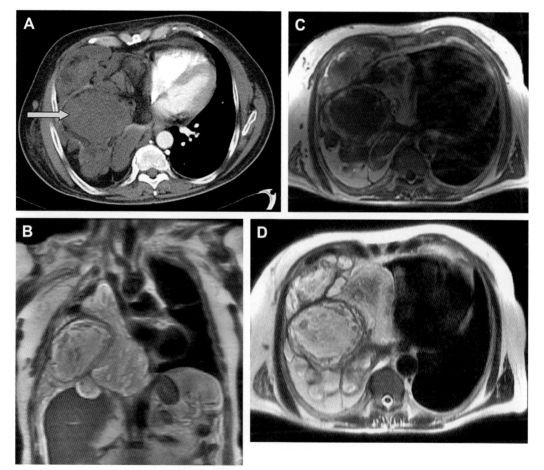

Fig. 7. Liposarcoma metastatic to the right pleura. (*A*) Axial CT image shows a fat-containing tumor (*arrow*) encasing the right lung. (*B*) T1-weighted coronal image shows that the fat planes between mediastinal structures and the diaphragm to advantage compared with CT. (*C*) Axial T1-weighted image shows that the more poorly differentiated component is of low intensity, whereas the well-differentiated component is hyperintense. (*D*) Axial T1-weighted contrast-enhanced axial image shows isointense to hyperintense heterogeneous pleural tumor.

lipomas. They appear as heterogeneous masses on CT with soft tissue and fat components, measuring less than 50 HU (mean CT values) on pre- and postintravenous contrast-enhanced images. On MR imaging, liposarcomas often show high signal intensity on T2-weighted sequences because of the presence of myxoid degeneration, whereas low signal is common on T1-weighted sequences, with variable enhancement following intravenous contrast administration (**Fig. 7**).[18]

Diffuse Benign Pleural Thickening

Diffuse pleural thickening primarily involves the visceral pleura and usually is preceded by pleural effusion and subsequent fibrosis that adheres to the parietal pleura. On CT, diffuse pleural thickening is defined as a continuous sheet of thickening of at least 5 cm in lateral extent, with a 3-mm thickness.[19] Prior *Mycobacterium tuberculosis* infection (MTB), empyema, trauma, drug exposure, collagen vascular disease, and asbestos exposure may result in diffuse pleural thickening (see **Table 1**).

Asbestos-related diffuse pleural thickening
Unlike asbestos-related pleural plaques, diffuse pleural thickening rarely calcifies, and it is generally associated with a restrictive pattern on pulmonary function testing.[20]

Occasionally, round atelectasis may be encountered in the setting of asbestos-related pleural disease, but may be seen with pleural thickening related to trauma, chronic infections, and collagen vascular disease. Round atelectasis represents juxtapleural lung collapse resulting from cicatrized pleural disease.[21] On CT and MR, the classic comet tail sign corresponds to vessels and bronchi curving into the round, oval, or wedge-shaped mass, and has signal intensity similar to liver on T1-weighted sequences.[21]

Non–asbestos-related benign pleural thickening
The appearance of benign pleural thickening unrelated to asbestos exposure on imaging studies may reflect the underlying cause. In patients who had prior MTB, unilateral, sheetlike calcification with marked volume loss associated with

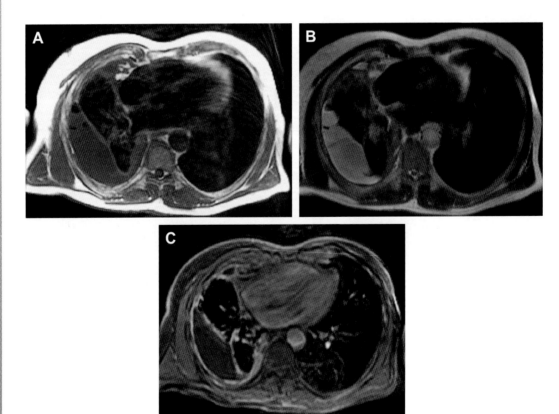

Fig. 8. Pleural metastasis from adenocarcinoma of the colon. (*A*) Axial T1-weighted image shows an isointense loculated right pleural effusion associated with pleural thickening. (*B*) Axial T2-weighted image shows that the loculated pleural effusion is predominantly hyperintense. (*C*) Axial contrast-enhanced 3D gradient echo image shows intense pleural enhancement.

parenchymal findings related to prior MTB infection are also seen. In posttraumatic or postsurgical hemothoraces, the process is usually unilateral and may be associated with calcification, multiple rib fractures, or prior sternotomy. Talc and chemical pleurodesis can also result in diffuse thickening, with or without calcification or high attenuation.

Diffuse Malignant Pleural Thickening

Metastatic pleural disease is the most common cause of malignant pleural thickening: bronchogenic carcinoma accounts for 40% of cases, followed by breast cancer (20%), lymphoma (10%), and gastric and ovarian cancer (5%).[22] Metastasizing thymoma and thymic carcinoma may spread to the pleural space in a contiguous or multifocal pattern, with drop metastases to the pleura following biopsy or surgery. Sarcomas rarely metastasize to the pleura, and when they do, they generally occur after surgical resection of pulmonary nodules. Primary pleural lymphoma is rare and usually presents as disease recurrence or as contiguous extension from the mediastinum.[23] Differentiation of metastatic pleural disease from mesothelioma on chest radiography is usually not possible; history of a potential primary source

of malignancy or pleural biopsy is typically needed to arrive at the diagnosis (**Figs. 8 and 9**).

Contrast-enhanced CT is the imaging modality of choice for differentiating between benign and malignant causes of pleural thickening. Several studies have shown that in malignant pleural thickening, the parietal pleura is more than 1 cm thick, with nodular and circumferential pleural thickening and involvement of the mediastinal and diaphragmatic surfaces of the pleura. In a series by Leung and colleagues,[1] the specificities of these findings were 94%, 94%, 100%, and 88%, respectively. CT may also demonstrate the primary tumor and distant metastases to the liver and the adrenal glands.

Several studies have assessed the role of MR in distinguishing benign from malignant pleural disease. In two reports, pleural thickening greater than 1 cm was described in benign and malignant disease.[24] When morphologic features and signal intensity characteristics were combined, MR imaging was superior to CT, with a sensitivity of 98% to 100% and specificity of 87% to 92% for detecting malignant pleural thickening.[24] Falaschi and colleagues[25] reported that pleural signal hypointensity relative to the intercostal muscles on T2-weighted sequences was a reliable predictor of benign disease.

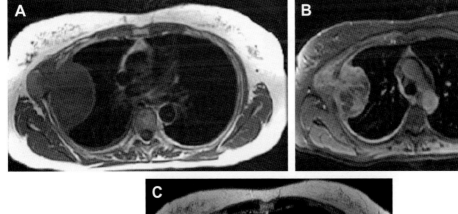

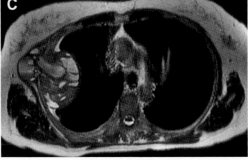

Fig. 9. Right pleural metastasis from synovial sarcoma invading the chest wall. (*A*) Axial T1-weighted image shows that the right pleural-based mass is isointense with muscle, with central low attenuation areas representing necrosis. (*B*) Axial fat saturation contrast-enhanced image shows that the mass has intense enhancement with central necrosis. (*C*) Axial T2-weighted imaging shows heterogeneous areas of signal abnormality with regions of hyperintensity and fluid levels.

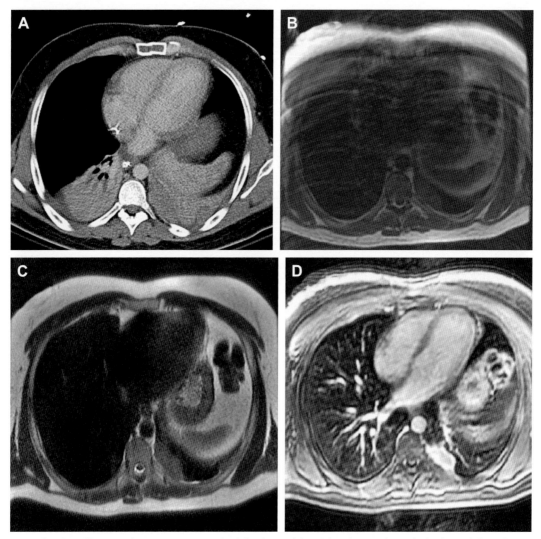

Fig. 10. Thymic malignancy drop metastases to the left pleura. (*A*) Axial CT image through the lower lobes, showing pleural nodularity in the left lower pleura, somewhat difficult to distinguish from adjacent atelectasis. (*B*) Axial T1-weighted image shows hypointense pleural nodularity in the left base. (*C*) Axial T2-weighted image shows that the left pleural abnormality is predominantly isointense. (*D*) Axial contrast-enhanced 3D gradient echo image shows intense enhancement, with a pattern and intensity similar to the mediastinal mass, consistent with known thymic neoplasia.

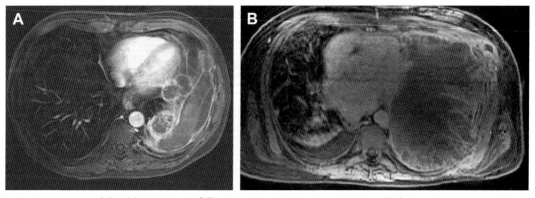

Fig. 11. Osteosarcoma. (*A*) Axial LAVA image following chemotherapy shows lobulated left pleural metastases with only one area of peripheral enhancement showing good response to chemotherapy, with less than 20% viable tumor seen along the medial aspect with more nodular peripherally enhancing component. (*B*) Axial 3D gradient echo image following pneumonectomy shows tumor recurrence along the lateral aspect of the pneumonectomy space.

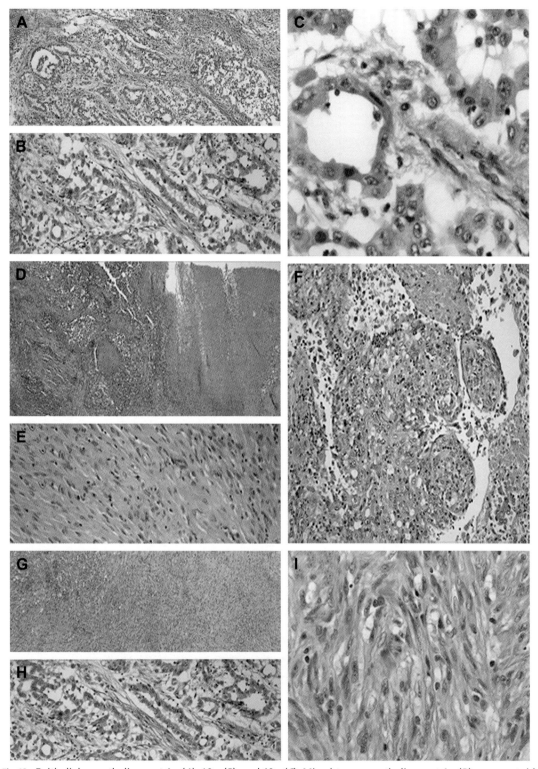

Fig. 12. Epithelial mesothelioma at 4× (A), 10× (B), and 40× (C). Mixed-type mesothelioma at 4× (D), sarcomatoid-mixed 20× (E), and epithelioid-mixed 20× (F). Sarcomatoid mesothelioma at 4× (G), 10× (H) and 40× (I). (*Courtesy of* Robert Padera, MD, PhD, Boston, MA.)

Table 2
New international staging system for diffuse malignant pleural mesothelioma

	Stage	Definition
T1	T1a	Tumor limited to the ipsilateral parietal pleura, including mediastinal and diaphragmatic pleura: no involvement of the visceral pleura.
	T1b	Tumor involving the ipsilateral parietal pleura, including mediastinal and diaphragmatic pleura; scattered foci of tumor also involving the visceral pleura.
T2		Tumor involving each of the ipsilateral pleural surfaces (parietal, mediastinal, diaphragmatic, and visceral pleura). Involvement of diaphragmatic muscle. Confluent visceral pleural tumor (including the fissures) or extension of tumor from visceral pleura into the underlying pulmonary parenchyma.
T3		Describes locally advanced but potentially resectable tumor. Tumor involving all of the ipsilateral pleural surfaces (parietal, mediastinal, diaphragmatic, and visceral pleura) with at least one of the following features: Involvement of the endothoracic fascia. Extension into the mediastinal fat. Solitary, completely resectable focus of tumor extending into the soft tissues of the chest wall. Nontransmural involvement of the pericardium.
T4		Describes locally advanced technically unresectable tumor. Tumor involving all of the ipsilateral pleural surfaces (parietal, mediastinal, diaphragmatic, and visceral) with at least one of the following features: Diffuse extension or multifocal masses of tumor in the chest wall, with or without associated rib destruction. Direct transdiaphragmatic extension of tumor to the peritoneum. Direct extension of tumor to the contralateral pleura. Direct extension of tumor to one or more mediastinal organs. Direct extension of tumor into the spine. Tumor extending through to the internal surface of the pericardium with or without a pericardial effusion, or tumor involving the myocardium.

N		
	NX	Regional lymph nodes cannot be assessed.
	N0	No regional lymph node metastases.
	N1	Metastases in the ipsilateral bronchopulmonary or hilar lymph nodes.
	N2	Metastases in the subcarinal or ipsilateral mediastinal lymph nodes, including the ipsilateral internal mammary nodes.
	N3	Metastases in the contralateral mediastinal, contralateral internal mammary, ipsilateral, or contralateral supraclavicular lymph nodes.
M		
	MX	Presence of distant metastases cannot be assessed.
	M0	No distant metastasis.
	M1	Distant metastasis present.
Stage I	Ia	T1aN0M0
	Ib	T1bN0M0
Stage II		T2N0M0
Stage III		Any T3M0
		Any N1M0
		Any N2M0
Stage IV		Any T4
		Any N3
		Any M1

Data from Rusch VW, Group TIMI. A proposed new international TNM staging system for malignant pleural mesothelioma from the International Mesothelioma Interest Group. Chest 1995;108:16.

Table 3
The revised Brigham and Women's Hospital staging system for malignant pleural mesothelioma

Stage No.	Definition
I	Disease confined within capsule of the parietal pleura: ipsilateral pleura, lung, pericardium, diaphragm, or chest wall disease limited to previous biopsy sites.
II	All of stage I with positive intrapleural (N1) lymph nodes.
III	Local extension of disease into chest wall or mediastinum; heart, or through diaphragm, peritoneum; with or without extrapleural (N2) or contralateral (N3) lymph node involvement.
IV	Distant metastatic disease.

Data from Sugarbaker DJ, Flores RM, Jaklitsch MT, et al. Resection margins, extrapleural nodal status, and cell type determine postoperative long-term survival in trimodality therapy of malignant pleural mesothelioma: results in 183 patients. J Thorac Cardiovasc Surg 1999;117(1):54–63.

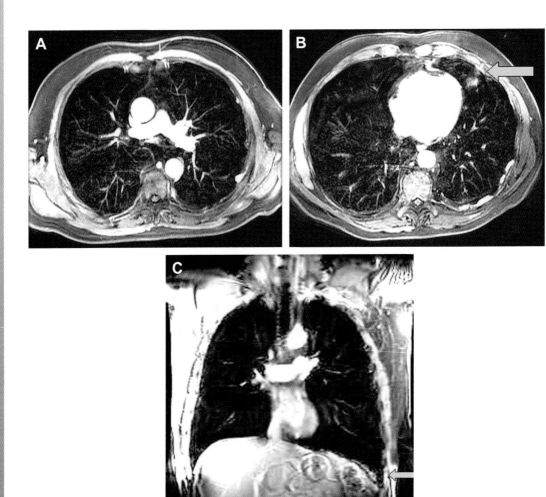

Fig. 13. MR imaging of epithelial mesothelioma. (*A* and *B*) Axial and (*C*) contrast-enhanced LAVA images show enhancing circumferential pleural nodularity on the left and in the posterior costophrenic sulcus extending along the major fissure without evidence of diaphragmatic or chest wall invasion. Note the preserved smooth left diaphragm on the coronal image.

MR imaging is usually performed in problematic cases and for surgical planning. It allows for excellent soft tissue contrast, and multiplanar imaging helps in determining invasion of adjacent structures. MR imaging is superior to CT in determining direct intra-abdominal or diaphragmatic extension.[26] Contrast-enhanced T1-weighted sequences are best for depicting pleural abnormalities. Contrast-enhanced, 3D gradient echo images may be performed on patients who have malignant pleural disease before intervention and following intervention to assess treatment response, and are especially useful following radiofrequency ablation and chemotherapy. CT has a limited role in these patients because of the generally relatively poor contrast enhancement of pleural malignancy (**Figs. 10 and 11**).

PET is a useful noninvasive functional imaging modality for the diagnosis and staging of malignant pleural disease. Several studies have examined the role of PET in distinguishing malignant from benign pleural thickening, with sensitivities greater than 96% and a negative predictive value of less than 92% for differentiating between benign and malignant causes of pleural thickening.[27,28] False-positive scans after infectious and uremic pleuritis and pleurodesis can occur, however, and false-negative scans can be seen with solitary fibrous tumor of the pleura and low-grade lymphoma.[28]

Malignant Pleural Mesothelioma

Malignant pleural mesothelioma (MPM) is a rare and aggressive malignant neoplasm that arises mainly from the pleura [29] and is often associated with asbestos exposure. Although MPM was once uncommon, its incidence is increasing worldwide as a result of widespread exposure to asbestos. Three distinct histologic subtypes of MPM are recognized: (1) the epithelial variant, (2) the sarcomatoid (sarcomatous) variant, and (3) a mixed (biphasic) variant (**Fig. 12**). In addition, desmoplastic MPM has been described as a rare subtype of sarcomatoid mesothelioma.[30]

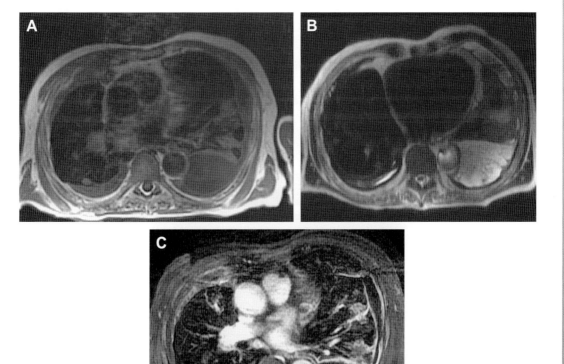

Fig. 14. Advanced-stage epithelial mesothelioma with bilateral lung nodules. (*A*) Axial T1-weighted image shows hypointense bilateral pleural effusion. (*B*) Axial T2-weighted image shows hyperintense bilateral pleural effusions. (*C*) Axial contrast-enhanced 3D gradient echo image shows nodular enhancement of the left pleura.

Staging

Preoperative staging of MPM is extremely difficult. The International Mesothelioma Interest Group proposed a tumor-node-metastasis (TNM) staging system for MPM (**Table 2**).[31]

Sugarbaker and colleagues[32] evaluated 183 patients who had MPM treated with extrapleural pneumonectomy followed by adjuvant chemotherapy and radiotherapy, and concluded that patients who had epithelial tumor histology, margin-negativ, extrapleural node-negative status had extended survival. The revised Brigham and Women's Hospital surgical staging system has been shown to successfully stratify survival of MPM patients; this staging system considers resectability, tumor histology, and nodal status with definition of four stages (**Table 3**).[32]

Malignant Pleural Mesothelioma and Imaging

CT has been widely used as the primary imaging modality for the diagnosis, staging, and monitoring of therapeutic response in MPM. The spectrum of findings ranges from unilateral pleural effusion, circumferential nodular pleural thickening, and invasion of adjacent structures. Biphasic mesothelioma and sarcomatoid subtypes have more aggressive behavior, and can present with distant and osseous metastases in early stages of the disease. Pleural thickening or effusions are the most common CT findings in patients who have MPM.[33] In most patients who have MPM, pleural thickening presents as circumferential (rindlike) pleural involvement, which is frequently nodular.[34]

CT tends to underestimate early chest wall invasion and peritoneal involvement, and has well-known limitations for the evaluation of lymph node metastases. Blood flow, blood volume, and capillary permeability can be assessed by perfusion CT.[35] Perfusion CT can be performed using sequential acquisitions during contrast administration before and after treatment, thereby providing information regarding tumor or tissue

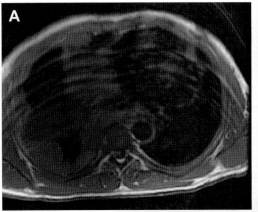
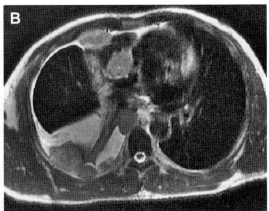
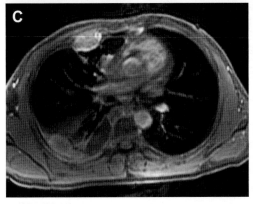

Fig. 15. Biphasic mesothelioma, with focal sarcomatoid component along the anterior aspect. (*A*) Axial T1-weighted image shows circumferential pleural nodularity with a focal anterior solid component with possible chest wall invasion. (*B*) Axial T2-weighted image shows the pleural masses are hypointense in comparison to the pleural fluid, which is hyperintense. (*C*) Axial contrast-enhanced 3D gradient echo image shows that the masses and the pleural thickening and nodularity enhance.

microvascularity, which can be used to assess treatment response. Although perfusion CT is widely available and the concept is simple, the high radiation exposure and side effects related to iodinated contrast material limit its use.[36]

Because of its excellent contrast resolution, MR imaging is superior to CT in the differentiation of malignant from benign pleural disease and the assessment of chest wall and diaphragmatic involvement in patients who have MPM.[37] In addition, perfusion MR imaging is promising technique for evaluating angiogenesis in MPM.[36]

Compared with adjacent chest wall musculature, MPM has intermediate or slightly higher signal intensity on T1-weighted images, and moderately high signal intensity on T2-weighted images.[24,38,39] MPM signal is enhanced with the use of gadolinium-based contrast material (Gd-CM).[24,38,39] MR imaging is useful to confirm and characterize CT findings, particularly diffuse pleural thickening, pleural effusion, and involvement of adjacent structures. Pleural effusion is readily identified by very high signal intensity on T2-weighted images (**Fig. 13**).[37]

Using morphologic features in combination with signal intensity information, the sensitivity and specificity of MR imaging for the detection of pleural malignancy and staging of pleural malignancy improves further.[26] In addition, contrast-enhanced T1-weighted fat-suppressed sequences are the most sensitive sequences for detecting enhancement of the interlobar fissures and for the detection of tumor invasion of adjacent structures (**Fig. 14**).[37]

The excellent contrast resolution of MR imaging can improve the evaluation of tumor invasion, especially extension of tumor into the chest wall or diaphragm, resulting in better prediction of overall resectability when compared with CT.[37] MR imaging can reliably differentiate involvement of both diaphragmatic surfaces, and is the modality of choice in determining secondary involvement of

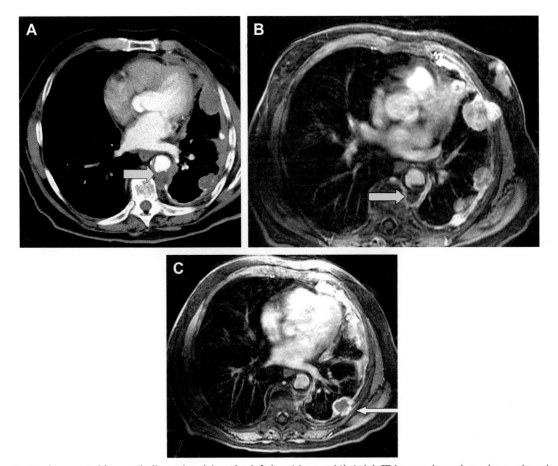

Fig. 16. Sarcomatoid mesothelioma involving the left hemithorax. (*A*) Axial CT image shows hypodense pleural thickening encasing the left lung, inseparable from the descending thoracic aorta. Aortic pseudoaneurysm (*arrow*) is visible. (*B*) and (*C*) Axial 3D gradient echo postcontrast images show possible invasion of the aorta with a pseudoaneurysm (*blue arrow*) and pathologic rib fracture and chest wall metastases (*white arrow*).

the chest by peritoneal mesothelioma by way of direct diaphragmatic spread (**Fig. 15**). Patz and colleagues[26] compared the value of CT versus MR for predicting MPM resectability. The sensitivity was high for both CT and MR imaging for evaluating the resectability of MPM along the diaphragm and the chest wall (sensitivity = 94% and 93% for MPM at the diaphragm and chest wall, respectively, for CT, and 100% and 100% for MR imaging).[26] CT and MR imaging provided similar information in most cases. In difficult cases, however, important complementary anatomic information was derived only from MR imaging. Heelan and colleagues[37] found MR imaging superior to CT in revealing invasion of the diaphragm (55% accuracy for CT versus 82% for MR imaging) and in showing endothoracic fascia or solitary resectable foci of chest wall invasion (46% accuracy for CT versus 69% for MR imaging).

MPM can invade visceral and parietal pleura and frequently extends to involve adjacent structures, such as the chest wall, mediastinum, and diaphragm. Parallel MR imaging allows for a quantitative assessment of tumor mobility and local lung motion.[40] Lymph node spread or metastases to distant organs, such as the lungs, liver, kidneys, and adrenal glands, can occur. It has been shown that the overall survival in MPM is related to the extent of the primary tumor (see **Fig. 15**; **Figs. 16 and 17**).[37]

Conventional therapies, such as surgery, radiotherapy, and chemotherapy, do not necessarily improve the overall survival.[37] Advances in the understanding of molecular biologic features of MPM have shown that angiogenesis is directly associated with the prognosis in MPM. Zucali and Giaccone[38] recently published a review on management of MPM with antiangiogenesis agents.

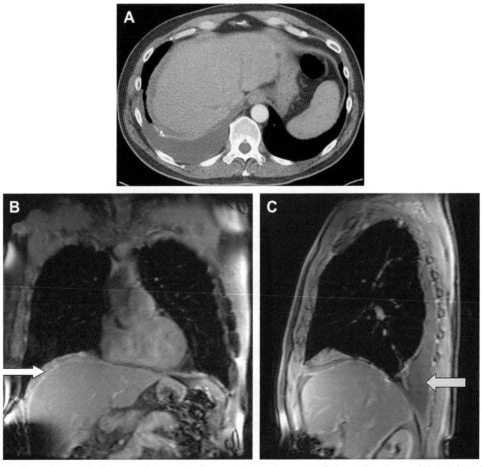

Fig. 17. Peritoneal mesothelioma with transdiaphragmatic involvement of the right pleura. (*A*) Axial CT image shows right pleural effusion and perihepatic ascites. Coronal (*B*) and sagittal MR (*C*) contrast-enhanced LAVA images show pleural enhancement (*blue arrow* in *C*) and pleural effusion, with subtle enhancement involving both surfaces of the diaphragm and peritoneum (*white arrow*) and ascites.

Imaging may play an important role in identifying the candidates for antiangiogenesis therapy and in documenting early response. Perfusion MR imaging using Gd-CM can be used to assess perfusion and tumor vascularity in patients who have MPM.[1,36,41–43] Currently, perfusion MR imaging is being used in clinical trials to evaluate response to antiangiogenic therapy.[35,36,44] After the administration of Gd-CM, sequential images with a temporal resolution of 1 second are acquired through the tumor tissue, and the pharmacokinetic analysis can provide information about tumor microvascularity.[36,41–43]

Gd-CM diffuses passively from the blood vessel into the extracellular space, and diffuses back to the vascular space without binding.[35] A two-compartment pharmacokinetic model can thus be used to calculate amplitude (amp), redistribution rate constant (kep), and elimination rate constant (kel).[36,41] Dynamic contrast-enhanced MR imaging can be used to map the heterogeneity of microcirculation in MPM; kep and kel can help predict therapeutic response and stratify survival.[36] Giesel and colleagues[36] found that patients who had MPM who did not respond to chemotherapy had higher kep value (3.6 minutes) than clinical responders (2.6 minutes), which was correlated to shorter survival (460 days versus 780 days), thereby implying that a high pretherapeutic kep value correlated with a poor overall response to chemotherapy. Perfusion MR imaging can be an invaluable tool to select patients for chemotherapeutic trials; however, this concept requires evaluation in a larger population. In addition, direct comparison between perfusion MR imaging parameters and angiogenesis factors, such as VEGF expression, is necessary. Furthermore, the ability of perfusion MR imaging to monitor the therapeutic effect of combination chemotherapy and antiangiogenesis drugs remains to be assessed.

The advantages of integrated PET/CT imaging for staging and assessing resectability of MPM have recently been reported by Erasmus and colleagues.[45] These authors concluded that PET/CT increased the accuracy of overall staging of patients who had MPM and improved the selection of patients for extrapleural pneumonectomy. PET/CT was superior to other imaging modalities because it detected more extensive disease involvement and identified occult distant metastases not suspected after conventional imaging. The main limitation of PET is its limited anatomic landmarks, especially in the setting of MPM.[44,46–48] It still remains to be shown if the use of PET/CT and fusion imaging could improve the assessment of local invasion into the chest wall, pericardium,

and diaphragm during the initial staging of patients who have MPM. PET-CT currently serves as an adjunct to MR imaging for the selection of a biopsy site.

SUMMARY

CT plays a primary role in the diagnosis, staging, and posttreatment management of pleural diseases and malignancies.

MR imaging and PET offer complementary information that balances some of the limitations observed with CT. An understanding of the potential MR imaging options enables formulation of and more efficient application of MR imaging strategies to the study of benign and malignant pleural disease.

When properly performed, MR imaging greatly enhances surgical planning for patients who have MPM, enhancing patient survival.

Newer technological developments in hardware and techniques, such as 3D MR imaging and parallel imaging, are useful for assessing lung perfusion and tumor mobility and invasion of adjacent structures.

REFERENCES

1. Leung A, Muller NL, Miller RR. CT in differential diagnosis of diffuse pleural disease. AJR Am J Roentgenol 1990;154(3):487–92.

2. McLoud TC. CT and MR in pleural disease. Clin Chest Med 1998;19(2):261–76.

3. Wilson AG. Pleura and pleural disorders. In: Armstrong P, Wilson AG, Dee P, et al. editors. Imaging of diseases of the chest. London: Mosby; 1995. p. 641–716.

4. Maskell NA, Butlan RJ. BTS guidelines for the investigation a unilateral pleural effusion in adults. Thorax 2003;58(Suppl 2):ii8–17.

5. Davis SD, Henschke CI, Yankelevitz DF, et al. MR imaging of pleural effusions. J Comput Assist Tomogr 1990;14(2):192–8.

6. Baysal T, Bulut T, Gokimak M, et al. Diffusion weighted MR imaging of pleural fluid; differentiation of transudative vs exudative pleural effusions. Eur Radiol 2004;14(5):890–6.

7. Qureshi NR, Geeson FV. Imaging of pleural disease. Clin Chest Med 2006;27(2):193–213.

8. Hahn PF, Stark DD, Vici LG, et al. Duodenal hematoma: the ring sign in MR imaging. Radiology 1986;159(2):379–82.

9. McLoud TC, Flower CD. Imaging the pleura: sonography, CT and MR imaging. AJR Am J Roentgenol 1991;156:1145–53.

10. Rockoff SD, Kagan E, Schwartz A, et al. Visceral pleural thickening in asbestos exposure: the occurrence and implications of thickened interlobar fissures. J Thorac Imaging 1987;2(4):58–66.

11. Proto AV. Conventional chest radiographs: anatomic understanding of newer observations. Radiology 1992;183:593–603.

12. Weber MA, Bock M, Plathow C, et al. Asbestos-related pleural disease: value of dedicated magnetic resonance imaging techniques. Invest Radiol 2004;39(9):554–64.

13. Theros EG, Feigin DS. Pleural tumors and pulmonary tumors: differential diagnosis. Semin Roentgenol 1977;12:239–47.

14. Rosado-de-Christenson ML, Abbott GF, McAdams HP, et al. Localized fibrous tumor of the pleura. Archives of the AFIP. Radiographics 2003; 23:759–83.

15. Tateishi U, Nishihara H, Morikawa T, et al. Solitary fibrous tumor of the pleura: MR appearance and enhancement pattern. J Comput Assist Tomogr 2002;26(2):174–9.

16. Williford ME, Hidalgo H, Putman CE, et al. Computed tomography of pleural disease. AJR Am J Roentgenol 1983;140(5):909–14.

17. Davies C, Gleeson FV. Diagnostic radiology. In: Light RW, Lee YC, editors. Textbook of pleural diseases. London: Arnold; 2003. p. 210–37.

18. Sung MS, Kang HS, Suh JS, et al. Myxoid liposarcoma appearance at MR imaging with histologic correlation. Radiographics 2000;20(4):1007–19.

19. Lynch DA, Gamsu G, Ray CS, et al. Asbestos related focal lung masses; manifestations on conventional and high resolution CT scans. Radiology 1988;169:603–7.

20. Copley SJ, Wells AJ, Rueben MB, et al. Functional consequences of pleural disease evaluated with chest radiography and CT. Radiology 2001;220(1): 237–43.

21. McHugh K, Blaquiere RM. CT features of round atelectasis. AJR Am J Roentgenol 1989;153:257–60.

22. Henschke CI, Yankelevitz DF, Davis SD. Pleural diseases: multimodality imaging and clinical management. Curr Probl Diagn Radiol 1991;20:155–81.

23. Shuman LS, Libshitz HI. Solid pleural manifestations of lymphoma. AJR Am J Roentgenol 1984;142: 269–73.

24. Hierholzer J, Lou L, Bittner RC, et al. MRI and CT in the differential diagnosis of malignant from benign pleural disease. Clin Med J (Engl) 2001; 114:645–9.

25. Falaschi F, Battola L, Zampa V, et al. Comparison of computerized tomography and magnetic resonance in the assessment of benign and malignant pleural diseases. Radiol Med (Torino) 1996;92:713–8.

26. Patz EF, Shaffer K, Piwnica-Worms DR, et al. Malignant pleural mesothelioma: value of CT and MR imaging in predicting resectability. AJR Am J Roentgenol 1992;159(5):961–6.

27. Kramer H, Pieteman RM, Slebos DJ, et al. PET for the evaluation of pleural thickening observed on CT. J Nucl Med 2004;45:995–8.

28. Duysinx B, Nguyen D, Louis R, et al. Evaluation of pleural disease with 18-flourodeoxyglucose positron emission tomography imaging. Chest 2004;125: 489–93.

29. Yamamuro M, Gerbaudo VH, Gill RR, et al. Morphologic and functional imaging of malignant pleural mesothelioma. Eur J Radiol 2007;64(3):356–66 [Epub Oct 22, 2007].

30. Corson JM. Pathology of mesothelioma. Thorac Surg Clin 2004;14(4):447–60.

31. Rusch VW. A proposed new international TNM staging system for malignant pleural mesothelioma. From the International Mesothelioma Interest Group. Chest 1995;108(4):1122–8.

32. Sugarbaker DJ, Flores RM, Jaklitsch MT, et al. Resection margins, extrapleural nodal status, and cell type determine postoperative long-term survival in trimodality therapy of malignant pleural mesothelioma: results in 183 patients. J Thorac Cardiovasc Surg 1999;117(1):54–63.

33. Kawashima A, Libshitz HI. Malignant pleural mesothelioma: CT manifestations in 50 cases. AJR Am J Roentgenol 1990;155(5):965–9.

34. Metintas M, Ucgun I, Elbek O, et al. Computed tomography features in malignant pleural mesothelioma and other commonly seen pleural diseases. Eur J Radiol 2002;41(1):1–9.

35. Drevs J, Schneider V. The use of vascular biomarkers and imaging studies in the early clinical development of anti-tumor agents targeting angiogenesis. J Intern Med 2006;260(6):517–29.

36. Giesel FL, Bischoff H, von Tengg-Kobligk H, et al. Dynamic contrast-enhanced MRI of malignant pleural mesothelioma: a feasibility study of noninvasive assessment, therapeutic follow-up, and possible predictor of improved outcome. Chest 2006;129(6): 1570–6.

37. Heelan RT, Rusch VW, Begg CB, et al. Staging of malignant pleural mesothelioma: comparison of CT and MR imaging. AJR Am J Roentgenol 1999; 172(4):1039–47.

38. Zucali PA, Giaccone G. Biology and management of malignant pleural mesothelioma. Eur J Cancer 2006; 42(16):2706–14.

39. Wang ZJ, Reddy GP, Gotway MB, et al. Malignant pleural mesothelioma: evaluation with CT, MR imaging, and PET. Radiographics 2004;24(1): 105–19.

40. Plathow C, Klopp M, Fink C, et al. Quantitative analysis of lung and tumour mobility: comparison of two time-resolved MRI sequences. Br J Radiol 2005;78: 836–40.

41. Brix G, Semmler W, Port R, et al. Pharmacokinetic parameters in CNS Gd-DTPA enhanced MR imaging. J Comput Assist Tomogr 1991;15(4):621–8.

42. Hatabu H, Gaa J, Kim D, et al. Pulmonary perfusion: quantitative assessment with dynamic contrast-enhanced MRI using ultra-short TE and invasion recovery turbo FLASH. Magn Reson Med 1996;36:503–8.

43. Ohno Y, Hatabu H, Takenaka D, et al. Solitary pulmonary nodules; potential role of dynamic MR imaging in management—initial experience. Radiology 2002; 224:503–11.

44. Bénard F, Sterman D, Smith RJ, et al. Metabolic imaging of malignant pleural mesothelioma with fluorodeoxyglucose positron emission tomography. Chest 1998;114(3):713–22.

45. Erasmus JJ, Truong MT, Smythe WR, et al. Integrated computed tomography-positron emission tomography in patients with potentially resectable malignant pleural mesothelioma: staging implications. J Thorac Cardiovasc Surg 2005;129(6): 1364–70.

46. Gerbaudo VH, Sugarbaker DJ, Britz-Cunningham S, et al. Assessment of malignant pleural mesothelioma with ^{18}F-FDG dual-head gamma-camera coincidence imaging: comparison with histopathology. J Nucl Med 2002;43:1144–9.

47. Gerbaudo VH, Britz-Cunningham S, Sugarbaker DJ, et al. Metabolic significance of the pattern, intensity and kinetics of 18F-FDG uptake in malignant pleural mesothelioma. Thorax 2003;58(12): 1077–82.

48. Gerbaudo VH. 18F-FDG imaging of malignant pleural mesothelioma: scientiam impendere vero.... Nucl Med Commun 2003;24(6):609–14.

MR Imaging of the Thoracic Inlet

Ellen E. Parker, MD*, Christine M. Glastonbury, MBBS

KEYWORDS

- Thoracic inlet • MR imaging

The thoracic inlet serves as the central connecting pathway between the head and upper neck and the chest. It is the sole conduit of all the vital organ systems passing from the neck to the chest or from the chest to the neck: the gastrointestinal and respiratory tracts, the peripheral nervous system, major arm and neck vascular structures, and central body lymphatics. The literature is confusing regarding the terminology and true definition of this area. Many different terms are used as synonyms for the thoracic inlet, such as thoracic outlet, root of the neck, cervical inlet, cervical outlet, or superior thoracic aperture; however, they will not be used here. This article first covers the pertinent normal anatomic boundaries, landmarks, and traversing structures of the thoracic inlet, with discussion also of the infrahyoid neck and superior thorax. The authors also mention selected examples of pathologic conditions affecting this area, illustrating key imaging features to help evaluate these lesions. Although the thyroid and parathyroid glands are typically located above the thoracic inlet proper, their proximity to, and not infrequent extension into, the thoracic inlet warrant their inclusion in this discussion.

ANATOMIC BOUNDARIES AND DEFINITIONS

The thoracic inlet is best described as a thin axial plane of tissue best defined by its osseous boundaries: the body of the first thoracic vertebra posteriorly and superiorly, the first pair of ribs and their costal cartilages bilaterally, and the superior border of the manubrium anteriorly and inferiorly.[1] The inlet slopes anteroinferiorly, paralleling the obliquity of the first pair of ribs, so that the lung apices are located at the posterior aspect of the inlet, whereas the major traversing structures are located more anteriorly. Such traversing structures include the esophagus; the trachea; lymphatic structures, such as the thoracic duct; vascular structures, including the major aortic arch branches; and paired neural structures, including the sympathetic chains and brachial plexuses. The superior border of the manubrium is usually located at the level of T2–3; therefore, on true axial imaging, the thoracic inlet spans multiple slices from the T1 through T3 levels. On true axial imaging through the level of T1, the manubrium and clavicles are usually not visible. Images through the level of T3 must be reviewed to cover the thoracic inlet.

FASCIAL SPACES OF THE INFRAHYOID NECK AND THORACIC INLET

The spaces of the infrahyoid neck are anatomically demarcated by layers of the deep cervical fascia.[2] Many of these spaces traverse the thoracic inlet into the mediastinum. **Figs. 1A and 1B** are axial diagrams of the lower neck (at the level of C7) and the thoracic inlet (at the level of T1). The boundaries and contents of spaces associated with the thoracic inlet are also summarized in **Table 1**. At the level of the thoracic inlet, the visceral space is divided into the pretracheal space anteriorly and the retrovisceral space posteriorly. The "pretracheal" or "paratracheal" space extends from the level of the hyoid into the superior mediastinum and terminates just posterior to the manubrium. It contains the larynx, trachea, thyroid gland, parathyroid glands, recurrent laryngeal nerve, sympathetic trunk, level VI lymph nodes, thyroid arteries, and fat.

Division of Neuroradiology, University of California, San Francisco, 505 Parnassus Avenue, L 358, San Francisco, CA 94143-0628, USA

* Corresponding author.

E-mail address: ellen.parker@radiology.ucsf.edu (E.E. Parker).

Magn Reson Imaging Clin N Am 16 (2008) 341–353

doi:10.1016/j.mric.2008.02.018

1064-9689/08/$ – see front matter

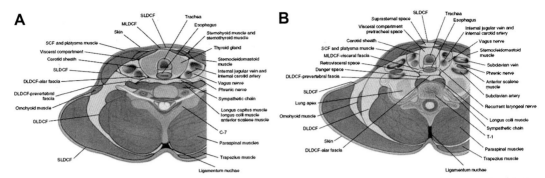

Fig. 1. (*A*) Axial diagram through the level of C7, just above the level of the thoracic inlet, illustrates the relationships of the thyroid, trachea, and esophagus. Note the common visceral space at this anatomic level (ie, the pretracheal and retrovisceral spaces freely communicate). (*B*) Axial diagram through the level of T1, at the level of the thoracic inlet. Because of the anterior-inferior slope of the thoracic inlet, the clavicles and manubrium are absent on this true axial section. The superior margin of the manubrium would be visible on a section through the level of T2–3. DLDCF, deep layer deep cervical fascia; MLDCF, middle layer deep cervical fascia; SCF, superficial cervical fascia; SLDCF, superficial layer deep cervical fascia. (*From* Som PM, Curtin HD. Head and neck imaging. 4th edition. St Louis (MO): Mosby; 2003. p. 1822; with permission.)

The retrovisceral space extends from the skull base into the middle mediastinum (**Fig. 2**). At the level of the thoracic inlet, the retrovisceral space contains the esophagus and fat. Above the level of the inferior thyroid artery, the pretracheal and retrovisceral components of the visceral space communicate freely. Caudal to the inferior thyroid artery, the pretracheal and retrovisceral compartments are separated by a layer of deep cervical fascia. Pathologic processes involving the retrovisceral space (eg, retropharyngeal abscess) can thus involve the thyroid secondarily (see **Fig. 2A**). Conversely, because the extension of the pretracheal space into the superior mediastinum terminates at the level of the manubrium, primary space-occupying lesions of the pretracheal space (such as multinodular goiters or large thyroid carcinomas) tend to spread into the middle mediastinum along the retrovisceral space (**Fig. 3A**).

Two other spaces with a parallel craniocaudal course are located posterior to the retrovisceral space. The more ventral is the danger space, which runs from the skull base into the posterior mediastinum and terminates just superior to the diaphragms. The danger space is a potential space with no intrinsic contents and no communication with adjacent spaces; however, pathologic conditions such as infection may gain access to the danger space by breaching the fascia. Once within the danger space, no barrier exists to infection spreading superiorly to the skull base or inferiorly into the posterior mediastinum. Dorsal to the danger space is the prevertebral space, which runs from the skull base to the coccyx. The prevertebral space contains the anterior longitudinal ligament, cervical vertebrae and discs, longus colli and longus capitis muscles, phrenic nerves, and fat.

The carotid spaces, located lateral to the visceral space, contain the common carotid arteries, internal jugular veins, and vagus nerves. The paravertebral spaces, lateral to the carotid spaces, contain roots of the brachial plexus, vertebral arteries and veins, fat, and several neck muscles: the scalenes, the levator scapulae, and splenius capitis and cervicis.

The posterior cervical spaces, which correspond to the anatomic posterior triangles, are posterolateral to the paravertebral spaces. The posterior cervical spaces contain fat, level V lymph nodes, spinal accessory nerve, brachial plexus (trunks, divisions, and cords), dorsal scapular and long thoracic nerves, and cutaneous nerves of the cervical plexus.

STRUCTURES TRAVERSING THE THORACIC INLET

Multiple structures traverse the thoracic inlet within these fascially defined spaces and are best described by organ system.

Respiratory and Digestive Tracts: Trachea and Esophagus

The respiratory and digestive tracts traverse the thoracic inlet within the visceral space. The trachea is anterior to the esophagus. Posteriorly, the esophagus is bounded by the retrovisceral space, with the danger space dorsal to this. At the level of the thoracic inlet, the esophagus is usually located to the left of midline, and the anterior cervical esophageal wall is closely associated

Table 1
Spaces of the infrahyoid neck at its junction with the thoracic inlet

Space	Relationships	Normal Contents	Important Concepts
Carotid space	Lateral to visceral space	Carotid artery, internal jugular vein, vagus (cranial nerve 10)	The patency of arteries and veins should always be confirmed on imaging studies.
Pretracheal space (anterior aspect of visceral space)	Medial to carotid spaces	Larynx, trachea, thyroid gland, parathyroid glands, level VI lymph nodes, fat, recurrent laryngeal nerve, sympathetic trunk.	The bulk of lower neck pathology pertains to this space. Although the nerves cannot be seen, their locations can be inferred using known anatomic landmarks.
Retrovisceral space (posterior aspect of visceral space)	Between pretracheal space (anterior) and danger space (posterior)	Esophagus, fat	This space is contiguous with retropharyngeal space superiorly. It terminates inferiorly between levels of C6–7 and T4.
Danger space	Between retrovisceral space (anterior) and prevertebral space (posterior)	None (the danger space is a potential space)	Pathologic conditions enter this space by way of direct extension through fascia and can then extend up to skull base or down to posterior mediastinum.
Prevertebral space	Posterior to danger space	Anterior longitudinal ligament, cervical vertebrae and discs, longus colli and longus capitis muscles, phrenic nerve, fat	This space is the site of anterior extension of diskitis (prevertebral abscess) or vertebral body metastases. It is not otherwise a common site of neck pathology.
Paravertebral space	Lateral to carotid spaces	Brachial plexus roots, vertebral artery, vertebral veins, fat, and muscles: scalenes, levator scapulae, splenius capitis, and splenius cervicis	Little primary or secondary pathology is seen in this space. Muscle groups are sometimes mistaken for lymph nodes.
Posterior cervical space	Posterolateral to paravertebral space	Level V lymph nodes, fat and nerves: CN11; brachial plexus trunks, divisions, and cords; dorsal scapular and long thoracic nerves; cutaneous nerves of cervical plexus	This space clinically corresponds to posterior triangle. It is a common site for adenopathy in the neck, especially with lymphoma and scalp tumors.

with the posterior membranous tracheal wall. On CT or MR imaging, these walls are often impossible to distinguish. Visualization of fat planes lateral to the lower cervical esophagus on MR imaging is more reliable.[3] Any obscuration of periesophageal fat planes in the setting of documented or suspected malignancy must be viewed with suspicion. The recurrent laryngeal nerves (RLNs) ascend from the thoracic inlet within the tracheoesophageal grooves on their course to the larynx.

The pathologic processes that commonly involve the trachea and esophagus include infectious/inflammatory, posttraumatic (including iatrogenic), and neoplastic processes. Primary cases

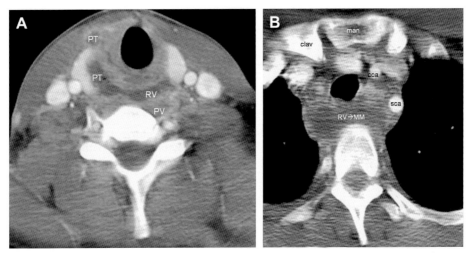

Fig. 2. A 17-year-old man who has sore throat and fever. (*A*) Axial contrast-enhanced CT at the level of the thyroid. Low-density infection is demonstrated in the retrovisceral space (RV), with direct extension into the pretracheal space (PT) medial and anterior to the right thyroid lobe, and into the prevertebral space (PV). (*B*) Axial contrast-enhanced CT at the level of the inferior thoracic inlet. Low-density infection is demonstrated at the level of the claviculomanubrial junction, which demarcates the inferior margin of the thoracic inlet and the site of transition of the retrovisceral space into the middle mediastinum (RV→MM). cca, common carotid artery; clav, clavicle; man, manubrium; RV→MM, site of transition of retrovisceral space into middle mediastinum; sca, subclavian artery.

of tracheal malignancy are rare, with the most common being squamous cell carcinoma, followed by adenoid cystic carcinoma.[4] It is more common for the trachea to be secondarily involved by malignancy originating from an adjacent structure such as the thyroid, the esophagus, or lung (**Fig. 3**B). In addition to malignancy, benign processes such as multinodular goiter can compress the trachea, resulting in significant airway compromise. The most common primary tumors

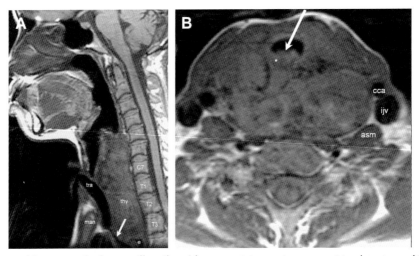

Fig. 3. A 59-year-old woman who has papillary thyroid cancer, status post–emergent tracheostomy. (*A*) Sagittal T1 noncontrast image. Note that the thyroid mass (thy) extends superior and inferior to the expected level of the thyroid bed within the retrovisceral space. The arrow denotes significant substernal narrowing of the airway due to the mass. Note that the superior border of the manubrium (man) is at the level of T2–3. e, air-filled esophageal lumen at inferior aspect of mass; tra, tracheostomy. (*B*) Axial T1 noncontrast image, just above the level of the tracheostomy. Arrow indicates endoluminal component of the thyroid mass invading the trachea. Asterisk (*) indicates subtle loss of fat plane surrounding the trachea. asm, anterior scalene muscle; cca, common carotid artery; ijv, internal jugular vein.

of the cervicothoracic portion of the esophagus are cell carcinoma, followed by adenocarcinoma.

Acquired tracheoesophageal fistula may be iatrogenic or may occur with primary malignancy in either the esophagus or the trachea.[5] Instrumentation, indwelling foreign bodies including endotracheal and feeding tubes, and irradiation can all result in an acquired fistulous communication between the esophagus and trachea (**Fig. 4**). The much rarer and often lethal tracheoinnominate (artery) fistula can also occur as a complication of endotracheal intubation or tracheostomy.[6] Although the role of CT and MR imaging is limited in the acute diagnosis and management of these fistulae, careful attention to the relationship of indwelling tubes and catheters to the walls of the trachea and esophagus and adjacent structures on "routine" studies may allow the radiologist to alert the referring physician to impending danger.

Lymphatic Channels and Nodal Groups

The lymphatic channels draining the body converge and drain into the venous system at the level of the thoracic inlet within the paravertebral space.[7] Although great variability in lymphatic anatomy exists, typically, the right lymphatic duct receives lymphatic drainage from the right jugular trunk (draining the right head and neck), the right subclavian trunk (draining the right upper extremity), and the right bronchomediastinal trunk (draining the right chest, right lung, right heart, and convex portion of the liver). The right lymphatic duct then empties into the lateral aspect of the confluence of the right subclavian and internal jugular veins. The thoracic duct receives all of the lymphatic drainage from the body that is not directed to the right lymphatic duct, but again, is subject to some variability. Typically the thoracic duct receives contributions from the left jugular trunk, the left subclavian trunk, and the left bronchomediastinal trunk before emptying into the lateral aspect of the confluence of the left subclavian and left internal jugular veins. The normal thoracic duct may be identified in 55% of cases on routine CT of the neck; the normal right lymphatic duct is identified less reliably.[8] On MR imaging, the thoracic duct is seen as a T2 hyperintense linear structure coursing posterior to the carotid sheath in the lower neck (**Fig. 5**). The only normal structure between the left anterior scalene muscle and the left jugular vein is the thoracic duct. The

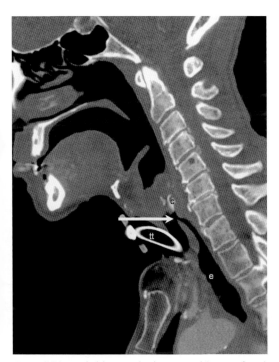

Fig. 4. A 61-year-old man who has a past history of neck irradiation and no evidence of recurrent head and neck cancer by endoscopy or imaging. Sagittal reformation of contrast-enhanced multidetector CT of the neck. Arrow indicates subcricoid fistula between the trachea and esophagus, which is presumably radiation induced in the absence of recurrent tumor. c, cricoid; e, esophagus; tt, tracheostomy tube.

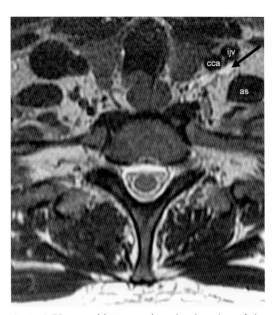

Fig. 5. A 59-year-old man undergoing imaging of the thoracic spine. Axial T2 image at the level of the T1 vertebral body demonstrates the normal thoracic duct (*arrow*) as a linear T2 hyperintense structure coursing posterior to the common carotid artery (cca) and internal jugular vein (ijv). The anterior scalene muscle (as) is posterior.

thoracic duct can be mistaken for a level IV lymph node if it appears distended (**Fig. 6**).

The level IV or "lower jugular chain" nodes are located within the carotid space inferior to the lower aspect of the cricoid cartilage and superior to the upper margin of the manubrium. They lie anteromedial or deep to the sternocleidomastoid muscle. The level V or "posterior triangle" nodes are located within the paravertebral space, posterolateral to a line between the posterolateral margins of the sternocleidomastoid and anterior scalene muscles. When a portion of the clavicle is visible on the same axial image as a level V node, then that node is generally referred to as "supraclavicular."[2] Level VI or "visceral" nodes are located medial to the carotid arteries between the levels of the hyoid bone and the manubrium. Superior mediastinal nodes are sometimes designated as level VII, and are located between the carotid arteries below the manubrium and above the left innominate vein.

Isolated left supraclavicular lymphadenopathy is much more commonly metastatic from chest, abdominal, or pelvic malignancies or from lymphoma, rather than from a primary head and neck malignancy.[9] The association of a pathologic left supraclavicular node with abdominal or pelvic malignancy is known as a Virchow's node, after its description in 1848 in German, or as Troisier's sign, after its description in French in 1886.[10]

Vascular Structures

In most patients, the aortic arch has three branches: the brachiocephalic artery (innominate artery), which divides into the right subclavian and common carotid arteries; the left common carotid artery; and left subclavian artery. The right internal jugular vein joins with the right subclavian vein to form the short-segment right brachiocephalic (innominate) vein, which empties into the superior vena cava. The left internal jugular vein joins with the left subclavian vein to form the left brachiocephalic (innominate) vein, which courses anterior to the aortic arch before emptying into the superior vena cava. The carotid and jugular vessels are located within the carotid space. The subclavian and vertebral vessels are located within the paravertebral space.

The anterior scalene muscle is a useful landmark for identifying the subclavian vein, which lies anterior to the muscle, and the subclavian artery, which lies posterior to the muscle. The anterior scalene muscles are frequently mistaken for lower neck adenopathy, but their symmetry and muscle signal intensity or density should be guiding clues to their nature. The level IV lymph nodes lie immediately anterior to the anterior scalene muscle between the muscle and the jugular vein. On the left side, the only normal structure between the anterior scalene muscle and the jugular vein is the thoracic duct.

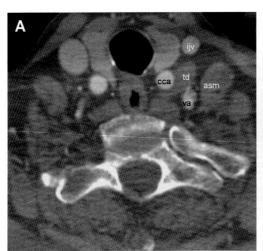 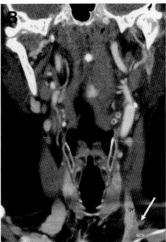

Fig. 6. A 70-year-old man who has a history of lymphoma undergoing surveillance imaging. (*A*) Axial contrast-enhanced multidetector CT through the level of T1 demonstrates an ovoid nonenhancing density lateral to the common carotid artery suspicious for a level 4 lymph node. Scrolling through axial images confirms that this structure is, in fact, the thoracic duct, which is often dilated just proximal to its termination at the venous confluence because of the presence of valves. (*B*) Coronal reformatted image confirms emptying of the nonenhancing thoracic duct into the confluence of the internal jugular and subclavian veins. The arrow indicates termination of the thoracic duct at the venous confluence. asm, anterior scalene muscle; cca, common carotid artery; ijv, internal jugular vein; scv, subclavian vein; td, thoracic duct; va, vertebral artery.

The aberrant right subclavian artery arises from the aortic arch distal to the left subclavian artery and courses posterior to the esophagus (**Fig. 7**A). Even if the origin of the right subclavian artery is not included in the imaging field of view, an aberrant right subclavian artery may be identified by examining the relationship of the right subclavian artery to a coronal plane defined by the posterior wall of the trachea (**Fig. 7**B). An artery lying completely posterior to this plane must be retroesophageal in origin; an artery transected by the plane or lying anterior to this plane originates in typical fashion from the brachiocephalic (innominate) artery.[11] Recognition of an aberrant right subclavian artery, with an incidence in the general population of 1% to 3%, is important for its association with a nonrecurrent course of the right RLN.[12–14]

Neural Structures

Knowledge of the typical locations of peripheral neural structures traversing the thoracic inlet allows the radiologist to predict involvement of these structures by pathologic processes. Elements of the brachial plexus may sometimes be identified on routine imaging and, with high-resolution dedicated imaging, the brachial plexus may be studied directly. The vagus nerves, RLNs, phrenic nerves, and sympathetic chains are rarely directly discernible, even on high-resolution imaging, although their location may be inferred by recognizing anatomic landmarks of their expected course. For example, the anterior margins of the proximal subclavian arteries mark the locations of the phrenic nerves as they pass through the thoracic inlet, and the inferior cervical ganglia/stellate ganglia are located at the posterior aspect of the origins of the vertebral arteries from the subclavian arteries (**Fig. 8**).

Vagus and Recurrent Laryngeal Nerves

The right and left vagus nerves exit the skull base through the jugular foramina and travel within their respective carotid sheaths between the carotid artery and internal jugular vein. At the level of the thoracic inlet, the vagus nerves are lateral to their respective carotid arteries and at the posteromedial aspect of the internal jugular vein. The superior laryngeal nerves arise from the vagi well above the level of the thoracic inlet and have a horizontal course from the vagus to the larynx. The inferior laryngeal nerves (ILNs), which are most commonly referred to as the RLNs, typically arise from the vagi at, or just below, the level of the thoracic inlet.

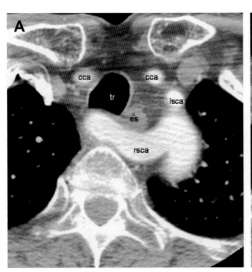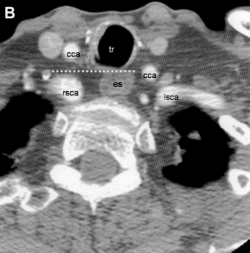

Fig. 7. An 81-year-old man who has a history of papillary thyroid carcinoma and surgically proved nonrecurrent right inferior laryngeal nerve. (*A*) Axial CT image at the level of the origin of the right subclavian artery distal to the origin of the left subclavian artery clearly shows its aberrant retroesophageal course. (*B*) Axial CT at the level of T1, above the level of *A*. Note that the rsca lies completely posterior to a coronal plane (*dotted lines*) defined by the posterior membranous wall of the trachea. A right subclavian artery lying completely posterior to this plane is retroesophageal in origin; an artery transected by the plane or lying anterior to this plane originates in typical fashion from the brachiocephalic (innominate) artery. The aberrant retroesophageal course of the right subclavian artery is associated with the nonrecurrent right inferior laryngeal nerve, which is more prone to injury during surgery. Note that the normal left subclavian artery lies posterior to this plane. cca, common carotid artery; es, esophagus; lsca, left subclavian artery; rsca, right subclavian artery; tr, trachea.

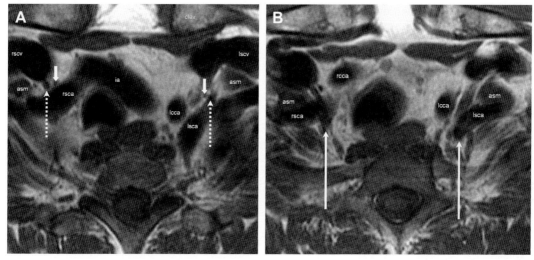

Fig. 8. A 44-year-old man who has a history of squamous cell carcinoma of the right nasal ala, status postsurgery and local irradiation, undergoing MR imaging for restaging. (*A*) Short block arrows indicate the locations of the phrenic nerves as they pass anterior to the subclavian arteries, just medial to the origins of the internal mammary arteries (*long dashed arrows*). (*B*) Long solid arrows indicate the locations of the stellate ganglia/inferior cervical ganglia, just posterior to the origins of the vertebral arteries. asm, anterior scalene muscle; clav, clavicle; ia, innominate (brachiocephalic) artery; lcca, left common carotid artery; lsca, left subclavian artery; lscv, left subclavian vein; rcca, right common carotid artery; rsca, right subclavian artery; rscv, right subclavian vein.

The RLNs then recur around vascular structures before ascending to the larynx within the pretracheal space.

The right RLN typically recurs under the right subclavian artery before ascending in the right tracheoesophageal groove to the larynx. However, in the approximately 1% to 3% of the population with an aberrant right subclavian artery, the right ILN has a nonrecurrent course and is called a nonrecurrent inferior laryngeal nerve (NRILN); its course arises from the right vagus at the level of the larynx and it courses in a transverse fashion to the larynx just below, and parallel to, the superior laryngeal nerve. An NRILN is more susceptible to injury during surgery than an RLN.[12] Identification and reporting of an aberrant right subclavian artery and its association with a right NRILN will aid surgeons in operative planning, reducing risk to the nerve.

The left RLN typically arises from the left vagus and courses inferomedially under the aortic arch before ascending in the left tracheoesophageal groove to the larynx. A nonrecurrent course of the left ILN is rare, reported to occur only in cases of right aortic arch with situs inversus and aberrant left subclavian artery.[15]

Phrenic Nerves

The paired phrenic nerves, which are typically the sole motor supply to the diaphragm, receive contributions from C3, C4, and C5. From its origin, each phrenic nerve courses in an oblique superolateral-to-inferomedial orientation along the superficial surface of the anterior scalene muscle. Each nerve then passes medial to the anterior scalene muscle and courses along the anterior surface of the subclavian artery (at the level of the origin of the internal mammary artery) as it passes through the thoracic inlet to travel inferiorly along the lateral mediastinal pleura.[16] The phrenic nerve is at risk for injury during cardiac bypass surgery using the internal mammary artery. It may also be compromised by tumors of the pulmonary apex. Reports of phrenic nerve dysfunction due to intrinsic nerve sheath tumor are exceedingly rare (**Fig. 9**).[17]

Sympathetic Chain

The paired sympathetic chains, a fundamental component of the autonomic nervous system, extend from the skull base through the sacrum. At the level of the thoracic inlet, the cervical sympathetic chains are located anterior to the prevertebral muscles, immediately posterior to the carotid sheath. Each inferior cervical ganglion, located at the level of C7, is found immediately posterior to the origin of the vertebral artery from the subclavian artery.[16] In 80% of the population, the first thoracic ganglion and inferior cervical ganglion are fused, yielding a "stellate ganglion" at the level of C7–T1. The lung apex is located

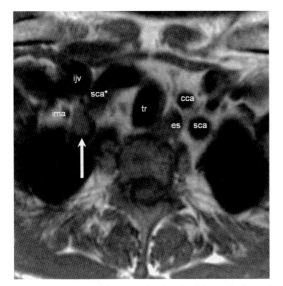

Fig. 9. A 44-year-old man who has incidentally found right hemidiaphragm paralysis and no history of malignancy. Axial T1 imaging reveals a 1.2-cm mass (*arrow*) at the anterior-superior surface of the right subclavian artery (sca) immediately adjacent to the origin of the right internal mammary artery (ima). This mass demonstrated postcontrast enhancement and is thought to represent a nerve sheath tumor arising from the right phrenic nerve. This site would be unusual for lymphadenopathy. cca, common carotid artery; es, esophagus; ijv, internal jugular vein; tr, trachea.

immediately inferior to this stellate ganglion. Percutaneous anesthetic blockade of the stellate ganglion may be beneficial in the diagnosis and treatment of pain syndromes of the head and neck and upper extremity related to sympathetic dysfunction.[18]

The cervical sympathetic chain at the level of the thoracic inlet is an important part of the oculosympathetic pathway. Lesions of this pathway may result in Horner syndrome, which is described as the classic triad of meiosis, ptosis, and anhidrosis. The meiosis and ptosis occur with lesions at any level; presence or absence of anhidrosis and certain diagnostic maneuvers (eg, use of pharmacologic eye drops) allows the clinician to determine the location of the lesion.[19] Congenital Horner syndrome is often associated with birth trauma and concomitant injury to the lower brachial plexus. An acquired Horner syndrome in an adult must be considered malignant until proven otherwise and is most commonly caused by squamous cell carcinoma of the lung apex (Pancoast's tumor) or lymphadenopathy in the lower neck. An acquired Horner syndrome in a child must raise the suspicion of neuroblastoma.

Brachial Plexus

The brachial plexus is a complex, interwoven web of nerves arising from the neural foramina of C5 through to T1 that provides motor and sensory innervation to the shoulder and arm. As the brachial plexus passes through the lower neck to the axilla, it is enveloped in a fascial sheath derived from the deep layer of deep cervical fascia. Traditionally the plexus is described in terms of five anatomic components: the roots, trunks, divisions, cords, and proximal branches (**Fig. 10**A). Clinically and surgically however, the plexus can be divided into three anatomic portions, based on its relationship to the clavicle (**Fig. 10**B). The clavicle obliquely crosses the path of the plexus, which accords division of the brachial plexus into the "supraclavicular" (roots and trunks), "retroclavicular" (divisions), and "infraclavicular" (cords and branches) portions. This simplified approach to brachial plexus anatomy is less unwieldy and promotes a more dedicated imaging study. With good clinical history, MR imaging can be tailored to the area of greatest concern, allowing a dedicated high-resolution examination.

The supraclavicular plexus consists of the exiting C5 through T1 nerve roots and the upper, middle, and lower trunks. The roots are derived from the ventral rami that arise after union of dorsal (sensory) and ventral (motor) roots of the spinal cord at the dorsal root ganglia. The corresponding dorsal rami from C5–T1 supply the posterior neck muscles and skin. Unusual variations in the plexus neural connections are the "prefixed" and "postfixed" plexus. The prefixed plexus has a major contribution from the C4 root with absent or reduced input from T1, whereas the postfixed plexus has a major contribution from the T2 root and minimal contribution from the C5 root.[20]

After exiting the neural foramina, the C5–C8 nerve roots have a downward and anterolateral converging course. The T1 root has the least direct path, because it initially curves superiorly and anteriorly over the lung apex from its more posteroinferior dorsal root ganglia. It is important to obtain more posterior coronal images to appreciate the full course of this root. In the absence of cervical ribs, the C8 and T1 roots are identified on the oblique sagittal images as coursing above and below the first rib, respectively. The five nerve roots converge between the anterior and middle scalene muscles in the interscalene triangle to form the three trunks of the brachial plexus: the upper, middle, and lower trunks. C5 and C6 unite to form the upper trunk, C8 and T1 form the lower trunk, and the C7 root remains independent as the middle trunk. The supraclavicular plexus lies

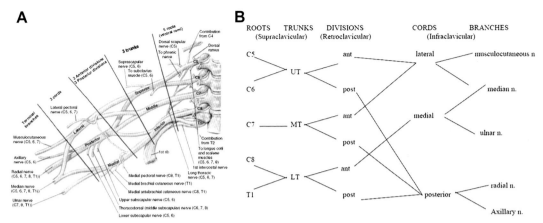

Fig. 10. The anterior and middle scalene muscles form the interscalene triangle in the sagittal plane with the first rib as its base. The roots (C5–T1) and trunks (upper, middle, and lower) of the supraclavicular plexus pass though the triangle adjacent to the subclavian artery. The subclavian vein and nodes pass anterior to the triangle. The anterior and posterior divisions (retroclavicular plexus) arise where the clavicle passes obliquely anterior to the plexus and first rib. The anterior cords supply the flexors of the arm, and the posterior cords supply the extensors. The axillary artery commences at the outer margin of the first rib, with the vein initially anterior and inferior to the artery. The cords are named by their position, with reference to the axillary artery (medial, lateral, and posterior). At the outer margin of pectoralis minor (at the level of the coracoid process), the branches arise from the cords (together, infraclavicular plexus). (*A*) Traditional anatomic diagram of the roots, trunks, cords, divisions, and branches of the brachial plexus. Note the unusual composition shown. The prefixed plexus has a large C4 contribution but lacks T1; the postfixed plexus lacks C5 but has T2 contribution. (*From* Som PM, Curtin HD. Head and neck imaging. 4th edition. St Louis (MO): Mosby; 2003. p. 2218; with permission.) (*B*) Simplified schematic diagram of the supraclavicular, retroclavicular, and infraclavicular components of the brachial plexus. ant, anterior; LT, lower trunk; MT, middle trunk; n, nerve; post, posterior; UT, upper trunk.

above and behind the subclavian artery, as it passes through the interscalene triangle.

The retroclavicular plexus is formed as each trunk branches into anterior and posterior divisions behind the clavicle. The lower trunk is usually the last to divide.[2] The posterior divisions of the trunks form the posterior cord, and supply the extensor muscles of the arm. The anterior divisions of the three trunks innervate the arm flexor muscles.

The infraclavicular plexus is composed of three cords and their peripheral nerve branches. The cords are the longest segment of the brachial plexus, extending from the level of the clavicle to the lateral margin of the pectoralis minor muscle. Lateral to the first rib, the subclavian artery becomes the axillary artery and the plexus cords are closely related to this vessel. The anterior divisions of the upper trunk and middle trunk converge to form the lateral cord, and the anterior division of the lower trunk becomes the medial cord. The posterior divisions of all three trunks form the posterior cord. The cords are named according to their relationship to the axillary artery in the anatomic plane; however, with cross-sectional imaging, this nomenclature becomes confusing. On sagittal images, the lateral cord lies superoanterior to the axillary artery, the posterior cord lies superoposterior, and the medial cord lies posterior

and sometimes slightly inferior to the artery (**Fig. 11**). Through the length of the infraclavicular plexus, the axillary vein lies anteroinferior to the artery, moving more superficially as the plexus courses deeper within axillary tissue.

An additional useful landmark in plexus imaging is the pectoralis minor muscle, which arises from the anterior aspect of the third to fifth ribs (and fascia over the intervening intercostal muscles), and inserts on the coracoid process. At the lateral border of this muscle, the plexus cords divide into peripheral terminal branches. Branches also arise from the brachial plexus more proximally, with four branches arising from the roots, two branches arising from the trunks, and seven smaller branches arising from the cords. Each cord, however, has two dominant branches, resulting in five terminal nerves of the brachial plexus, which may be demonstrated with high-resolution MR imaging. The posterior cord divides into the axillary nerve and radial nerve, the lateral cord produces the musculocutaneous nerve and the lateral root of the median nerve, and the medial cord has the medial root of the median nerve and the ulnar nerve. Because of the complex intertwining of nerves from the roots to these terminal branches, they have a contribution from several or all of the cervicothoracic brachial plexus roots. For

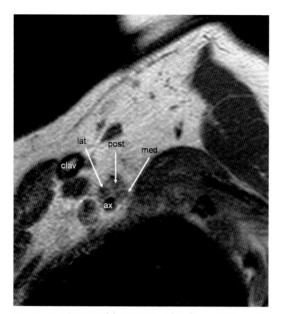

Fig. 11. A 43-year-old woman who has right upper extremity pain. Normal brachial plexus neurogram. Sagittal T1 image demonstrates the relationships of the infraclavicular cords to the axillary artery (ax). The lateral cord (lat) lies superoanterior, the posterior cord (post) lies superoposterior, and the medial cord (med) lies posterior and sometimes slightly inferior to the artery. clav, clavicle.

example, the radial nerve is derived from C5, C6, C7 and T1, the median nerve has supply from C6 through to T1, and the axillary nerve receives fibers from only C5 and C6.

The possible causes of brachial plexopathy are myriad. About one half of cases are posttraumatic and are most often caused by fractures of the cervical spine or clavicle, nerve root avulsion with or without an associated pseudomeningocele, soft-tissue edema, or hematoma.[2] Nontraumatic causes include primary neural tumors, such as meningiomas and schwannomas; metastatic disease primary tumors, including neuroblastoma and small round blue cell tumors (**Fig. 12**); Pancoast's tumor; postirradiation injury (**Fig. 13**); radiculopathy secondary to disk disease; and bony abnormalities, such as cervical ribs.

Endocrine Structures

The thyroid gland is located within the pretracheal compartment of the visceral space. The isthmus lies above the level of the thoracic inlet, at, or just below, the level of the cricoid cartilage. The right and left lobes of the thyroid lie on each side of the trachea, and although they typically terminate above the clavicle, they may extend substernally into the thoracic inlet proper, when enlarged.[21]

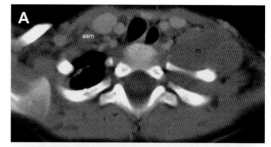

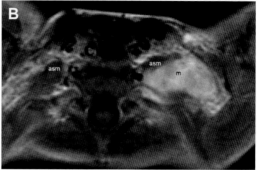

Fig. 12. A 2-year-old boy presenting with left neck and chest mass and a history of minor trauma. (A) Axial CT obtained as part of initial evaluation reveals a mass (m) involving the left lung apex and supraclavicular region extending toward the axilla. The right anterior scalene muscle (asm) is well defined; the left anterior scalene muscle is difficult to distinguish from the mass. (B) Subsequent MR imaging (axial T1 postcontrast with fat saturation) reveals that this enhancing mass (m) is located within the interscalene space, with anterior displacement and distortion of the left anterior scalene muscle. Compare with normal-appearing right anterior scalene muscle. Biopsy revealed small round blue cell tumor with involvement of the brachial plexus.

The thyroid gland may be affected by congenital anomalies, autoimmune diseases and thyroiditis, benign nodular enlargement (thyroid goiter), and benign and malignant neoplasms. Primary thyroid malignancies include papillary carcinoma, follicular carcinoma, Hurthle cell tumors, medullary carcinoma, anaplastic carcinoma, and primary lymphoma. The thyroid gland may also be involved secondarily by lymphoma or metastatic disease.

Primary imaging for most suspected thyroid disorders includes nuclear scintigraphy and ultrasound. MR imaging is most often used to address specific questions regarding nodular or neoplastic disease, such as the substernal extension of a multinodular goiter, or invasion of adjacent structures such as the trachea (see **Fig. 3**B), esophagus, and prevertebral musculature by thyroid malignancy.[22]

The parathyroid glands are also typically located in the pretracheal compartment. Most individuals have four glands, although the number ranges

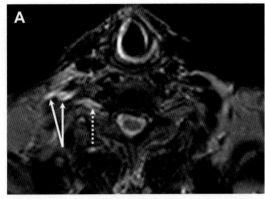
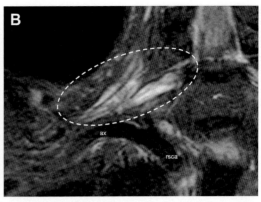

Fig. 13. A 59-year-old man status postchemoradiation for base of tongue squamous cell carcinoma, with a 6-month history of progressive numbness and weakness of the right upper extremity. (*A*) Routine MR imaging of the neck to evaluate for tumor recurrence (T2 with fat saturation) reveals asymmetric bright signal within the roots (*dashed arrow*), and trunks and divisions (*solid arrows*), of the right brachial plexus. Imaging revealed no evidence of tumor recurrence. (*B*) Dedicated right brachial plexus neurogram (coronal short tau inversion recovery) better demonstrates abnormal bright signal and enlargement of the roots, trunks, divisions, and cords of the right brachial plexus (*within the dashed oval*). No focal mass exists to suggest tumor recurrence and these findings are most compatible with radiation plexitis. ax, axillary artery; rsca, right subclavian artery.

from four to six. The superior pair of parathyroid glands is typically located posterior to the upper or lower third of the thyroid. The inferior pair of glands is more variable in its location: 50% occur lateral to the lower pole, 15% may be found within 1 cm of the inferior thyroid pole, and the remainder may be found anywhere along the thyrothymic tract, encompassing an area from the angle of the mandible into the lower aspect of the superior mediastinum.[23] Imaging of parathyroid hyperplasia is variable, with many institutions relying primarily on ultrasound or nuclear imaging, often only after initial surgical exploration has failed to resolve parathormone abnormalities. MR imaging may be of benefit as an adjunct for workup of refractory hyperparathyroidism.[22]

SUMMARY

The thoracic inlet is really best considered as a plane connecting the neck and chest but through which traverses crucial digestive, respiratory, vascular, lymphatic, and neural structures. Endocrine tissues located in the lower neck (the thyroid and parathyroid glands) may also extend into the thoracic inlet.

Knowledge of the fascial spaces of the infrahyoid neck is helpful for understanding and predicting patterns of spread of tumor or infection through the thoracic inlet and into the mediastinum.

Isolated left supraclavicular adenopathy is most often due to metastasis from an abdominal or pelvic primary malignancy, rather than due to primary head and neck malignancy or lymphoma.

Although neural structures are rarely directly visualized, even with high-resolution MR imaging, anatomic landmarks can be used to determine their location.

An aberrant retroesophageal right subclavian artery, found in up to 3% of the general population, is associated with a nonrecurrent course of the right ILN, which is more susceptible to injury during neck surgery.

Complex brachial plexus anatomy is best simplified for radiologic interpretation by considering it in terms of its supraclavicular, retroclavicular, and infraclavicular components. The supraclavicular portion traverses the thoracic inlet, between the anterior and middle scalene muscles, and is intimately related to the subclavian artery.

REFERENCES

1. Moore KL, Dalley AF, Agur AMR. Clinically oriented anatomy. Philadelphia: Lippincott Williams & Wilkins; 2006.
2. Som PM, Curtin HD. Head and neck imaging. 4th edition. St Louis (MO): Mosby; 2003. 1 CD-ROM.
3. Schmalfuss IM, Mancuso AA, Tart RP. Postcricoid region and cervical esophagus: normal appearance at CT and MR imaging. Radiology 2000;214:237–46.
4. Webb BD, Walsh GL, Roberts DB, et al. Primary tracheal malignant neoplasms: the University of Texas

MD Anderson Cancer Center experience. J Am Coll Surg 2006;202:237–46.

5. Reed MF, Mathisen DJ. Tracheoesophageal fistula. Chest Surg Clin N Am 2003;13:271–89.

6. Siobal M, Kallet RH, Kraemer R, et al. Tracheal-innominate artery fistula caused by the endotracheal tube tip: case report and investigation of a fatal complication of prolonged intubation. Respir Care 2001;46:1012–8.

7. Dalley RW. Lesions and nodes of the thoracic inlet. Semin Ultrasound CT MR 1996;17:576–604.

8. Liu ME, Branstetter BF 4th, Whetstone J, et al. Normal CT appearance of the distal thoracic duct. AJR Am J Roentgenol 2006;187:1615–20.

9. Cervin JR, Silverman JF, Loggie BW, et al. Virchow's node revisited. Analysis with clinicopathologic correlation of 152 fine-needle aspiration biopsies of supraclavicular lymph nodes. Arch Pathol Lab Med 1995;119:727–30.

10. Morgenstern L. The Virchow-Troisier node: a historical note. Am J Surg 1979;138:703.

11. Watanabe A, Kawabori S, Osanai H, et al. Pre-operative computed tomography diagnosis of non-recurrent inferior laryngeal nerve. Laryngoscope 2001;111:1756–9.

12. Toniato A, Mazzarotto R, Piotto A, et al. Identification of the nonrecurrent laryngeal nerve during thyroid surgery: 20-year experience. World J Surg 2004; 28:659–61.

13. Hermans R, Dewandel P, Debruyne F, et al. Arteria lusoria identified on preoperative CT and nonrecurrent inferior laryngeal nerve during thyroidectomy: a retrospective study. Head Neck 2003;25:113–7.

14. Coady MA, Adler F, Davila JJ, et al. Nonrecurrent laryngeal nerve during carotid artery surgery: case report and literature review. J Vasc Surg 2000;32: 192–6.

15. Henry JF, Audiffret J, Denizot A, et al. The nonrecurrent inferior laryngeal nerve: review of 33 cases, including two on the left side. Surgery 1988;104: 977–84.

16. Reede DL. The thoracic inlet: normal anatomy. Semin Ultrasound CT MR 1996;17:509–18.

17. Mevio E, Gorini E, Sbrocca M, et al. Unusual cases of cervical nerves schwannomas: phrenic and vagus nerve involvement. Auris Nasus Larynx 2003;30:209–13.

18. Vallejo R, Plancarte R, Benyamin RM, et al. Anterior cervical approach for stellate ganglion and T2 to T3 sympathetic blocks: a novel technique. Pain Pract 2005;5:244–8.

19. Lee JH, Lee HK, Lee DH, et al. Neuroimaging strategies for three types of Horner syndrome with emphasis on anatomic location. AJR Am J Roentgenol 2007;188:W74–81.

20. Johnson EO, Vekris MD, Zoubos AB, et al. Neuroanatomy of the brachial plexus: the missing link in the continuity between the central and peripheral nervous systems. Microsurgery 2006;26:218–29.

21. Loevner LA. Imaging of the thyroid gland. Semin Ultrasound CT MR 1996;17:539–62.

22. Gotway MB, Higgins CB. MR imaging of the thyroid and parathyroid glands. Magn Reson Imaging Clin N Am 2000;8:163–82 ix.

23. Loevner LA. Imaging of the parathyroid glands. Semin Ultrasound CT MR 1996;17:563–75.

MR Imaging Evaluation of Disorders of the Chest Wall

Theodore J. Lee, MD[a,b,*], Jeremy Collins, MD[c]

KEYWORDS
- Chest wall • MR imaging • Sarcoma

Diseases of the chest wall are uncommon in comparison with those of the heart and lungs. When the chest wall is abnormal, the unique tissue- and spatial-resolving capabilities of MR imaging are useful in characterizing the anatomic extent and tissue composition of lesions. MR imaging is complementary to radiographic and CT techniques. The authors review the uses of MR imaging in evaluating lesions of the chest wall, and describe characteristic MR imaging findings in common and unusual diseases. The thoracic inlet and brachial plexus are discussed in an article by Parker and colleagues elsewhere in this issue.

IMAGING TECHNIQUE

Selection of the appropriate MR imaging technique begins with an assessment of the extent of the suspected disease process. The patient's history should be reviewed, as should prior imaging. The size and location of suspected lesions guide the choice of field of view and coil types. When possible, dedicated surface coils should be used, and smaller palpable lesions marked at the overlying skin.

Prone imaging has been proposed as a means of minimizing respiratory motion for anterior chest wall lesions. Respiratory gating is useful for limiting breathing artifacts during image acquisition. Cardiac gating for chest wall lesions is less critical than with assessment of mediastinal structures. Although selection of imaging sequences should be tailored to the suspected disease, in general, axial and sagittal or coronal images are acquired using T1- and T2-weighted sequences. Fat-saturation sequences are useful for confirming macroscopic fat and should also be used on enhanced images. Gadolinium administration is an important part of MR imaging technique, and patients should be screened for contraindications to administration. In patients who have diminished renal function, informed consent should be obtained if gadolinium administration is required. Typically, a dose of 0.1 mmol/kg of intravenous gadolinium is administered.[1,2]

SOFT TISSUES OF THE CHEST WALL
Cellulitis, Necrotizing Fasciitis

Infections of chest wall soft tissues range from cellulitis to infections of deeper soft tissues, including myositis, osteomyelitis, abscess, and necrotizing fasciitis. Cellulitis often appears more extensive on MR imaging than on other imaging modalities because of MR imaging's sensitivity for tissue edema. Cellulitis is characterized by high T2 signal in subcutaneous soft tissues (**Fig. 1**A), sometimes with thickening of the skin or small fluid collections, with diffuse enhancement after gadolinium administration (**Fig. 1**B). MR imaging is helpful in detecting the enhancing rim of an abscess, although, because some tumors demonstrate similar appearance when centrally necrotic, correlation with clinical findings is important.[3–5]

[a] Department of Radiology, University of California, San Francisco, San Francisco, California 94143, USA
[b] Thoracic Radiology, San Francisco General Hospital, 1001 Potrero Avenue, San Francisco, CA 94110, USA
[c] Department of Radiology, Diagnostic Radiology Residency Program, University of California, San Francisco, 505 Parnassus Avenue, Box 0628, San Francisco, CA 94143-0628, USA
* Corresponding author. Department of Radiology, 1x57, San Francisco General Hospital, 1001 Potrero Avenue, San Francisco, CA 94110.
E-mail address: theodore.lee@radiology.ucsf.edu (T.J. Lee).

Magn Reson Imaging Clin N Am 16 (2008) 355–379
doi:10.1016/j.mric.2008.03.001

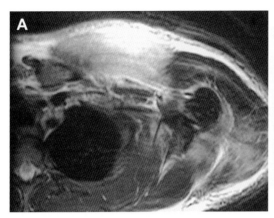
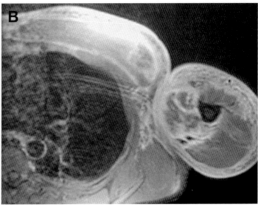

Fig. 1. Necrotizing fasciitis. (A) Axial T2-weighted image from a 35-year-old injection drug user demonstrates diffuse edema of the subcutaneous tissues, pectoralis major, and proximal arm muscles. (B) Axial T1-weighted image following intravenous administration of gadolinium shows fascial enhancement surrounding these muscle groups and also extending into the axilla.

Necrotizing fasciitis is a soft tissue infection typically caused by group A *Streptococci* that involves superficial and deep fascia with extensive tissue edema and enhancement. Soft tissue fluid collections and gas may be present, although gas is more readily discerned on CT. In the absence of deep fascial involvement on MR imaging, necrotizing fasciitis is unlikely.[4]

Muscle Lesions

Muscles of the chest wall are a frequent site of traumatic injury and inflammation. MR imaging is superior to CT and ultrasound (US) in assessment of muscle injury and pyomyositis, because of its tissue sensitivity and multiplanar capability, although CT and ultrasonography are more useful for guiding tissue biopsies or other interventions.[5–7] Muscle strains, ruptures, and hematomas are often seen as a result of sports injuries and trauma, frequently involving the pectoralis muscles. Strains are characterized by edema and perimuscular fluid, with high signal on T2-weighted imaging sequences. When hematoma is present, the muscle may be diffusely enlarged, with heterogeneous high T1 and T2 signal intensity varying as the hematoma evolves (**Fig. 2**). Muscle hematomas typically resolve in 6 to 8 weeks, although fibrosis may develop.[7–9] Pyomyositis is a bacterial infection of the skeletal muscles, typically presenting with muscle pain and fever. Its incidence is increasing in the United States, particularly among patients who have diabetes or HIV infection. The causative organism is typically *Staphylococcus aureus*, *Streptococcus* species, or gram-negative bacteria. MR imaging typically demonstrates muscle enlargement, edema with T2 hyperintensity, and diffuse or heterogeneous

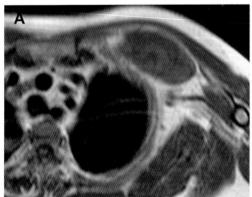
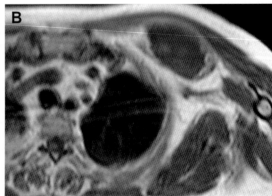

Fig. 2. Intramuscular hematoma. (A) Axial T1-weighted image demonstrates a circumscribed low signal intensity hematoma in the pectoralis minor muscle in this patient on anticoagulation therapy. (B) Axial T1-weighted image following intravenous administration of gadolinium shows peripheral nodular enhancement.

enhancement after gadolinium administration. Abscesses are frequently seen in later stages of the disease.[10–12] MR imaging is also being explored as an aid in the assessment of neuromuscular disease. Chronic denervation results in volume loss and fatty infiltration seen as an increase in T1 signal. Acute denervation results in increased T2 signal intensity on T2-weighted sequences such as short tau inversion recovery (STIR). Acute denervation is also associated with diffuse muscle enhancement following gadolinium administration. MR imaging has been used to identify hereditary myopathies and to measure changes in muscle volume, and may allow assessment of metabolic changes in affected muscle by way of MR spectroscopy.[13–16]

Soft Tissue Tumors

Lipoma

Lipomas are the most common tumors of soft tissue, most frequently seen in patients older than 50. They are benign masses composed predominantly of adipocytes, although connective tissue septa, calcification, and other nonadipose tissue are seen in about one third of lesions.[17,18] On MR imaging, lipomas are characterized by a predominance of adipose tissue, generally 75% or more by volume, and often show homogeneously fat signal on MR imaging (**Fig. 3**),[17] although biochemical differences have been demonstrated between lipomas and other adipose tissue.[19] The adipocytes do not enhance following gadolinium contrast administration. A thin capsule is frequently seen, but lipomas may also infiltrate within adjacent tissues without a defined capsule.[20] Thin septa measuring less than 2 mm in thickness are often visible within the mass, and these may enhance weakly.[1,17,18] Lipomas of the chest wall are often large, and generally present as a gradually enlarging mass. They may be found superficially in subcutaneous tissue or deep within the chest wall. Among deeply located lipomas, the chest wall is the most frequent location. Lipomas may also occur within other structures, such as bone and muscle.[1,17,18]

Hibernoma

Hibernomas are benign tumors of brown fat. Hibernomas present as slow-growing, painless subcutaneous masses, with peak incidence before the age of 50. Lesions are composed of brown fat, although normal adipose may be interspersed within the lesions. Signal characteristics on MR imaging relate to the histologic components, with those with a higher proportion of brown fat demonstrating lower signal on T1 sequences and higher signal on T2 or STIR sequences. The typical appearance of hibernomas on MR imaging is T1 hyperintensity, less than that of normal adipose tissue, with diffuse enhancement following administration of gadolinium contrast. Tortuous vessels and septa may be found, particularly in lesions with a higher proportion of brown fat. The appearance of these lesions on gross examination is characteristic, with rust-brown to tan coloration. The radiologic appearance overlaps that of lipomas and liposarcomas.[18,21–24]

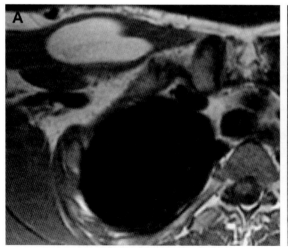 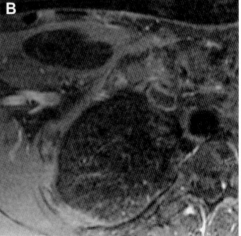

Fig. 3. Intrapectoral lipoma. (*A*) Axial T1-weighted image demonstrates a smoothly circumscribed area of high signal fat without visible septation within the pectoralis major muscle of this 56-year-old patient. (*B*) T1-weighted postcontrast fat saturation shows no evidence of enhancement. Note the uniform loss of signal due to the use of fat-saturation technique.

Liposarcoma

Liposarcomas are the second most common chest wall soft tissue sarcoma behind malignant fibrous histiocytoma, accounting for 10% to 35% of cases.[25,26] Liposarcomas are histologically and radiographically diverse. The World Health Organization recognizes five histologic types: well-differentiated, dedifferentiated, myxoid, pleomorphic, and mixed, with the well-differentiated type being most common.[27] As with lipoma, most patients present with an enlarging mass. Occurrence in the thorax is rare, in comparison with the extremities and retroperitoneum, and predominantly affects the shoulder. Descriptions of tumor appearance are largely found in the musculoskeletal radiology literature. Although some have reported possible cases of malignant transformation of lipomas into liposarcomas, this transformation is not generally accepted as a pathway for development.[26,28]

The imaging appearance of liposarcoma varies substantially, based on subtype. Well-differentiated liposarcomas may appear predominantly fatty, and the overlap in their imaging presentation is a known radiologic challenge. MR imaging features that most suggest a well-differentiated liposarcoma over a lipoma have been described, and include the presence of internal septations greater than 2 mm in thickness, mass-like or nodular areas of nonadipose tissue, and a decreased proportion of fat to nonadipose tissue.[17,28,29] Additional features that may help suggest liposarcoma include large size (particularly larger than 10 cm in greatest dimension), male sex, increased patient age, and hyperintense septa or nodules on T2-weighted imaging.[28,30] A soft tissue mass adjoining an apparently well differentiated liposarcoma should raise the possibility of a dedifferentiated liposarcoma.[26,28]

More aggressive liposarcomas may lack any identifiable fat on MR imaging in up to one half of cases and are generally less than 25% fat by volume. Myxoid liposarcomas, typically presenting as rounded intermuscular masses, often have high T2 signal intensity caused by high water content. Rarely, lesions may mimic cysts, and therefore, gadolinium administration is useful to demonstrate characteristic enhancement. Non–fat-containing liposarcomas may not be reliably distinguished from other malignant soft tissue tumors.[26,28,31,32]

Neurogenic Lesions

Neurogenic tumors originate in cells derived from the embryonic neural crest. Most thoracic neural tumors originate in the mediastinum, with only about 5% originating from the intercostal nerves.[33,34] The most common chest wall lesions are the benign peripheral nerve sheath tumors, neurofibromas, and schwannomas. A schwannoma, also known as a neurilemoma, typically affects young adults and presents as a painless, slowly growing ovoid or fusiform mass involving intercostal nerves or spinal nerve roots. Malignant transformation is rare. Multiple schwannomas may occasionally be seen, with a slight association with neurofibromatosis type I. Schwannomas are typically isointense to muscle on T1-weighted imaging, with high signal on T2-weighted imaging. Lesions tend to enhance avidly after gadolinium administration. Larger lesions may demonstrate cystic degeneration, a feature that may help distinguish a schwannoma from a neurofibroma. Biopsy, as with other nerve sheath tumors, is characteristically painful. The nerve of origin can typically be dissected free from the tumor at the time of surgical resection.[1,35,36]

Neurofibromas may be found incidentally or because of local or radiating pain. An intercostal or paraspinous location is the most common. Most often, neurofibromas are localized, and most are not associated with neurofibromatosis, unlike plexiform neurofibromas, which are strongly associated with neurofibromatosis type I. In cases of localized neurofibroma, treatment is surgical excision, generally requiring sacrifice of the involved nerve.[35] At imaging, neurofibromas may be indistinguishable from schwannomas (**Fig. 4**). MR imaging demonstrates a lobulated mass of low T1 signal intensity (**Fig. 4**B) and high T2 signal intensity, often with the "target sign" of central low signal intensity on T2-weighted images (**Fig. 4**C). Gadolinium enhancement is typically avid but may be heterogeneous (**Fig. 4**D).[35–38] Large neurofibromas may, on occasion, cause considerable chest wall deformity.[39,40]

Neurofibrosarcomas are sarcomas of the intercostal nerves, spinal nerve roots, or brachial plexus, and may be found in the chest wall and thoracic inlet as enlarging painful masses (**Fig. 5**). These tumors, also known as malignant peripheral nerve sheath tumors, typically arise from neurofibromas, and thus, have a strong association with neurofibromatosis. A change in the appearance of a neurofibroma should raise concern for sarcomatous degeneration, with increasing heterogeneity seen on T1- and T2-weighted MR imaging.[41]

Malignant Fibrous Histiocytoma and Other Sarcomas

Primary soft tissue sarcomas of the chest wall are rare. Malignant fibrous histiocytoma is the most

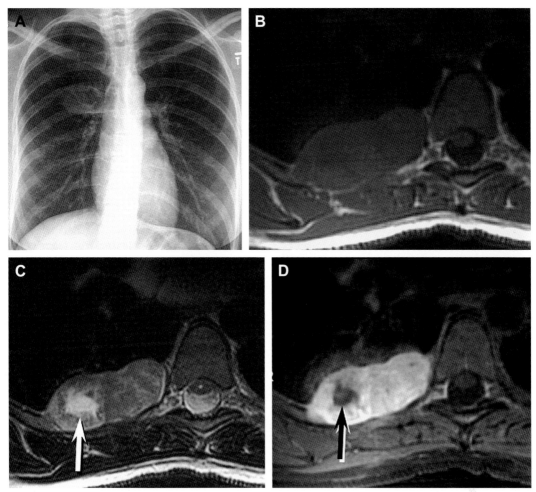

Fig. 4. Neurofibroma. A 20-year-old woman presents with 2 years of pain radiating around her right chest wall. (*A*) Frontal chest radiograph shows smooth rib erosion in association with a lobulated intercostal mass projected over the right hilum. (*B*) Axial T1-weighted image shows a soft tissue mass, isointense to muscle, arising from the intercostal space. (*C*) Axial T2-weighted image shows inhomogeneous signal intensity, with most of the mass mildly hyperintense to muscle, but with one focal area of prominent T2 prolongation (*arrow*). (*D*) T1-weighted postcontrast image shows diffuse intense enhancement of the mass, with diminished enhancement in the small region of intense T2 signal (*arrow*), likely reflecting the presence of cystic change.

common soft tissue sarcoma (**Fig. 6**) and is typically seen in the deep fascia or muscles of older adults.[41,25] On MR imaging, most tumors are isointense to muscle on T1-weighted sequences (**Fig. 6**A), with intensity greater than fat on T2-weighted sequences (**Fig. 6**B). As on CT, heterogeneous enhancement is seen following gadolinium contrast administration (**Fig. 6**C).[42] Invasion of intercostal muscles is frequently identified, and better defined on MR imaging than on CT.[43] Other sarcomas, including fibrosarcoma, angiosarcoma, leiomyosarcoma, rhabdomyosarcoma, synovial sarcoma, neurofibrosarcoma, and poorly differentiated liposarcoma, share similar MR imaging characteristics, and differentiation of

one sarcoma type from another frequently requires biopsy.[44]

Elastofibroma

Elastofibromas represent common soft tissue masses of the posterolateral chest wall, most frequently found in older women, and are composed of elastic fibers and collagen, with interspersed fat. Elastofibromas are typically semilunar in shape, and are found adjacent to the scapula in the subscapular, or infrascapular, chest wall. Smaller lesions are frequently overlooked at imaging.[45] MR imaging typically demonstrates areas of poorly circumscribed tissue isointense to muscle, with linear or focal areas of internal fat being

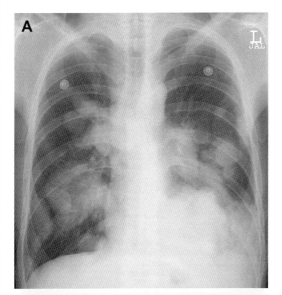

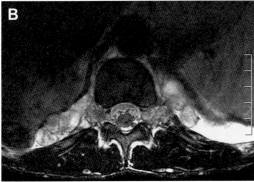

Fig. 5. Neurofibrosarcoma in a 32-year-old man with neurofibromatosis. (*A*) Frontal chest radiograph demonstrates numerous lung parenchymal, pleural, and chest wall masses, consistent with metastatic neurofibrosarcoma. (*B*) Axial T2-weighted image at the level of the diaphragm shows lobulated paraspinous masses extending from the neural foramina and left pleural effusion.

a characteristic finding (**Fig. 7**). Lesions are frequently bilateral, which helps exclude malignant considerations. Diagnosis in equivocal cases may be confirmed by biopsy to demonstrate positive elastin stains. Malignant transformation has not been reported, although lesions may recur following surgical excision.[45–47]

Desmoid

Desmoid tumors are dense, often large fibromatous tumors found on rare occasions in the axilla, shoulder girdle, and intercostal musculature. Masses are hypointense-to-isointense to muscle on T1-weighted images (**Fig. 8**A) and moderate-to-high signal intensity on T2 (**Fig. 8**B), and may show avid enhancement with contrast (**Fig. 8**C).

Management typically involves wide surgical resection. The incidence of local recurrence is high (37.5% reported in one series of 53 patients treated at the Mayo Clinic), particularly in the setting of positive margins; thus, preoperative imaging to determine tumor extent is warranted.[44,48,49]

Lymphangioma

Lymphangioma is a congenital lesion consisting of dilated lymphatics with occasional smooth muscle that may be found in any tissue but is most commonly found at the cervicothoracic junction in children and in the mediastinum in adults. It is a rare lesion, even in children. Occasional cases of adults with isolated axillary or chest wall lymphangiomas or mediastinal lymphangiomas extending to the chest wall have been reported, but no large series has been reviewed. MR imaging of these lesions typically demonstrates T1 signal isointense to muscle, with bright T2 signal within cystic portions (**Fig. 9**). The margins of the lesion enhance following gadolinium administration.[50–57]

Hemangioma

Hemangioma is another congenital lesion predominantly found in children that may be found, on occasion, in the adult chest wall. Hemangiomas consist of dilated tortuous blood vessels, and are typically found in subcutaneous tissue, although intramuscular and intraosseous lesions have been reported.[58–60] Lesions in adults are typically cavernous hemangiomas, as distinct from the capillary hemangiomas of infancy.[52] Chest radiography or thoracic CT may demonstrate central phleboliths, which are not well demonstrated on MR imaging. The presence of internal fat is a characteristic feature and helps differentiate hemangiomas from lymphangiomas. T1-weighted MR imaging typically shows regions isointense to muscle and fat because of vascular tissue intermixed with variable, and sometimes substantial, amounts of fat (**Fig. 10**A). Flow-related signal voids may be present. T2-weighted images typically show high signal intensity (**Fig. 10**B). Following gadolinium contrast administration, heterogeneously bright enhancement is expected (**Fig. 10**C).[1,38,44,48,61]

Lymphoma

Axillary and peripectoral lymph nodes are well assessed by CT and MR imaging in patients who have lymphoma. Chest wall invasion occurs in about 2% to 5% of patients who have thoracic lymphoma. MR imaging shows greater sensitivity than CT for evaluating chest wall involvement in lymphoma. T2-weighted imaging sequences such as STIR are the most sensitive to chest wall invasion. MR imaging should be considered if

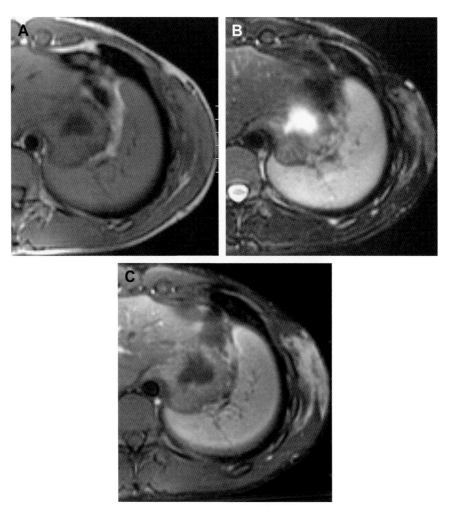

Fig. 6. Malignant fibrous histiocytoma. (*A*) Axial T1-weighted, (*B*) axial T2-weighted, and (*C*) T1-weighted contrast-enhanced images show an infiltrative enhancing mass in the left chest wall in a patient who has vague chest pain and palpable mass. Biopsy demonstrated malignant fibrous histiocytoma, for which the patient underwent surgical chest wall resection with reconstruction.

chest wall involvement is suspected, because it has been shown to alter treatment planning.[62–64]

CHEST WALL POSTPROCEDURAL FINDINGS

MR imaging is occasionally used for evaluation of the postoperative chest wall, typically to evaluate for potential complications or to search for the causes of persistent symptoms such as pain or fever. The use of MR imaging for the evaluation of patients who have undergone sternotomy has been described, although MR imaging of the chest wall is limited by artifact from sternal wires.[65] MR imaging findings have also been reported in rare cases of plombage, complicated oleothorax, and retained foreign body.[44,66,67] MR imaging has also been used to evaluate thoracic wall reconstruction, most notably breast reconstruction,

with the transverse rectus abdominis myocutaneous flap.[68–70]

Vascular Collaterals, Arteriovenous Malformations, and Aneurysms

Prominent vascular collaterals are occasionally found on MR imaging of the chest wall. Intercostal arterial collaterals are well known in the setting of aortic coarctation, and may cause rib notching on chest radiographs (**Fig. 11**A). MR imaging and MR angiography offer noninvasive assessment of the size and extent of collaterals (**Fig. 11**B, C), which may not be possible because of tight coarctation limiting catheter access. Visual estimation of collateral circulation correlates with quantitative MR imaging flow calculation. Intercostal aneurysms and enlarged collateral vessels

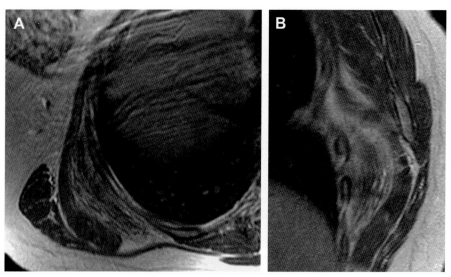

Fig. 7. Elastofibroma in a 55-year-old woman. (*A*) Axial and (*B*) sagittal T1-weighted images centered at the level of the angle of the scapula show a heterogeneous striated-appearing mass along the chest wall, consistent with elastofibroma. Note the linear areas of increased T1 signal comparable to subcutaneous fat.

may also occur, with a prevalence of about 10%.[71–73]

THE OSSEOUS THORAX
Benign Osseous Tumors

Primary osseous tumors of the chest wall are uncommon, accounting for 5% to 8% of all skeletal lesions.[74] Approximately 95% of these lesions are located within the ribs. Most of the remainder are found within the sternum.[75] Rib lesions are equally likely to be benign or malignant, whereas sternal lesions are usually malignant, exclusive of imaging appearance.[76]

Fibrous dysplasia

The most common primary bone tumor of the chest wall, fibrous dysplasia accounts for approximately 30% of all benign chest wall bone lesions.[77] This entity is congenital, originating from bone-forming mesenchyme where osteoblasts fail to differentiate and mature.[78] Osseous involvement is either monostotic or polyostotic. Monostotic disease accounts for 70% to 80% of cases; lesions are typically found incidentally, with age at presentation ranging from 10 to 70 years, and prevalence peaking at 20 to 30 years of age.[1,79] Not uncommonly, patients present with pain or pathologic fracture. Polyostotic disease is seen in the remainder and is usually unilateral; when bilateral, lesions are distributed asymmetrically. Patients who have polyostotic fibrous dysplasia are more commonly symptomatic and present before age 10. Pathologic fracture is the

presenting symptom in 85%. Polyostotic involvement is associated with cafe-au-lait spots and precocious puberty in the McCune-Albright syndrome.[79,80]

Lesions involve the ribs, proximal humeri, and clavicles in decreasing order of frequency.[1] Typical findings at radiography include an expansile, lytic lesion that scallops the endosteal cortex with a sharp zone of transition. CT demonstrates an osteoid ground glass matrix to better advantage. MR imaging demonstrates a sharply defined, lobulated lesion with a low signal intensity rim because of sclerotic margins. On T1- and proton density–weighted images, fibrous dysplasia lesions are characterized by intermediate signal intensity, less intense than adjacent normal marrow. Fibrous dysplasia has a variable appearance on T2-weighted images, with signal intensity ranging from low to intermediate, depending on the presence of intralesional bony trabeculae. Postgadolinium enhancement is noted in most.[81,82] Intermediate signal is present on proton density–weighted imaging. Malignant transformation to osteosarcoma or fibrosarcoma is rare and, when it occurs, a history of irradiation can usually be elicited.

Aneurysmal bone cyst

The aneurysmal bone cyst was initially recognized as a distinct entity in 1942 by Jaffe and Lichtenstein,[83] who described it as "a peculiar blood-containing cyst of large size." Aneurysmal bone cysts are rare, accounting for 1% to 6% of all primary bone tumors, with a slight female predominance.[84]

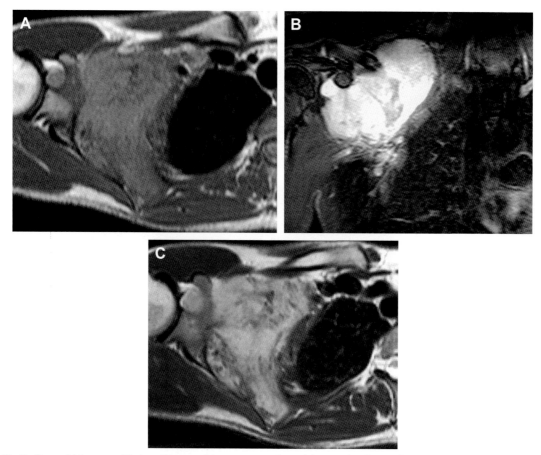

Fig. 8. Desmoid tumor axilla in a 25-year-old man presenting with an enlarging axillary mass, initially thought to represent a sarcoma. (*A*) Axial and (*B*) coronal contrast-enhanced T1-weighted and (*C*) axial T2-weighted images obtained following intravenous administration of gadolinium demonstrate typical signal characteristics in the bulky mass that extends from the supraclavicular fossa to the axilla. Tissue is moderately bright on T2-weighted images, with strong enhancement following gadolinium administration.

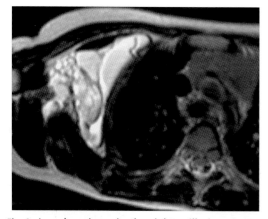

Fig. 9. Lymphangioma in the right axilla in a 9-year-old girl. Axial T2-weighted image shows a septated mass in the right axilla, consistent with a large lymphangioma.

Average age at presentation is 13 to 18, with nearly all patients younger than 30. Presenting symptoms are varied and include pain and soft tissue swelling. Pathologic fracture is found at presentation in 8% to 21% of patients. Although benign, this lesion can present as a rapidly enlarging, locally aggressive process. Aneurysmal bone cysts have a predilection for the posterior elements of the spine, followed by the proximal humerus.[85] At radiography, an aneurysmal bone cyst appears as an expansile, lytic lesion with well-defined inner margins. CT clearly demarcates the intraosseous extension. MR imaging demonstrates a lobulated lesion with low signal intensity peripherally on all pulse sequences (**Fig. 12**).[86,87] The lesion is characterized by heterogeneous signal intensity on T1- and T2-weighted imaging. The visualization of fluid–fluid levels on T2-weighted imaging is highly suggestive of the diagnosis, representing

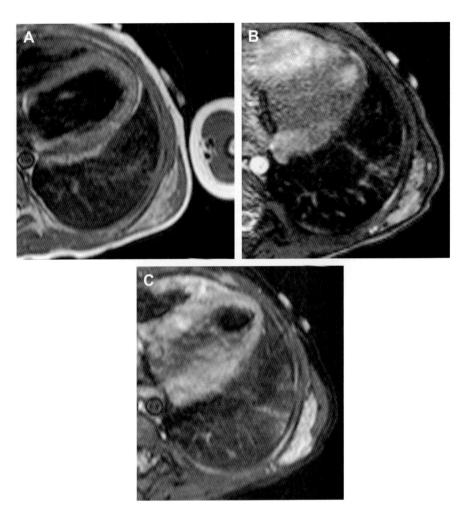

Fig. 10. Hemangioma in a 17-year-old patient with a chest wall mass. (*A*) Axial T1-weighted image shows high signal consistent with intralesional fat, although no flow voids are seen. (*B*) Axial T2-weighted and (*C*) contrast-enhanced images show high signal intensity and enhancement characteristic of a hemangioma.

cysts with hemorrhagic contents. Postgadolinium enhancement is noted within lesion septa.[88] Aneurysmal bone cysts do not undergo malignant degeneration. However, these lesions can be secondary, arising in pre-existing malignant lesions such as giant cell tumors or osteosarcomas.[89,90] Aneurysmal bone cysts are usually treated by intralesional curettage; local recurrence has been noted.

Enchondroma

Enchondromas are benign cartilaginous neoplasms characterized histologically as ectopic hyaline cartilage rests within intramedullary bone. The lesions likely arise from displaced cartilage from nearby growth plates. Enchondromas account for 12% to 14% of benign bone tumors. These lesions are rare in the chest; 3% occur in the ribs or sternum. Enchondromas are detected

incidentally, or patients present with pathologic fracture between the third and fifth decades.[91,92] Multiple lesions suggest the diagnosis of Ollier's or Maffucci's syndrome. Enchondromas are expansile at radiography, showing a partially calcified chondroid matrix, classically demonstrating "ring and arc" calcifications (**Fig. 13**A). Chondroid-type matrix calcifications are better assessed by CT. Lesions are well demarcated at MR imaging, with a lobulated appearance, low signal intensity relative to surrounding marrow on T1-weighted imaging (**Fig. 13**B), and high signal intensity on T2-weighted and STIR imaging (**Fig. 13**C). Enchondromas demonstrate focal, septal, and peripheral nodular enhancement (**Fig. 13**D). The absence of surrounding marrow or soft tissue signal abnormality helps exclude gross malignant transformation. The development of pain in a pre-existing enchondroma without

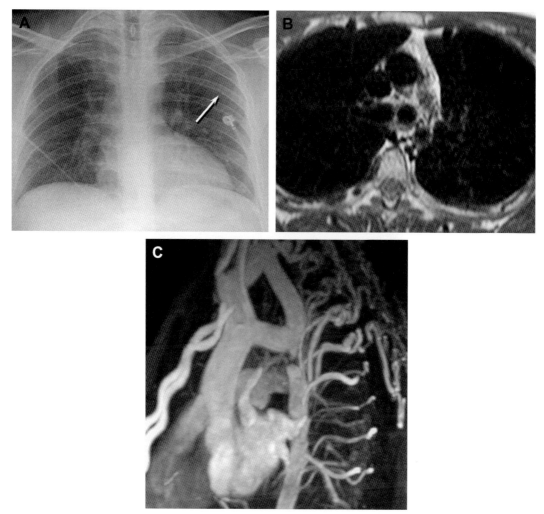

Fig. 11. Coarctation with intercostal collateral vessels in a 27-year-old man evaluated for a ruptured aneurysm. (*A*) Frontal chest radiograph shows rib notching (*arrow*) and abnormal contour of the thoracic aorta. (*B*) Axial T1 image shows large paraspinous and intercostal collaterals with associated flow-related signal voids. (*C*) Oblique sagittal maximum-intensity projected image shows severe coarctation of the thoracic aorta with large intercostal and internal thoracic collateral vessels.

obvious pathologic fracture is concerning for transformation to chondrosarcoma.[93]

Cavernous hemangioma

Hemangiomas consist of a hamartomatous proliferation of vascular tissue containing endothelium-lined cavities. The thoracic vertebral column is the most common site of intraosseous involvement, followed by the lumbar spine, although ribs can sometimes be involved. Hemangiomas constitute less than 1% of all primary bone tumors but were found to be present in 12% to 14% of patients in autopsy series.[94–96] Hemangiomas are noted incidentally in most patients. Patients may present with back pain, myelopathy, or radiculopathy.[97] Lesions with lower proportions of fat-containing

elements are more likely to be symptomatic. Hemangiomas are well-circumscribed lesions with the classic CT finding of thickened trabeculae demonstrating a "polka-dot" configuration on axial imaging.[97,98] MR imaging findings of hemangiomas include high signal on T1- and T2-weighted imaging, reflecting the presence of fatty elements. Increased T2 signal may also be related to edema or slow blood flow. Hemangiomas demonstrate diffuse enhancement following gadolinium administration. Atypical, symptomatic hemangiomas (**Fig. 14**) are fat poor and demonstrate low signal on T1-weighted imaging. High signal persists on T2-weighted imaging, however. Atypical hemangiomas have increased vascularity and enlarged supplying vessels, and are more likely to involve

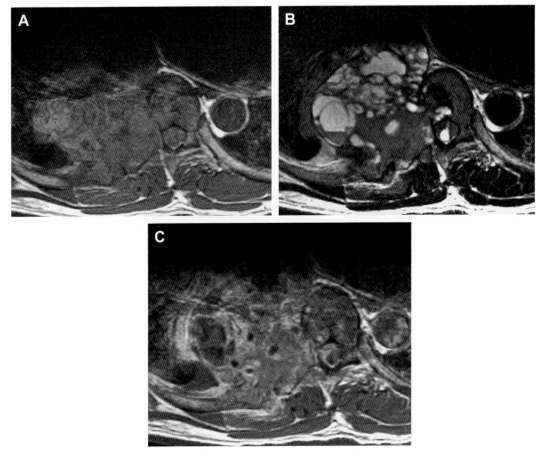

Fig. 12. Thoracic spine aneurysmal bone cyst in a 45-year-old man. (*A*) Axial T1-weighted, (*B*) axial T2-weighted, and (*C*) contrast-enhanced axial T1-weighted images show an expansile cystic lesion involving the right aspect of a lower thoracic spine vertebral body, extending into the posterior elements and the vertebral canal.

the entire vertebral body. Preservation of vertebral body height is useful for differentiating this entity from other aggressive osseous lesions.

Brown tumor

Brown tumors are giant cell-containing tumors that arise secondary to underlying hyperparathyroidism. Brown tumors occur in patients who have secondary hyperparathyroidism from end-stage renal disease, with a prevalence of 1.5 to 1.7%.[99,100] Asymptomatic presentation is the rule. Radiographic findings demonstrate a well-defined lytic lesion on a background of osteopenia.[101] Subperiosteal resorption may be seen in the distal clavicle. Brown tumors are circumscribed at MR imaging, with low signal on T1-weighted imaging and high signal on T2-weighted imaging. Occasionally, lesions demonstrate T2 hypointensity because of blood components. Brown tumors enhance following gadolinium administration. Healing at MR

imaging is manifest with T2 shortening and reduced enhancement.

Malignant Osseous Tumors

Osteosarcoma

Osteosarcoma is a malignant mesenchymal tumor that rarely occurs in the thorax.[42] Intraosseous and extraosseous osteosarcomas appear clinically and therapeutically distinct.[102] Intraosseous lesions primarily occur in patients younger than 30 years of age, and commonly involve the ribs, scapula, or clavicle. Extrapleural masses are not uncommon. Compared with extremity lesions, chest wall lesions have a greater propensity for lung and regional lymph node metastasis. Extraosseous lesions are rare, with only 300 cases reported in the literature. This subtype presents in patients over the age of 50. Both present clinically with an enlarging, painful chest wall mass. Osteosarcomas present radiographically with a destructive mass, a wide zone of transition,

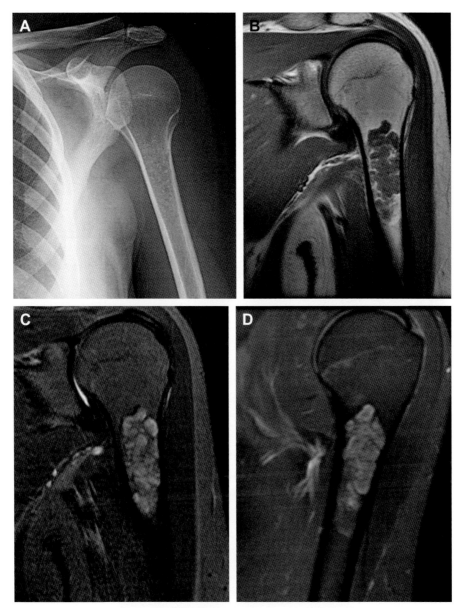

Fig. 13. Humeral enchondroma in a 32-year-old woman with an enchondroma of the proximal left humerus. (*A*) Left shoulder radiograph shows a subtle circumscribed lesion with chondroid matrix. (*B*) Coronal T1-weighted, (*C*) coronal STIR, and (*D*) coronal postgadolinium T1-weighted images acquired on a 3T system show decreased T1-weighted signal intensity with areas of T2 prolongation; septa within the lesion are hypointense on T2-weighted imaging. Intense enhancement is seen following contrast administration.

and an osteoid matrix (**Fig. 15**A).[103] The osteoid matrix can be better appreciated at CT. These lesions demonstrate calcification that is greater at the center of the mass. MR imaging depicts the full extent of osseous and soft tissue extension.[104] Osteosarcomas demonstrate T1 shortening and T2 prolongation (**Fig. 15**B, C), and enhance homogeneously. Because of cystic spaces and blood products, lesions may be heterogeneous on T1-weighted sequences. A distinct histologic and clinical entity, telangiectatic osteosarcoma is predominantly lytic and characterized by rapid enlargement. This lesion demonstrates multiple cystic spaces with fluid–fluid levels and may be indistinguishable at MR imaging from an aneurysmal bone cyst. Pain without pathologic fracture supports the diagnosis of telangiectatic osteosarcoma over aneurysmal bone cyst.

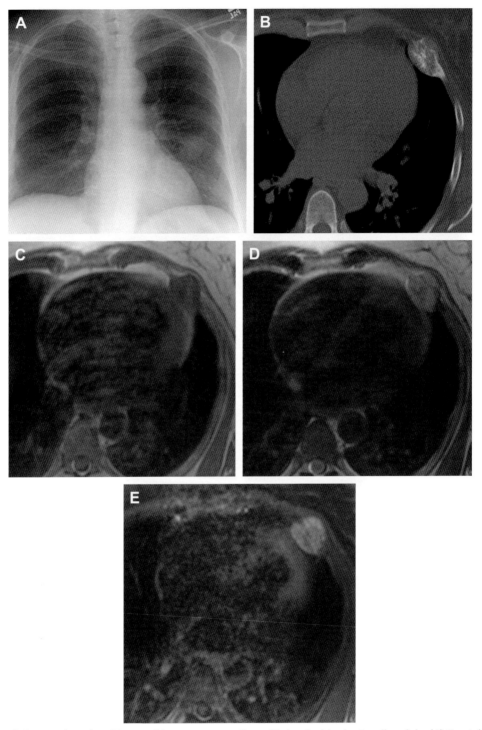

Fig. 14. Rib hemangioma in a 50-year-old woman presenting with a palpable chest wall nodule. (A) Frontal chest radiograph shows a sclerotic lesion within the left anterior fourth rib. (B) Axial thoracic CT shows a lytic component evident on CT, with prominent spicules of bone radiating from the center of the lesion. (C) Axial T1-weighted, (D) axial T2-weighted, and (E) contrast-enhanced T1-weighted images show decreased signal on T1-weighted images, with mixed signal intensity (central areas of low signal related to internal bone) and intense contrast enhancement, the latter sparing the radiating spicules of bone.

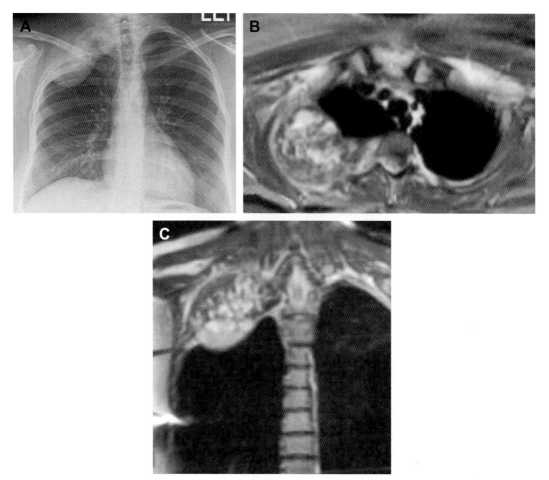

Fig. 15. Osteosarcoma in a 22-year-old woman who has right apical osteosarcoma. (*A*) Frontal chest radiograph shows a large extrapleural mass with osteoid matrix arising from the second rib. The first and third ribs demonstrate periostitis. Axial (*B*) and coronal (*C*) T2-weighted images show a mixed-intensity right apical chest wall mass with multiple cystic regions.

Ewing's sarcoma

Characterized histologically by small cells with scant cytoplasm, Ewing's sarcoma was initially classified as a primitive neuroectodermal tumor.[105] Both entities have a characteristic balanced translocation between chromosomes 11 and 22 - t(11;22) (q24;q12). In the thorax, Ewing's sarcoma presents in children and adolescents as either a solitary mass or multiple masses.[103] Typical locations include the clavicle, sternum, scapula, and ribs; a paravertebral location is common with neural foraminal extension. Occasional extraosseous origin is present, presumably from ectopic rests of neural crest cells. Ewing's sarcoma displaces, rather than invades, adjoining structures.[42] However, lesions can directly invade the lung and may cause pneumothoraces. At radiography, Ewing's lesions are permeative mixed lytic and sclerotic lesions.[103]

CT demonstrates osseous destruction to advantage and may show cystic areas with scattered dystrophic calcifications. Small lesions are hyperintense to muscle on T1-weighted imaging. Foci of hemorrhage and necrosis are common in larger lesions and create heterogeneous signal at T1-weighted imaging (**Fig. 16**A). Ewing's sarcoma is heterogeneously bright on T2-weighted imaging (**Fig. 16**B), with avid enhancement (**Fig. 16**C). MR imaging demonstrates better the full extent of tumor involvement.[106,107]

Chondrosarcoma

The most common primary malignant tumor of the chest wall, chondrosarcoma accounts for 33% of primary rib tumors.[108] Lesions predominate within the anterior osseous chest wall, most frequently involving the upper five ribs near the costochondral junction. Patients may present with pain,

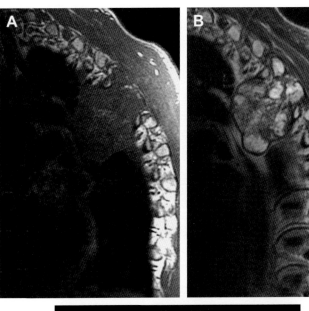

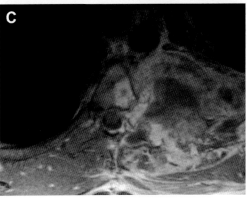

Fig. 16. Ewing's sarcoma in the thoracic spine of a 21-year-old man presenting with vertebral body compression fracture and a kyphotic deformity. Sagittal T1-weighted (*A*), T2-weighted (*B*), and axial postgadolinium (*C*) images show heterogeneous enhancement of the bulky mass, with extension into the spine.

a palpable mass, or swelling. Primary chondrosarcoma is uncommon, arises centrally in bone, and is seen in children. Secondary lesions arise from enchondromas or osteochondromas. Patients who have multiple exostoses, a type of chondrodysplasia, have a risk of malignant degeneration to chondrosarcoma of between 0.5% and 2%.[109] Development of an osteochondroma with cartilage cap thicker than 2 cm is suspicious for malignant degeneration. Chondrosarcoma prevalence peaks at under 20 years of age, with a second peak in patients older than 50. Radiographically, chondrosarcoma presents as a mass with a wide zone of transition, a cortical breakthrough, and a chondroid matrix classically exhibiting ring and arc or stippled calcifications. Secondary lesions may have a primarily lytic appearance. MR imaging is useful in delineating all compartments of involvement (**Fig. 17**). Chondrosarcomas are lobulated on T1-weighted imaging, with signal intensity similar to muscle, and signal intensity similar to, or

brighter than, fat on T2-weighted imaging. Enhancement is heterogeneous (see **Fig. 17**C).[110,111] Metastases are unusual. Myxoid chondrosarcoma is a distinct entity without chondroid calcification.[42] This lesion demonstrates marked T2 prolongation.

Myeloma/solitary plasmacytoma

Myeloma is the second most common lytic osseous lesion in the chest wall. This entity has a range of disease presentation, ranging from extraosseous and intraosseous plasmacytoma to diffuse infiltration of the bone marrow with focal mass-like lytic areas, termed multiple myeloma.[112]

Solitary intraosseous plasmacytoma (SIP) is usually diagnosed in the sixth decade of life with a 2:1 male predominance. The most common presenting symptom is pain. In the chest, the thoracic vertebrae are involved in 80% of cases, followed by the rib, sternum, clavicle, or scapula.[113] SIP progresses to multiple myeloma in 50% to 60%

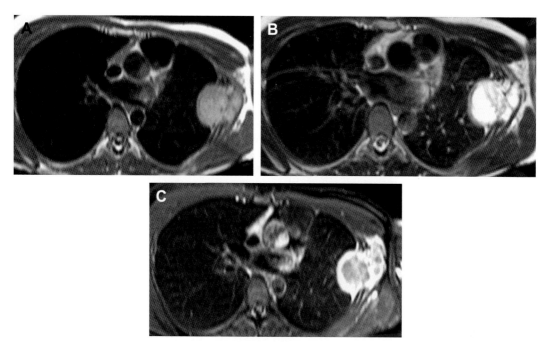

Fig. 17. Chondrosarcoma in a 34-year-old woman with multifocal chondrosarcoma involving the left apex and left lateral chest wall. Axial T1-weighted (*A*), T2-weighted (*B*), and contrast-enhanced T1-weighted (*C*) images show intrinsically increased T1 and T2 signal with intense contrast enhancement.

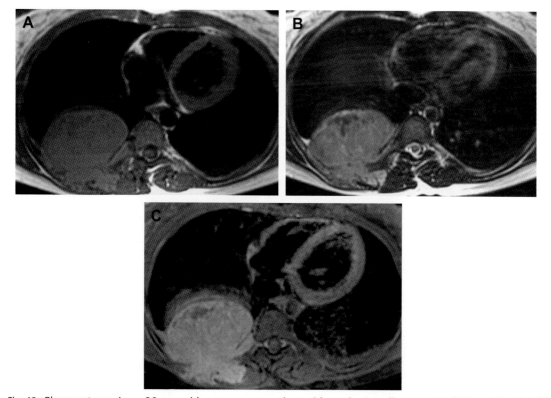

Fig. 18. Plasmacytoma in a 36-year-old woman presenting with a chest wall mass. Axial T1-weighted (*A*), T2-weighted (*B*), and T1-weighted contrast-enhanced fat-suppression (*C*) images show a heterogeneous right posterior chest wall mass arising from the right seventh, eighth, and ninth ribs. Note prominent enhancement.

of cases.[114] Radiography demonstrates a lytic, usually well circumscribed lesion. Occasionally, sclerosis can be seen in the absence of pathologic fracture or treatment. The classic MR imaging "brain within a brain" appearance is lobulated and well circumscribed within a thoracic vertebra. Low signal intensity septa extend into the lesion on all sequences. SIP lesions are homogeneous in appearance, with T2 shortening and T1 prolongation, and enhance after gadolinium administration.[103]

Multiple myeloma is a malignant tumor of plasma cells and usually presents in patients aged 50 to 70, 5 to 10 years after the diagnosis of a plasmacytoma.[112,115] Patients can present insidiously or have symptoms referable to the monoclonal gammopathy, marrow infiltration, or extraosseous extension. In the thorax, myeloma is characterized by predilection for the vertebral bodies, ribs, and clavicles. Findings at radiography are nonspecific, with multiple, poorly marginated lytic lesions and osteopenia. Diffuse low marrow signal may be seen on T1-weighted imaging, suggestive of marrow infiltration.[116] When focal, lesions demonstrate low signal on T1-weighted sequences, high signal on T2-weighted

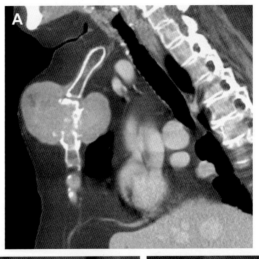

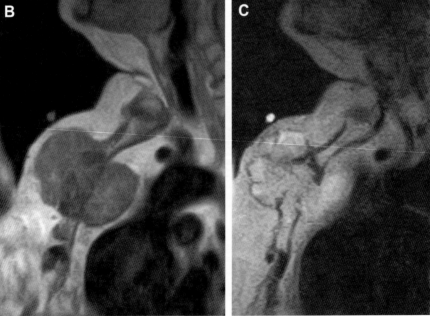

Fig. 19. Sternal metastasis in a 65-year-old woman with pheochromocytoma metastatic to the sternum. Sagittal reformat from CT (A), sagittal T1 (B), and T2-weighted (C) images shows a large mass arising from the sternum.

sequences, and enhance (**Fig. 18**). MR imaging is useful for detecting complications, such as epidural extension with cord compression, which occurs in 10% to 20% of cases.

Osseous metastases

Metastases frequently account for osseous chest wall lesions. Breast, lung, thyroid, prostate, and renal tumors commonly metastasize to bone and account for 80% of cell types found at biopsy.[117,118] In the thorax, lesions are commonly seen in the vertebra, ribs, and proximal humerus. Although the imaging appearance of osseous metastases is highly variable, specific cell types commonly present with osteolytic, sclerotic, or mixed density patterns.[119] Thyroid and renal tumors are invariably osteolytic and may be expansile; most lung cancer metastases are osteolytic. Prostate metastases are invariably sclerotic, whereas breast lesions vary from mixed density to sclerotic. Radiography and CT are insensitive for lytic and mixed density osseous metastases because loss of 40% to 50% of bone trabecula is necessary for detection.[120] Bone scintigraphy is sensitive but not specific in the detection of metastases. Osteolytic and mixed-density lesions demonstrate low signal on T1-weighted sequences and intermediate-to-high signal on T2-weighted sequences (**Fig. 19**).[119,121] Sclerotic lesions usually demonstrate low signal on T1- and T2-weighted sequences. Postgadolinium enhancement is usually seen before treatment. Surrounding bone marrow edema and extraosseous extension are suggestive secondary findings.

Trauma

Sternomanubrial dislocation

A rare injury, sternomanubrial dislocation is associated with high-energy trauma.[122] Because of the high-energy mechanism, coexistent intrathoracic or intra-abdominal injury is common.[123,124] Two types have been described, based on the relative position of the sternum to the manubrium (**Fig. 20**). Type I injuries are associated with direct trauma to the sternum, causing the sternum to be displaced posterior to the manubrium. Type II injuries are associated with thoracic spine hyperflexion injury with manubrial displacement posterior to the sternum. Thoracic spine and upper rib fractures are common with type II injuries.[125] Lateral chest radiographs or CT with sagittal reformatted images are usually diagnostic. MR imaging is often performed to assess for other thoracic injuries. Images acquired in the sagittal plane readily demonstrate the dislocation (see **Fig. 20**).

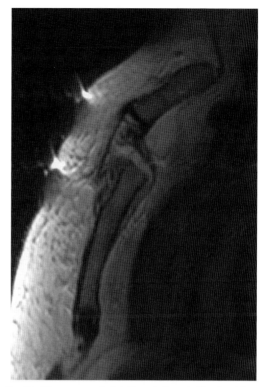

Fig. 20. Sternomanubrial dissociation. Following blunt trauma to the sternum in a motor vehicle accident, sagittal T2-weighted image through the anterior chest wall demonstrates displacement of the manubriosternal joint.

Scapulothoracic dissociation

Scapulothoracic dissociation (STD) is a type of closed forequarter amputation. In 1984, Oreck and colleagues[126] reported a series of patients who had closed forequarter amputation and coined STD to describe this entity. STD is associated with complete disruption of the osseous and musculotendinous scapulothoracic attachments. Osseous disruption occurs through acromioclavicular joint disruption, clavicular fracture, or sternoclavicular joint disruption, reported in 25%, 47%, and 28% of patients, respectively. Neurovascular injury is frequent and accounts for the high morbidity and mortality. Arterial injury is found in 88% of patients, with a spectrum of involvement ranging from dissection to frank disruption. Brachial plexus injury is seen in 94% of patients and is complete in 81%.[126–129]

A well-positioned frontal radiograph demonstrating disruption of the osseous or ligamentous attachment and lateral displacement of the scapula is highly suggestive of the diagnosis. MR imaging is useful in assessing the brachial plexus and demonstrating the extent and severity of soft tissue injuries. Direct evidence of preganglionic plexus injury includes nerve root avulsion from neural foramina. Indirect evidence includes a pseudomeningocele, cord edema, hemorrhage, or scar in the canal.[128,130,131] Direct evidence of postganglionic injury is plexus swelling on T1-weighted imaging, with increased signal on T2-weighted imaging. MR imaging has been shown to be accurate in predicting the level of plexus disruption. Absence of plexus injury at MR imaging is a good predictor of functional recovery.[129,132] Only 17% of patients have limited functional recovery.

Costochondral trauma

Traumatic costochondral injuries are an infrequent cause of chest pain in children and adults.[133] Often occult radiographically, these lesions present a diagnostic dilemma and may cause significant morbidity. An autopsy series of children who died from nonaccidental trauma demonstrated the anterior aspect of the ribs, near the costal junction, as a common site for fractures.[134] Although not a significant injury in isolation, these lesions can prove difficult to diagnose. Bone scintigraphy or MR imaging may be useful adjuncts. MR imaging findings include increased signal on T2-weighted imaging within the rib and adjacent costal cartilage and are best depicted in the coronal or axial planes (**Fig. 21**).

Osteomyelitis

Chest wall infections can spread from an adjoining focus of infection to involve the skeleton. Alternatively, infection can spread hematogenously from a remote, sometimes unclear, site. Risk factors

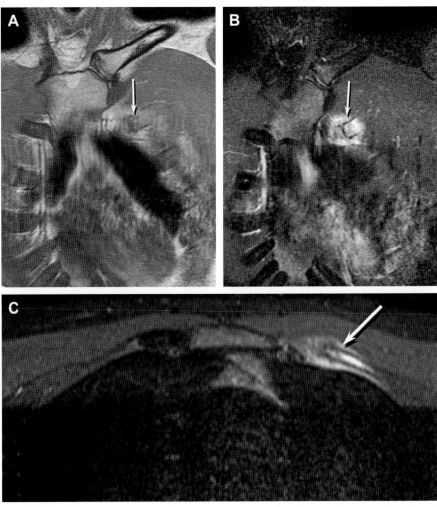

Fig. 21. Costochondral fracture in a 24-year-old man presenting with chest wall pain, localized to the left first costochondral junction. Coronal T1-weighted (*A*), coronal (*B*), and axial (*C*) STIR images show abnormal signal intensity (*arrows*), consistent with a nondisplaced left costochondral fracture.

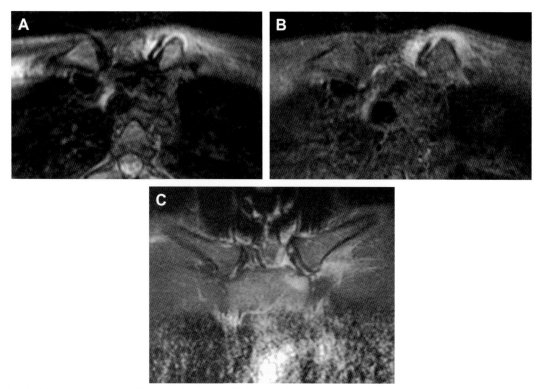

Fig. 22. Manubrial osteomyelitis in a 44-year-old injection drug user presenting with pain at the manubrioclavicular joint space. (*A*) Axial T2-weighted image shows surrounding soft tissue edema, with marrow edema in the left superior manubrium. Contrast-enhanced axial (*B*) and coronal (*C*) T1-weighted images show enhancement within the manubrium and surrounding soft tissues, consistent with osteomyelitis.

include immunosuppressed state, diabetes mellitus, and injection drug use.[108,135]

The sternoclavicular joint is an uncommon site for septic arthritis in the general population, accounting for 1% of infections.[136] However, it accounts for 17% of septic joint infections in injection drug users. A unique risk factor is an adjacent, long-standing central venous catheter. Patients typically present with localized pain, which may spread to the ipsilateral neck or shoulder. Symptoms are usually subacute, lasting approximately 14 days, in contradistinction to the typically acute symptoms seen with this entity in other joints.[137] The most commonly isolated organism is *Staphylococcus aureus*. Radiographs may be normal, although rarefaction of periarticular bone may be seen.[6] CT usually demonstrates loss of the fat plane surrounding the joint, with indistinct lytic changes in the adjoining manubrium and clavicle. MR imaging shows fluid within the sternoclavicular joint (**Fig. 22**). Diffuse periarticular intraosseous low signal is evident on T1-weighted imaging, with matched increased signal on T2-weighted imaging and avid postcontrast enhancement.

SUMMARY

- Lesions of the chest wall are uncommonly encountered in clinical practice, and may originate in various tissues, making evaluation of chest wall lesions a challenge for the radiologist.
- MR imaging can be useful in characterizing lesions, and familiarity with the signal characteristics of chest wall lesions can help guide construction of a focused differential.

REFERENCES

1. Tateishi U, Gladish GW, Kusumoto M, et al. Chest wall tumors: radiologic findings and pathologic correlation. Part 1. Benign tumors. Radiographics 2003;23:1477–90.
2. Landwehr P, Schulte O, Lackner K. MR imaging of the chest: mediastinum and chest wall. Eur Radiol 1999;9:1737–44.
3. Christian S, Kraas J, Conway WF. Musculoskeletal infections. Semin Roentgenol 2007;42(2):92–101.

4. Schmid MR, Kossmann T, Duewell S. Differentiation of necrotizing fasciitis and cellulitis using MR imaging. AJR Am J Roentgenol 1998;170: 615–20.

5. Wilson DJ. Soft tissue and joint infection. Eur Radiol 2004;14:E64–71.

6. Sharif HS, Clark DC, Aabed MY, et al. MR imaging of thoracic and abdominal wall infections: comparison with other imaging procedures. AJR Am J Roentgenol 1990;154:989–95.

7. Connell DA, Potter HG, Sherman MF, et al. Injuries of the pectoralis major muscle: evaluation with MR imaging. Radiology 1999;210:785–91.

8. Elsayes KM, Lammle M, Shariff A, et al. Value of magnetic resonance imaging in muscle trauma. Curr Probl Diagn Radiol 2006;35:206–12.

9. Carrino JA, Chandnanni VP, Mitchell DB, et al. Pectoralis major muscle and tendon tears: diagnosis and grading using magnetic resonance imaging. Skeletal Radiol 2000;29:305–13.

10. Drosos G. Pyomyositis. A literature review. Acta Orthop Belg 2005;71(1):9–16.

11. Crum NF. Bacterial pyomyositis in the United States. Am J Med 2004;117(6):420–8.

12. Yu C-W, Hsiao J-K, Hsu C-Y, et al. Bacterial pyomyositis: MRI and clinical correlation. Magn Reson Imaging 2004;22(9):1233–41.

13. Koltzenburg M, Yousry T. Magnetic resonance imaging of skeletal muscle. Curr Opin Neurol 2007; 20:595–9.

14. Mercuri E, Jungbluth H, Muntoni F. Muscle imaging in clinical practice: diagnostic value of muscle magnetic resonance imaging in inherited neuromuscular disorders. Curr Opin Neurol 2005;18: 526–37.

15. Mercuri E, Pichiecchio A, Allsop J, et al. Muscle MRI in inherited neuromuscular disorders: past, present, and future. J Magn Reson Imaging 2007; 25:433–40.

16. Kuo GP, Carrino JA. Skeletal muscle imaging and inflammatory myopathies. Curr Opin Rheumatol 2007;19:530–5.

17. Kransdorf MJ, Bancroft LW, Peterson JJ, et al. Imaging of fatty tumors: distinction of lipoma and well-differentiated liposarcoma. Radiology 2002; 224:99–104.

18. Bancroft LW, Kransdorf MJ, Peterson JJ, et al. Benign fatty tumors: classification, clinical course, imaging appearance, and treatment. Skeletal Radiol 2006;35:719–33.

19. Tos AD, Cin P. The role of cytogenetics in the classification of soft tissue tumors. Virchows Arch 1997; 431:83–94.

20. Roberts C, Liu P, Colby T. Encapsulated versus nonencapsulated superficial fatty masses: a proposed MR imaging classification. AJR Am J Roentgenol 2003;180:1419–22.

21. Anderson S, Schwab C, Staffer E, et al. Hibernoma: imaging characteristics of a rare benign soft tissue tumor. Skeletal Radiol 2001;30:590–5.

22. Ritchie D, Aniq H, Davies A, et al. Hibernoma - correlation of histopathology and magnetic-resonance-imaging features in 10 cases. Skeletal Radiol 2006;35:579–89.

23. Lee J, Gupta A, Saifuddin A, et al. Hibernoma: MRI features in eight consecutive cases. Clin Radiol 2006;61:1029–34.

24. Kallas K, Vaughan L, Haghighi P, et al. Hibernoma of the left axilla; a case report and review of MR imaging. Skeletal Radiol 2003;32:290–4.

25. Kransdorf M. Malignant soft tissue tumors in a large referral population: distribution of diagnosis by age, sex, and location. AJR Am J Roentgenol 1995;164:129–34.

26. Murphey MD, Arcara LK, Fanburg-Smith J. From the archives of the AFIP - imaging of musculoskeletal liposarcoma with radiologic-pathologic correlation. Radiographics 2005;25:1371–95.

27. Christopher D, Unni K, Mertens F. WHO classification of tumors. Pathology and genetics: tumors of soft tissue and bone. Lyon (France): IARC Press; 2002.

28. Peterson JJ, Kransdorf MJ, Bancroft LW, et al. Malignant fatty tumors: classification, clinical course, imaging appearance, and treatment. Skeletal Radiol 2006;32:493–503.

29. Hosono M, Kobayashi H, Fujimoto R, et al. Septum-like structures in lipoma and liposarcoma: MR imaging and pathologic correlation. Skeletal Radiol 1997;26(3):150–4.

30. Galant J, Marti-Bonmati L, Saez F, et al. The value of fat-suppressed T2 or STIR sequences in distinguishing lipoma from well-differentiated liposarcoma. Eur Radiol 2003;13:337–43.

31. Einarsdottir H, Soderlund V, Larson O, et al. MR imaging of lipoma and liposarcoma. Acta Radiol 1999;30:64–8.

32. Sung M-S, Kang HS, Suh JS, et al. Myxoid liposarcoma: appearance at MR imaging with histologic correlation. Radiographics 2000;20:1007–19.

33. Takeda S-i, Miyoshi S, Minami M, et al. Intrathoracic neurogenic tumors–50 years' experience in a Japanese institution. Eur J Cardiothorac Surg 2004;26: 807–12.

34. McClenathan JH, Bloom RJ. Peripheral tumors of the intercostal nerves. Ann Thorac Surg 2004;78: 713–4.

35. Murphey MD, Smith WS, Smith SE, et al. Imaging of musculoskeletal neurogenic tumors: radiologic-pathologic correlation. Radiographics 1999;19(5): 1253–80.

36. Pilavaki M, Chourmouzi D, Kiziridou A, et al. Imaging of peripheral nerve sheath tumors with pathologic correlation. Eur J Radiol 2004;52(3):229–39.

37. Jee W-H, Oh S-N, McCauley T, et al. Extraaxial neurofibromas versus neurilemmomas: discrimination with MRI. AJR Am J Roentgenol 2004;183: 629–33.

38. Papp DF, Khanna AJ, McCarthy EF, et al. Magnetic resonance imaging of soft-tissue tumors: determinate and indeterminate lesions. J Bone Joint Surg Am 2007;89(Suppl 3):103–15.

39. Margaritora S, Galetta D, Cesario A, et al. Giant neurofibroma of the chest wall. Eur J Cardiothorac Surg 2002;21(2):339.

40. Karaoglanoglu N, Kurkcuoglu IC, Eroglu A. Giant neurofibroma of the chest wall. Ann Thorac Surg 2004;78(2):718.

41. Gladish GW, Sabloff BM, Munden RF, et al. Primary thoracic sarcomas. Radiographics 2002;22: 621–37.

42. Tateishi U, Gladish GW, Kusumoto M, et al. Chest wall tumors: radiologic findings and pathologic correlation. Part 2. Malignant tumors. Radiographics 2003;23:1491–508.

43. Tateishi U, Kusumoto M, Hasegawa T, et al. Primary malignant fibrous histiocytoma of the chest wall: CT and MR appearance. J Comput Assist Tomogr 2002;26(4):558–63.

44. Jeung M-Y, Gangi A, Gasser B, et al. Imaging of chest wall disorders. Radiographics 1999;19:617–37.

45. Naylor M, Nascimento A, Sherrick A, et al. Elastofibroma dorsi: radiologic findings in 12 patients. AJR Am J Roentgenol 1996;167(3):683–7.

46. Yu J, Weis L, Vaughan L, et al. MRI of elastofibroma dorsi. J Comput Assist Tomogr 1995;19(4):601–3.

47. Kransdorf M, Meis J, Montgomery E. Elastofibroma: MR and CT appearance with radiologic-pathologic correlation. AJR Am J Roentgenol 1992;159:575–9.

48. O'Sullivan P, O'Dwyer H, Flint J, et al. Soft tissue tumours and mass-like lesions of the chest wall: a pictorial review of CT and MR findings. Br J Radiol 2007;80:574–80.

49. Abbas AE, Deschamps C, Cassivi SD, et al. Chest wall desmoid tumors: results of surgical intervention. Ann Thorac Surg 2004;78(4):1219–23.

50. Yacoub M, Lise M. Intrathoracic cystic hygromas. Br J Dis Chest 1969;63(2):107–11.

51. Shaffer K, Rosado-de-Christenson ML, Patz EF, et al. Thoracic lymphangioma in adults: CT and MR imaging features. AJR Am J Roentgenol 1994;162:283–9.

52. Watt AJB. Chest wall lesions. Paediatr Respir Rev 2002;3:328–38.

53. Yildirim E, Dural K, Kaplan T, et al. Cystic lymphangioma: a report of two atypical cases. Interact Cardiovasc Thorac Surg 2004;3(1):63–5.

54. Ardenghy M, Mirua Y, Kovach R, et al. Cystic hygroma of the chest wall: a rare condition. Ann Plast Surg 1996;37(2):211–3.

55. Brown L, Reiman H 3rd, E R, et al. Intrathoracic lymphangioma. Mayo Clin Proc 1985;61(11): 882–92.

56. Smith R, Sherk H, Kollmer C, et al. Cystic lymphangioma in the adult: an unusual axillary mass. Magn Reson Imag 1989;7(5):561–3.

57. Michail O, Michail P, Kyriaki D, et al. Rapid development of an axillary mass in an adult: a case of cystic hygroma. South Med J 2007;100(8):845–9.

58. Griffo S, Stassano P, Luca GD, et al. Intramuscular hemangioma of the chest wall: an unusual tumor. J Thorac Cardiovasc Surg 2007;134:1368–9.

59. Santiago Recuerda A, Corpa Rodrígues ME, García-Sánchez Girón J, et al. Vascular tumors arising from the chest wall: 25 years' experience. Arch Bronconeumol 2005;41(1):53–6.

60. Kinoshita S, Kyoda S, Tsuboi K, et al. Huge cavernous hemangioma arising in a male breast. Breast Cancer 2005;12(3):231–3.

61. Cohen E, Kressel Y, Perosio T, et al. MR imaging of soft-tissue hemangiomas: correlation with pathologic findings. AJR Am J Roentgenol 1988;150: 1079–81.

62. Bonomo L, Ciccotosto C, Guidotti A, et al. Staging of thoracic lymphoma by radiological imaging. Eur Radiol 1997;7:1179–89.

63. Bergin C, Healy M, Zincone G, et al. MR evaluation of chest wall involvement in malignant lymphoma. J Comput Assist Tomogr 1990;14(6):928–32.

64. Carlsen SE, Bergin CJ, Hoppe RT. MR imaging to detect chest wall and pleural involvement in patients with lymphoma: effect on radiation therapy planning. AJR Am J Roentgenol 1993;160:1191–5.

65. Randall PA, Trasolini NC, Kohman LJ, et al. MR imaging in the evaluation of the chest after uncomplicated median sternotomy. Radiographics 1993; 13(2):329–40.

66. Freedman BJ, McCarthy DM, Feldman F, et al. Fatty infiltration of osseous structures: a long-term complication of oleothorax - case report. Radiology 1999;210:515–7.

67. Vayre F, Richard P, Ollivier J. Intrathoracic gossypiboma: magnetic resonance features. Int J Cardiol 1999;70(2):199–200.

68. Gayer G, Yellin A, Apter S, et al. Reconstruction of the sternum and chest wall with methyl methacrylate: CT and MRI appearance. Eur Radiol 1998;8: 239–43.

69. Devon RK, Rosen MA, Mies C, et al. Breast reconstruction with a transverse rectus abdominis myocutaneous flap: spectrum of normal and abnormal MR imaging findings. Radiographics 2004;24: 1287–99.

70. Kang BJ, Jung JI, Park C, et al. Breast MRI findings after modified radical mastectomy and transverse rectus abdominis myocutaneous flap in patients

with breast cancer. J Magn Reson Imaging 2005; 21:784–91.

71. Haramati LB, Glickstein JS, Issenberg HJ, et al. MR imaging and CT of vascular anomalies and connections in patients with congenital heart disease: significance in surgical planning. Radiographics 2002;22(2):337–49.

72. Salanitri G. Intercostal artery aneurysms complicating thoracic aortic coarctation: diagnosis with magnetic resonance angiography. Australas Radiol 2007;51:78–82.

73. Holmqvist C, Stahlberg F, Hanseus K, et al. Collateral flow in coarctation of the aorta with magnetic resonance velocity mapping: correlation to morphological imaging of collateral vessels. J Magn Reson Imaging 2002;15:39–46.

74. Teitelbaum S. Twenty years' experience with intrinsic tumors of the bony thorax at a large institution. J Thorac Cardiovasc Surg 1972;63:776–82.

75. Waller D, Newman R. Primary bone tumors of the thoracic skeleton: an audit of the Leeds regional bone tumour registry. Thorax 1990;45:850–5.

76. Eng J, Sabanathan S, Pradhan G, et al. Primary bony chest wall tumours. J R Coll Surg Edinb 1990;35:44–7.

77. Anderson B, Burt M. Chest wall neoplasms and their management. Ann Thorac Surg 1994;58: 1774–81.

78. Resnick D, Greenway G. Tumors and tumor-like lesions of bone. In: Resnick D, editor. Bone and joint imaging. 2nd edition. Philadelphia: Saunders; 1996. p. 991–1075.

79. Scott W, Scott P, Trerotola S. Radiology of the thoracic skeleton. Philadelphia: Decker; 1991. p. 24–5.

80. Anand M. Fibrous dysplasia. Available at: eMedicine. com. Accessed January 8, 2008.

81. Kuhlman J, Bouchardy L, Fischman E, et al. CT and MR imaging evaluation of chest wall disorders. Radiographics 1994;14:571–95.

82. Jee W, Choi K, Choe B, et al. Fibrous dysplasia: MR imaging characteristics with radiopathologic correlation. AJR Am J Roentgenol 1996;167:1523–7.

83. Jaffe H, Lichtenstein L. Solitary unicameral bone cyst with emphasis on the roentgen picture, the pathologic appearance and the pathogenesis. Arch Surg 1942;44:1004–25.

84. Eastwood B. Aneurysmal bone cyst. Available at: eMedicine.com. Accessed January 8, 2008.

85. Schreuder H, Veth R, Pruszczynski M. Aneurysmal bone cysts treated by curettage, cryotherapy and bone grafting. J Bone Joint Surg Br 1997;79:20–5.

86. Beltran J, Simon D, Levy M, et al. Aneurysmal bone cysts: MR imaging at 1.5T. Radiology 1986;158: 689–90.

87. Zimmer W, Berquist T, Sim F, et al. Magnetic resonance imaging of aneurysmal bone cyst. Mayo Clin Proc 1984;59:633–6.

88. Murphey M, Andrews C, Flemming D. From the archives of the AFIP - primary tumors of the spine: radiologic-pathologic correlation. Radiographics 1996;16:1131–58.

89. Hudson T. Fluid levels in aneurysmal bone cysts: a CT feature. AJR Am J Roentgenol 1984;142: 1001–4.

90. Hudson T, Hamlin D, Fitzsimmons J. Magnetic resonance imaging of fluid levels in an aneurysmal bone cyst and in anticoagulated human blood. Skeletal Radiol 1985;13:267–70.

91. Teitelbaum S. Tumors of the chest wall. Surg Gynecol Obstet 1969;129:1059–73.

92. Unni K. General aspects and data on 11,087 cases. Dahlin's bone tumors. 5th edition. Philadelphia: Lippincott-Raven; 1996. p. 25–45.

93. Murphey M, Flemming D, Boyea S, et al. Enchondroma versus chondrosarcoma in the appendicular skeleton: differentiating features. Radiographics 1998;18:1213–37.

94. Chasi I. Hemangioma, bone. Available at: eMedicine. com. Accessed December 29, 2007.

95. Wilner D. Radiology of bone tumors and allied disorders. Philadelphia: Saunders; 1982. p. 664.

96. Ross J, Masaryk T, Modic M, et al. Vertebral hemangiomas: MR imaging. Radiology 1987;165: 165–9.

97. Friedman D. Symptomatic vertebral hemangiomas: MR findings. AJR Am J Roentgenol 1996;167: 359–64.

98. Baudrez V, Galant C, Vandeberg B. Benign vertebral hemangioma: MR-histological correlation. Skeletal Radiol 2001;30:442–6.

99. Griffiths H, Ennis J, Bailey G. Skeletal changes following renal transplantation. Skeletal Radiol 1984;30:442–6.

100. Katz A, Hampers C, Merrill J. Secondary hyperparathyroidism and renal osteodystrophy in chronic renal failure. Medicine 1969;38:333–74.

101. Mustonen A, Kiuru M, Stahls A, et al. Radicular lower extremity pain as the first symptom of primary hyperparathyroidism. Skeletal Radiol 2004;33: 472–6.

102. Ahmad S, Patel S, Ballo M, et al. Extraosseous osteosarcoma: response to treatment and long-term outcome. J Clin Oncol 2002;20:521–7.

103. Helms C. Malignant bone tumors. Fundamentals of skeletal radiology. 3rd edition. Philadelphia: Elsevier/Saunders; 2005.

104. Sundaram M, McGuire M, Herbold D. Magnetic resonance imaging of osteosarcoma. Skeletal Radiol 1987;16:23–9.

105. Dehner L. Primitive neuroectodermal tumor and Ewing's sarcoma. Am J Surg Pathol 1993;17: 1–13.

106. Winer-Muram H, Kauffman W, Gronemeyer S, et al. Primitive neuroectodermal tumors of the chest wall

(Askin tumors); CT and MR findings. AJR Am J Roentgenol 1993;161:265–8.

107. Boyko O, Cory D, Cohen M, et al. MR imaging of osteogenic and Ewing's sarcoma. Am J Roentgenol 1987;148:317–22.

108. Meyer C, White C. Cartilaginous disorders of the chest. Radiographics 1998;18:1109–23.

109. Wicklung C, Johnston P, Hecht J. Natural history study of hereditary multiple exostoses. Am J Med Genet 1995;55:43–6.

110. Varma D, Ayala A, Carrasco C, et al. Chondrosarcoma: MR imaging with pathologic correlation. Radiographics 1992;12:687–704.

111. Kransdorf M, Meis J. Extraskeletal osseous and cartilaginous tumors of the extremities. Radiographics 1993;13:853–84.

112. Bataille R, Sany J. Solitary myeloma: clinical and prognostic features of a review of 114 cases. Cancer 1981;48:845–51.

113. Burt M, Karpeh M, Ukoha O, et al. Medical tumors of the chest wall. Solitary plasmacytoma and Ewing's sarcoma. J Thorac Cardiovasc Surg 1993;105:89–96.

114. Soutar R, Lucraft H, Jackson G, et al. Guidelines on the diagnosis and management of solitary plasmacytoma of bone and solitary extramedullary plasmacytoma. Clin Oncol (R Coll Radiol) 2004;16:405–13.

115. Corwin J, Lindberg R. Solitary plasmacytoma of bone vs. extramedullary plasmacytoma and their relationship to multiple myeloma. Cancer 1979;43:1007–13.

116. Libshitz H, Malthouse S, Cunningham D, et al. Multiple myeloma: appearance at MR imaging. Radiology 1992;182:833–7.

117. Buckwalter J, Brandser E. Metastatic disease of the skeleton. Am Fam Physician 1997;55:1761–8.

118. Cancer facts and figures. Atlanta (GA): American Cancer Society; 1999.

119. Rosenthal D. Radiologic diagnosis of bone metastases. Cancer 1997;80(Suppl):1595–607.

120. Brage M, Simon M. Metastatic bone disease: evaluation, prognosis, and medical treatment considerations of metastatic bone tumors. Orthopedics 1992;15:589–96.

121. Hage W, Aboulafia A, Aboulafia D. Incidence, location, and diagnostic evaluation of metastatic bone disease. Orthop Clin North Am 2000;31:515–28.

122. Cheng S, Glickerman D, Karmy-Jones R, et al. Traumatic sternomanubrial dislocation with associated bilateral internal mammary artery occlusion. AJR Am J Roentgenol 2003;180:810.

123. Schwagten V, Beaucourt L, Schil PV. Traumatic manubriosternal joint disruption: case report. J Trauma 1994;36:747–8.

124. Hise MV, Primack S, Israel R, et al. CT in blunt chest trauma: indications and limitation. Radiographics 1998;18:1071–84.

125. Fowler A. Flexion-compression injury to the sternum. J Bone Joint Surg Br 1957;39:487–9.

126. Oreck S, Burgess A, Levine A. Traumatic lateral displacement of the scapula: a radiographic sign of neurovascular disruption. J Bone Joint Surg 1984;66A:758–63.

127. Rubenstein J, Ebraheim N, Kellam J. Traumatic scapulothoracic dissociation. Radiology 1985;157:297–8.

128. Lee G, Sush K, Choi J, et al. A case of scapulothoracic dissociation with brachial plexus injury: magnetic resonance imaging findings. Acta Radiol. 2007;48:1020–3.

129. Damschen D, Cogbill T, Siegel M. Scapulothoracic dissociation caused by blunt trauma. J Trauma 1997;42:537–50.

130. Rankine J. Adult traumatic brachial plexus injury. Clin Radiol 2004;59:767–74.

131. Todd M, Shah G, Mukherji S. MR imaging of the brachial plexus. Top Magn Reson Imaging 2004;15:113–25.

132. Hems T, Birch R, Carlstedt T. The role of magnetic resonance imaging in the management of traction injuries to the adult brachial plexus. J Hand Surg [Br] 1999;24:550–5.

133. Saltzman D, Schmitz M, Smith S, et al. The slipping rib syndrome in children. Paediatr Anaesth 2001;11:740–3.

134. Ng C, Hall C. Costochondral junction fractures and intra-abdominal trauma in non-accidental injury (child abuse). Pediatr Radiol 1998;28:671–6.

135. Sponseller P, Malech H Jr, E M, et al. Skeletal involvement in children who have chronic granulomatous disease. J Bone Joint Surg AM 1991;73:37–51.

136. Ross J, Shamsuddin H. Sternoclavicular septic arthritis: review of 180 cases. Medicine 2004;83(3):139–48.

137. Weston V, Jones A, Bradbury N, et al. Clinical features and outcomes of septic arthritis in a single UK health district 1982–1991. Ann Rheum Dis 1999;58:214–9.

Index

Note: Page numbers of article titles are in **boldface** type.

mri.theclinics.com